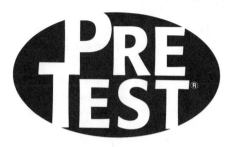

Surgery
PreTest® Self-Assessment and Review
Ninth Edition

PETER L. GELLER, M.D.

Associate Professor of Clinical Surgery
Columbia University College of Physicians & Surgeons
New York, New York

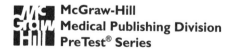 **McGraw-Hill**
Medical Publishing Division
PreTest® Series

NEW YORK   ST. LOUIS   SAN FRANCISCO   AUCKLAND
BOGATÁ   CARACAS   LISBON   LONDON   MADRID
MEXICO   CITY   MILAN   MONTREAL   NEW   DELHI
SAN JUAN   SINGAPORE   SYDNEY   TOKYO   TORONTO

McGraw-Hill

A Division of The **McGraw·Hill** Companies

Surgery: PreTest Self-Assessment and Review, Ninth Edition

Copyright © 2001, 1998, 1995, 1992, 1989, 1987, 1985, 1982, 1978 by The **McGraw-Hill Companies,** Inc. All rights reserved. Printed in the United States of America. Except as permitted under the United States Copyright Act of 1976, no part of this publication may be reproduced or distributed in any form or by any means, or stored in a data base or retrieval system, without the prior written permission of the publisher.

3 4 5 6 7 8 9 0   DOC/DOC   0 9 8 7 6 5 4 3 2

ISBN 0-07-135954-0

This book was set in Berkeley by North Market Street Graphics.
The editor was Catherine A. Wenz.
The production supervisor was Rohnda Barnes.
Project management was provided by North Market Street Graphics.
The text designer was Jim Sullivan / RepCat Graphics & Editorial Services.
The cover designer was Li Chen Chang / Pinpoint.
R.R. Donnelley & Sons was printer and binder.

This book is printed on acid-free paper.

Library of Congress Cataloging-in-Publication Data

Surgery : PreTest self-assessment and review. — 9th ed. / editor,
   Peter L. Geller; student reviewer, Jeffrey J. Anderegg.
         p.   cm.
      Includes bibliographical references.
      ISBN 0-07-135954-0 (pbk.)
      1. Surgery—Examinations, questions, etc.   I. Geller, Peter L.
   [DNLM: 1. Surgical Procedures, Operative—Examination
   Questions.   WO 18.2 S961 2000]
   RD37.2 .S97   2000
   617'.0076—dc21
                                        00-055444

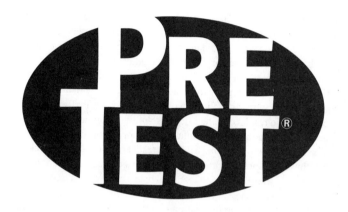

Surgery

PreTest® Self-Assessment and Review

NOTICE

Medicine is an ever-changing science. As new research and clinical experience broaden our knowledge, changes in treatment and drug therapy are required. The authors and the publisher of this work have checked with sources believed to be reliable in their efforts to provide information that is complete and generally in accord with the standards accepted at the time of publication. However, in view of the possibility of human error or changes in medical sciences, neither the authors nor the publisher nor any other party who has been involved in the preparation or publication of this work warrants that the information contained herein is in every respect accurate or complete, and they disclaim all responsibility for any errors or omissions or for the results obtained from use of the information contained in this work. Readers are encouraged to confirm the information contained herein with other sources. For example and in particular, readers are advised to check the product information sheet included in the package of each drug they plan to administer to be certain that the information contained in this work is accurate and that changes have not been made in the recommended dose or in the contraindications for administration. This recommendation is of particular importance in connection with new or infrequently used drugs.

CONTENTS

PREFACE

No longer can students assume that this kind of continuing education ends with the completion of formal training and the successful completion of licensing or certifying examinations. As of October 1979, all 22 member boards of the American Board of Medical Specialties committed themselves to the principle of periodic recertification of their members. Despite the Board's recognition that the cognitive skills measured in the objective examination do not assure clinical competence, recertification efforts—insofar as they involve examinations—are based on the assumption that knowledge of current information on which good clinical decisions should be made is worth cultivating; that, while such information does not guarantee competent practice, lack of it probably impedes competent practice, that this knowledge, unlike technical skills, is reasonably easy to assess; and that it can be acquired by well-motivated physicians. These assumptions all seem reasonable.

The questions presented in this book deal with issues of relative importance to medical students; other problem-oriented materials are becoming available that are aimed at more sophisticated audiences—groups that, within a very few years, will include the present generation of students. Regular review of such material is a habit worth developing. We hope that this edition of *Surgery: PreTest® Self-Assessment and Review* will justify your efforts in working through the problems by providing guidance for further study and by helping you to develop enduring learning habits.

PETER L. GELLER, M.D.

INTRODUCTION

Each question in *Surgery: PreTest® Self-Assessment and Review,* Ninth Edition, is accompanied by an answer, a paragraph explanation, and a specific page reference to either a current journal article, a textbook, or both. A bibliography, which lists all the sources used in the book, follows the last chapter.

Perhaps the most effective way to use this book is to allow yourself one minute to answer each question in a given chapter; as you proceed, indicate your answer beside each question. By following this suggestion, you will be approximating the time limits imposed by the board examinations.

When you have finished answering the questions in a chapter, you should then spend as much time as you need verifying your answers and carefully reading the explanations. Although you should pay special attention to the explanations for the questions you answered incorrectly, you should read every explanation. The authors of this book have designed the explanations to reinforce and supplement the information tested by the questions. If, after reading the explanations for a given chapter, you feel you need still more information about the material covered, you should consult and study the references indicated.

STUDENT REVIEWER

Jeffrey J. Anderegg
The University of Iowa College of Medicine
Iowa City, Iowa

PRE- AND POSTOPERATIVE CARE

Questions

DIRECTIONS: Each item below contains a question or incomplete statement followed by suggested responses. Select the **one best** response to each question.

1. A pregnant woman in her 32nd wk of gestation is given magnesium sulfate for pre-eclampsia. The earliest clinical indication of hypermagnesemia is

a. Loss of deep tendon reflexes
b. Flaccid paralysis
c. Respiratory arrest
d. Hypotension
e. Stupor

2. Five days after an uneventful cholecystectomy, an asymptomatic middle-aged woman is found to have a serum sodium level of 120 meq/L. Proper management would be

a. Administration of hypertonic saline solution
b. Restriction of free water
c. Plasma ultrafiltration
d. Hemodialysis
e. Aggressive diuresis with furosemide

3. A 50-year-old patient presents with symptomatic nephrolithiasis. He reports that he underwent a jejunoileal bypass for morbid obesity when he was 39. One would expect to find

a. Pseudohyperparathyroidism
b. Hyperuric aciduria
c. "Hungry bone" syndrome
d. Hyperoxaluria
e. Sporadic unicameral bone cysts

4. Following surgery, a patient develops oliguria. You believe the patient is hypovolemic, but before increasing intravenous fluids you seek corroborative data. This would include

a. Urine sodium of 28 meq/L
b. Urine chloride of 15 meq/L
c. Fractional excretion of sodium less than 1
d. Urine/serum creatinine ratio of 20
e. Urine osmolality of 350 mOsm/kg

5. A 45-year-old woman with Crohn's disease and a small intestinal fistula develops tetany during the 2nd wk of parenteral nutrition. The laboratory findings include Ca 8.2 meq/L; Na 135 meq/L; K 3.2 meq/L; Cl 103 meq/L; P_{O_4} 2.4 meq/L; albumin 2.4; pH 7.48; 38 kPa; P 84 kPa; bicarbonate 25 meq/L. The most likely cause of the patient's tetany is

a. Hyperventilation
b. Hypocalcemia
c. Hypomagnesemia
d. Essential fatty acid deficiency
e. Focal seizure

6. A patient with a nonobstructing carcinoma of the sigmoid colon is being prepared for elective resection. To minimize the risk of postoperative infectious complications, your planning should include

a. A single preoperative parenteral dose of antibiotic effective against aerobes and anaerobes
b. Avoidance of oral antibiotics to prevent emergence of Clostridium difficile
c. Postoperative administration for 2–4 days of parenteral antibiotics effective against aerobes and anaerobes
d. Postoperative administration for 5–7 days of parenteral antibiotics effective against aerobes and anaerobes
e. Operative time less than 5 h

7. A 70-year-old man with aortic and mitral valvular regurgitation undergoes an emergency sigmoid colectomy and end colostomy for perforated diverticulitis. His postoperative course is complicated by a myocardial infarction and atrial fibrillation. Four weeks later, he has improved and requests elective colostomy closure. You would recommend

a. Discontinuation of antiarrhythmic and antihypertensive medications on the morning of surgery
b. Discontinuation of beta-blocking medications on the day prior to surgery
c. Control of congestive heart failure with diuretics and digitalis in severe cases
d. Administration of prophylactic antibiotics, other than ampicillin and gentamicin, for patients with valvular heart disease who are undergoing gastrointestinal procedures
e. Postponement of elective surgery for 6–8 wk after a subendocardial myocardial infarction

Items 8–9

A previously healthy 55-year-old man undergoes elective right hemicolectomy for a Dukes A cancer of the cecum. His postoperative ileus is somewhat prolonged, and on the fifth postoperative day his nasogastric tube is still in place. Physical examination reveals diminished skin turgor, dry mucous membranes, and orthostatic hypotension. Pertinent laboratory values are as follows:

- Arterial blood gases: pH 7.56; P_{O_2} 85 kPa; P_{CO_2} 50 kPa

- Serum electrolytes (meq/L): Na^+ 132; K^+ 3.1; Cl^- 80; HCO_3- 42

- Urine electrolytes (meq/L): Na^+ 2; K^- 5; Cl^- 6

8. The values given above allow the descriptive diagnosis of

a. Uncompensated metabolic alkalosis
b. Respiratory acidosis with metabolic compensation
c. Combined metabolic and respiratory alkalosis
d. Metabolic alkalosis with respiratory compensation
e. "Paradoxical" metabolic respiratory alkalosis

9. The most appropriate therapy for the patient described would be

a. Infusion of 0.9% NaCl with supplemental KCl until clinical signs of volume depletion are eliminated
b. Infusion of isotonic (0.15 N) HCl via a central venous catheter
c. Clamping the nasogastric tube to prevent further acid losses
d. Administration of acetazolamide to promote renal excretion of bicarbonate
e. Intubation and controlled hypoventilation on a volume-cycled ventilator to further increase P_{CO_2}

Items 10–11

A 23-year-old woman is brought to the emergency room from a halfway house, where she apparently swallowed a handful of pills. The patient complains of shortness of breath and tinnitus, but refuses to identify the pills she ingested. Pertinent laboratory values are as follows:

- Arterial blood gases: pH 7.45; P_{O_2} 126 kPa; P_{CO_2} 12 kPa

- Serum electrolytes (meq/L): Na^+ 138; K^+ 4.8; Cl^- 102; HCO_3- 8

10. The patient's acid-base disturbance is best characterized by which of the following descriptions?

a. Acute respiratory alkalosis, compensated
b. Chronic respiratory alkalosis, compensated
c. Metabolic acids, compensated
d. Mixed metabolic acidosis and respiratory alkalosis
e. Mixed metabolic acidosis and respiratory acidosis

11. The most likely cause of the disturbance in this patient is an overdose of

a. Phenformin
b. Aspirin
c. Barbiturates
d. Methanol
e. Diazepam (Valium)

12. A 65-year-old man undergoes a technically difficult abdomino-perineal resection for a rectal cancer during which he receives three units of packed red blood cells. Four hours later in the intensive care unit he is bleeding heavily from his perineal wound. Emergency coagulation studies reveal normal prothrombin, partial thromboplastin, and bleeding times. The fibrin degradation products are not elevated but the serum fibrinogen content is depressed and the platelet count is 70,000/μL. The most likely cause of the bleeding is

a. Delayed blood transfusion reaction
b. Autoimmune fibrinolysis
c. A bleeding blood vessel in the surgical field
d. Factor VIII deficiency
e. Hypothermic coagulopathy

13. A 78-year-old man with a history of coronary artery disease and an asymptomatic reducible inguinal hernia requests an elective hernia repair. You explain to him that valid reasons for delaying the proposed surgery include

a. Coronary artery bypass surgery 3 mo earlier
b. A history of cigarette smoking
c. Jugular venous distension
d. Hypertension
e. Hyperlipidemia

14. A 68-year-old man is admitted to the coronary care unit with an acute myocardial infarction. His postinfarction course is marked by congestive heart failure and intermittent hypotension. On the fourth hospital day, he develops severe midabdominal pain. On physical examination, blood pressure is 90/60 mm Hg and pulse is 110 beats/min and regular; the abdomen is soft with mild generalized tenderness and distention. Bowel sounds are hypoactive; stool hematest is positive. The next step in this patient's management should be which of the following?

a. Barium enema
b. Upper gastrointestinal series
c. Angiography
d. Ultrasonography
e. Celiotomy

15. A 30-year-old woman in the last trimester of pregnancy suddenly develops massive swelling of the left lower extremity from the inguinal ligament to the ankle. The correct sequence of workup and treatment should be

a. Venogram, bed rest, heparin
b. Impedance plethysmography, bed rest, heparin
c. Impedance plethysmography, bed rest, vena caval filter
d. Impedance plethysmography, bed rest, heparin, warfarin (Coumadin)
e. Clinical evaluation, bed rest, warfarin

16. A 20-year-old woman is found to have an activated partial thromboplastin time (APTT) of 78/32 on routine testing prior to cholecystectomy. Further investigation reveals a prothrombin time (PT) of 13/12 (patient/control), a template bleeding time of 13 min, and a platelet count of 350 × 100/µL. Which one of the following characteristics of this woman's coagulopathy is true?

a. Infusion of purified factor VIII is usually required to normalize its concentration prior to surgery
b. Infusion of cryoprecipitate will not be followed by an improvement in coagulation
c. Most of these patients are, or become, seropositive for HIV
d. Epistaxis or menorrhagia is uncommon
e. Lack of platelet aggregation in response to ristocetin is a common feature of this disease

17. The chief surgical risk to which patients with polycythemia vera are exposed is that due to

a. Anemic disturbances
b. Hemorrhage
c. Infection
d. Renal dysfunction
e. Cardiopulmonary complications

18. A victim of blunt abdominal trauma requires a partial hepatectomy. He is rapidly transfused with 8 units of appropriately cross-matched packed red blood cells from the blood bank. He is noted in the recovery room to be bleeding from intravenous puncture sites and the surgical incision. His coagulopathy is likely due to thrombocytopenia and deficiencies of which clotting factors?

a. II only
b. II and VII
c. V and VIII
d. IX and X
e. XI and XII

19. Following celiotomy, normal bowel motility can ordinarily be presumed to have returned

a. In the stomach in 4 h, the small bowel in 24 h, and the colon after the first oral intake
b. In the stomach in 24 h, the small bowel in 4 h, and the colon in 3 days
c. In the stomach in 3 days, the small bowel in 3 days, and the colon in 3 days
d. In the stomach in 24 h, the small bowel in 24 h, and the colon in 24 h
e. In the stomach in 4 h, the small bowel immediately, and the colon in 24 h

20. A 65-year-old woman has a life-threatening pulmonary embolus 5 days following removal of a uterine malignancy. She is immediately heparinized and maintained in good therapeutic range for the next 3 days, then passes gross blood from her vagina and develops tachycardia, hypotension, and oliguria. Following resuscitation, an abdominal CT scan reveals a major retroperitoneal hematoma. You should now

a. Immediately reverse heparin by a calculated dose of protamine and place a vena cava filter (e.g., a Greenfield filter)
b. Reverse heparin with protamine, explore and evacuate the hematoma, and ligate the vena cava below the renal veins
c. Switch to low-dose heparin
d. Stop heparin and observe closely
e. Stop heparin, give fresh frozen plasma (FFP), and begin warfarin therapy

21. Which of the following surgical interventions is least likely to provide acceptable prolongation of life for patients with AIDS?

a. Splenectomy for AIDS-related idiopathic thrombocytopenic purpura
b. Colonic resection for perforation secondary to cytomegalovirus infection
c. Cholecystectomy for acalculous cholecystitis
d. Tracheostomy for ventilator-dependent patients with respiratory failure
e. Gastric resection for a bleeding gastric lymphoma or Kaposi's sarcoma

22. An elderly diabetic woman with chronic steroid-dependent bronchospasm has an ileocolectomy for a perforated cecum. She is taken to the ICU intubated and is maintained on broad-spectrum antibiotics, renal-dose dopamine, and a rapid steroid taper. On postoperative day 2 she develops a fever of 39.2°C (102.5°F), hypotension, lethargy, and laboratory values remarkable for hypoglycemia and hyperkalemia. The most likely diagnosis of this acute event is

a. Sepsis
b. Hypovolemia
c. Adrenal insufficiency
d. Acute tubular necrosis
e. Diabetic ketoacidosis

23. A cirrhotic patient with abnormal coagulation studies due to hepatic synthetic dysfunction requires an urgent cholecystectomy. A transfusion of fresh frozen plasma is planned to minimize the risk of bleeding due to surgery. The optimal timing of this transfusion would be

a. The day before surgery
b. The night before surgery
c. On call to surgery
d. Intraoperatively
e. In the recovery room

24. On postoperative day 3, an otherwise healthy 55-year-old man recovering from a partial hepatectomy is noted to have scant serosanguineous drainage from his abdominal incision. His skin staples are removed, revealing a 1.0-cm dehiscence of the upper midline abdominal fascia. Which of the following actions is most appropriate?

a. Removing all suture material and packing the wound with moist sterile gauze
b. Starting intravenous antibiotics
c. Placing an abdominal (Scultetus) binder
d. Prompt resuturing of the fascia in the operating room
e. Bed rest

25. Five days after a sigmoid colectomy for cancer, a patient's skin staples are removed and a large gush of serosanguineous fluid emerges. Examination of the wound reveals an extensive fascial dehiscence. The most appropriate management is

a. Wide opening of the wound to assure adequate drainage
b. Smear and culture of the fluid and appropriate antibiotics after the smear is reviewed
c. Careful reapproximation of the wound edges with tape
d. Immediate return to the operating room
e. Application of a Scultetus binder

26. Signs and symptoms of hemolytic transfusion reactions include

a. Hypothermia
b. Hypertension
c. Polyuria
d. Abnormal bleeding
e. Hypesthesia at the transfusion site

27. A patient suspected of having a hemolytic transfusion reaction should be managed with

a. Removal of nonessential foreign body irritants, e.g., Foley catheter
b. Fluid restriction
c. 0.1 M HCl infusion
d. Steroids
e. Fluids and mannitol

28. The surgeon should be particularly concerned about which coagulation function in patients receiving anti-inflammatory or analgesic medications?

a. APTT
b. PT
c. Reptilase time
d. Bleeding time
e. Thrombin time

29. The substrate depleted earliest in the postoperative period is

a. Branched-chain amino acids
b. Non-branched-chain amino acids
c. Ketone
d. Glycogen
e. Glucose

30. Diagnostic abdominal laparoscopy is contraindicated in which of the following patients?

a. A patient with rebound tenderness following a tangential gunshot wound to the abdomen
b. A stable patient with a stab wound to the lower chest wall
c. A patient with a mass in the head of the pancreas
d. A young female with pelvic pain and fever
e. An elderly patient in the intensive care unit suspected of having intestinal ischemia

31. A 23-year-old woman undergoes total thyroidectomy for carcinoma of the thyroid gland. On the second postoperative day, she begins to complain of tingling sensation in her hands. She appears quite anxious and later complains of muscle cramps. Initial therapy should consist of

a. 10 mL of 10% magnesium sulfate intravenously
b. Oral vitamin D
c. 100 μg of oral Synthroid
d. Continuous infusion of calcium gluconate
e. Oral calcium gluconate

32. Hypocalcemia is associated with

a. Acidosis
b. Shortened QT interval
c. Hypomagnesemia
d. Myocardial irritability
e. Hyperproteinemia

33. The enteric fluid with an electrolyte (Na^+, K^+, Cl^-) content similar to that of Ringer's lactate is

a. Saliva
b. Contents of small intestine
c. Contents of right colon
d. Pancreatic secretions
e. Gastric juice

34. Which of the following medications administered for hyperkalemia counteracts the myocardial effects of potassium without reducing the serum potassium level?

a. Sodium polystyrene sulfonate (Kayexalate)
b. Sodium bicarbonate
c. 50% dextrose
d. Calcium gluconate
e. Insulin

Items 35–37

An in-hospital workup of a 78-year-old, hypertensive, mildly asthmatic man who is receiving chemotherapy for colon cancer reveals symptomatic gallstones. Preoperative laboratory results are notable for a hematocrit of 24% and a urinalysis with 18–25 WBCs and gram-negative bacteria. On call to the operating room he receives intravenous penicillin. His abdomen is shaved in the operating room. An open cholecystectomy is performed and, despite a lack of indications, the common bile duct is explored. The wound is closed primarily with a Penrose drain exiting a separate stab wound. On postoperative day 3 the patient develops a wound infection.

35. Which of the following changes could make this wound a less favorable environment for infection?

a. Decreasing the operative time and wound contamination by omitting the common bile duct exploration
b. Placing a Penrose drain exiting directly through the lateral corner of the wound
c. Using oral rather than intravenous penicillin perioperatively
d. Leaving a seroma in the wound to prevent desiccation of the tissues
e. Reinforcing the wound closure with a sheet of prosthetic polypropylene mesh

36. Which of the following characteristics of this patient might increase the risk of a wound infection?

a. History of colon surgery
b. Hypertension
c. Male sex
d. Receipt of chemotherapy
e. Asthma

37. Which of the following changes in the care of this patient could decrease the chance of a postoperative wound infection?

a. Increasing the length of the preoperative hospital stay to prophylactically treat the asthma with steroids
b. Treating the urinary infection prior to surgery
c. Shaving the abdomen the night prior to surgery
d. Continuing the prophylactic antibiotics for three postoperative days
e. Use of a closed drainage system brought out through the operative incision

Items 38–39

The two solutions most commonly used to maintain fluid and electrolyte balance in the postoperative management of patients are 5% dextrose in 0.9% sodium chloride and lactated Ringer's solution.

38. A correct statement regarding 5% dextrose in 0.9% saline is which of the following?

a. It contains the same concentration of sodium ions as does plasma
b. It can be given in large quantities without seriously affecting acid-base balance
c. It is isosmotic with plasma
d. It has a pH of 7.4
e. It may cause a dilutional acidosis

39. Correct statements regarding lactated Ringer's solution include which of the following?

a. It contains a higher concentration of sodium ions than does plasma
b. It is most appropriate for replacement of nasogastric tube losses
c. It is isosmotic with plasma
d. It has a pH of less than 7.0
e. It may induce a significant metabolic acidosis

40. Four days after surgical evacuation of an acute subdural hematoma, a 44-year-old man becomes mildly lethargic and develops asterixis. He has received 2400 mL of 5% dextrose in water intravenously each day since surgery, and he appears well hydrated. Pertinent laboratory values are as follows:

- Serum electrolytes (meq/L): Na^+ 118; K^+ 3.4; Cl^- 82; HCO_3^- 24
- Serum osmolality: 242 mOsm/L
- Urine sodium: 47 meq/L
- Urine osmolality: 486 mOsm/L

A correct statement about this patient's fluid and electrolyte status is which of the following?

a. His low serum sodium indicates sodium deficiency, which should be treated with 3% saline infusion
b. He probably has the syndrome of inappropriate secretion of antidiuretic hormone
c. His blood glucose level should be checked because the hyponatremia may be artifactual
d. Water restriction is rarely effective in severe cases of hyponatremia
e. The underlying problem is the inappropriate excretion of sodium (renal sodium wasting)

41. A 43-year-old woman develops acute renal failure following an emergency resection of a leaking abdominal aortic aneurysm. Three days after surgery, the following laboratory values are obtained:

- Serum electrolytes (meq/L): Na^+ 127; K^+ 5.9; Cl^- 92; HCO_3- 15
- Blood urea nitrogen: 82 mg/dL
- Serum creatinine: 6.7 mg/dL

The patient has gained 4 kg since surgery and is mildly dyspneic at rest. Eight hours after these values are reported, the electrocardiogram shown below is obtained. The initial treatment for this patient should be

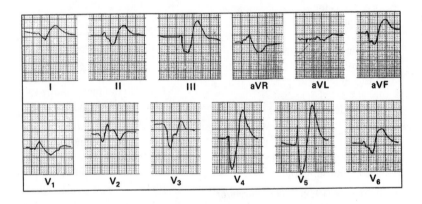

a. 10% calcium gluconate, 10 mL
b. Digoxin, 0.25 mg every 3 h for three doses
c. Oral Kayexalate
d. Lidocaine, 100 mg
e. Emergent hemodialysis

42. Prophylactic regimens of documented benefit in decreasing the risk of postoperative thromboembolism include

a. Early ambulation
b. External pneumatic compression devices placed on the upper extremities
c. Elastic stockings
d. Leg elevation for 24 h postoperatively
e. Dipyridamole therapy for 48 h postoperatively

43. Signs and symptoms associated with early sepsis include

a. Respiratory acidosis
b. Decreased cardiac output
c. Hypoglycemia
d. Increased arteriovenous oxygen difference
e. Cutaneous vasodilation

DIRECTIONS: Each group of questions below consists of lettered options followed by numbered items. For each numbered item, select the appropriate lettered option(s). Each lettered option may be used once, more than once, or not at all. **Choose exactly the number of options indicated following each item.**

Items 44–46

Match the gastrointestinal content at each site with its appropriate ionic composition (meq/L).

	Na	K	Cl	HCO$_3$
a.	140	5	104	30
b.	140	5	75	115
c.	60	10	130	0
d.	10	26	10	30
e.	60	30	40	50

44. Salivary (**SELECT 1 COMPOSITION**)

45. Stomach (**SELECT 1 COMPOSITION**)

46. Small bowel (**SELECT 1 COMPOSITION**)

Items 47–50

A 42-year-old man has a calculated resting energy expenditure of 1800 kcal/day (basal energy expenditure plus 10%). Match the following clinical situations with the appropriate daily energy requirement.

a. 1600
b. 2300
c. 2800
d. 3600
e. 4500

47. Sepsis (SELECT 1 EXPENDI-TURE)

48. Skeletal trauma (SELECT 1 EXPENDITURE)

49. Third-degree burns of 60% of body surface area (BSA) (SELECT 1 EXPENDITURE)

50. Prolonged starvation (SELECT 1 EXPENDITURE)

PRE- AND POSTOPERATIVE CARE

Answers

1. The answer is a. (*Schwartz, 7/e, pp 65–66.*) States of magnesium excess are characterized by generalized neuromuscular depression. Clinically, severe hypermagnesemia is rarely seen except in those patients with advanced renal failure treated with magnesium-containing antacids. Hypermagnesemia is produced intentionally, however, by obstetricians who use parenteral magnesium sulfate ($MgSO_4$) to treat preeclampsia. $MgSO_4$ is administered until depression of the deep tendon reflexes is observed, a deficit that occurs with modest hypermagnesemia (over 4 meq/L). Greater elevations of magnesium produce progressive weakness, which culminates in flaccid quadriplegia and in some cases respiratory arrest from paralysis of the chest bellows mechanism. Hypotension may occur because of the direct arteriolar relaxing effect of magnesium. Changes in mental status occur in the late stages of the syndrome and are characterized by somnolence that progresses to coma.

2. The answer is b. (*Schwartz, 7/e, pp 57–63.*) Acute severe hyponatremia sometimes occurs following elective surgical procedures. It is usually the result of the combination of appropriate postoperative stimulation of antidiuretic hormone and injudicious administration of excess free water in the first few postoperative days. Totally sodium-free intravenous fluids (e.g., dextrose and water) should be given with great caution postoperatively, since occasionally the resulting hyponatremia can be associated with sudden death from a flaccid heart or with severe permanent brain damage. The condition is usually best treated by withholding free water and allowing the patient to reequilibrate spontaneously. At levels below 115 meq/L, seizures or mental obtundation may mandate treatment with hypertonic sodium solutions. This must be done with extreme care because the risk of fluid overload with acute pulmonary or cerebral edema is high.

3. The answer is d. *(Sabiston, 15/e, p 931.)* Any patient who has lost much of the ileum (whether from injury, disease, or elective surgery) is at high risk of developing enteric hyperoxaluria if the colon remains intact. Calcium oxalate stones will develop in at least 10% of these patients. The condition results from excessive absorption of oxalate from the colon through two related synergistic mechanisms: unabsorbed fatty acids combine with calcium, which prevents the formation of insoluble calcium oxalate and allows oxalate to remain available for colonic absorption; and unabsorbed fatty acids and bile acids also increase the permeability of the colon to the oxalate.

4. The answer is c. *(Schwartz, 7/e, pp 452–455.)* When oliguria occurs postoperatively, it is important to differentiate between low output caused by the physiologic response to intravascular hypovolemia and that caused by acute tubular necrosis. The fractional excretion of sodium (FENa) is an especially useful test to aid in this differentiation. Values of FE < 1% in an oliguric setting indicate aggressive sodium reclamation in the tubules; values above this suggest tubular injury. The fractional excretion is a simple calculation: (urine Na × serum creatinine) ÷ (serum sodium × urinary creatinine). In the setting of postoperative hypovolemia, all findings would reflect the kidney's efforts to retain volume: the urine sodium would be below 20 meq/L, the urine chloride would not be helpful except in the metabolically alkalotic patient, the serum osmolality would be over 500 mOsm/kg, and the urine/serum creatinine ratio would be above 40.

5. The answer is c. *(Schwartz, 7/e, pp 64–66.)* Magnesium deficiency is common in malnourished patients and patients with large gastrointestinal fluid losses. The neuromuscular effects resemble those of calcium deficiency—namely, paresthesia, hyperreflexia, muscle spasm, and ultimately tetany. The cardiac effects are more like those of hypercalcemia. An electrocardiogram therefore provides a rapid means of differentiating between hypocalcemia and hypomagnesemia. Hypomagnesemia also causes potassium wasting by the kidney. Many hospital patients with refractory hypocalcemia will be found to be magnesium deficient. Often this deficiency becomes manifest during the response to parenteral nutrition when normal cellular ionic gradients are restored. A normal blood pH and arterial P_{CO_2} rule out hyperventilation. The serum calcium in this patient is normal when adjusted for the low albumin. Hypomagnesemia causes functional hypoparathyroidism, which can lower serum calcium and thus result in a combined defect.

6. The answer is c. (*Schwartz, 7/e, pp 143–149.*) Many clinical and experimental studies have looked at the optimum bowel preparation and preoperative regimen for elective colonic surgery to reduce the postoperative infectious complications of wound infection, intraabdominal abscess, and anastomotic leakage. Currently, a postoperative rate of wound infection of only 5% can be attained by combining mechanical cleansing, oral antibiotics, and perioperative parenteral antibiotics. The type of mechanical cleansing does not matter as long as it is effective. Preoperative oral antibiotics may be administered one or more days prior to surgery and should cover aerobes and anaerobes (e.g., neomycin-erythromycin). Parenteral antibiotics effective against aerobes and anaerobes (e.g., cefoxitin) should be administered on call to the operating room as a single dose and no more than 24 h postoperatively. Both antibiotic regimens yield maximum prophylaxis without fostering resistant transformation of microbes. Procedures that require operative time greater than 3 h or that involve the extraperitoneal rectum are associated with an increased risk of infectious complications.

7. The answer is c. (*Schwartz, 7/e, pp 462–465.*) There are several recommended interventions in cardiac patients who are undergoing noncardiac surgery. The two factors that correlate best with postoperative life-threatening or fatal cardiac complications are myocardial infarction (transmural or subendocardial) and uncontrolled congestive heart failure. Hence, delay of elective surgery for 6 mo after myocardial infarction and preoperative control of congestive heart failure with diuretics and digitalis, in severe cases, will have the greatest effect in decreasing the risks of surgery. A patient's cardiac medications should be continued preoperatively, including during the morning of surgery, to maintain adequate therapeutic levels. This is especially true for beta blockers, which can manifest withdrawal rebound hypertension and tachycardia approximately 24 h after discontinuation. Patients with prosthetic valves or valvular heart disease should be given prophylactic antibiotics to prevent seeding of their valves during episodes of significant bacteremia. This most commonly occurs during gastrointestinal or genitourinary procedures. Ampicillin and gentamicin cover the flora frequently encountered, including enterococci and gram-negative organisms.

8. The answer is d. (*Greenfield, 2/e, pp 259–266.*) Both the arterial pH and the P_{CO_2} are elevated in the patient presented in the question; the disturbance is alkalosis with hypoventilation. The P_{CO_2} typically increases by 0.5–1.0 pKa for each meq/L increase in serum bicarbonate. These findings suggest that the hypoventilation is compensatory rather than a primary phenomenon. This assumption is further supported by the absence of clinical lung disease.

9. The answer is a. (*Greenfield, 2/e, pp 259–266.*) The development of a clinically significant metabolic alkalosis in a patient requires not only the loss of acid or addition of alkali, but renal responses that maintain the alkalosis. The normal kidney can tremendously augment its excretion of acid or alkali in response to changes in ingested load. However, in the presence of significant volume depletion and consequent excessive salt and water retention, the tubular maximum for bicarbonate reabsorption is increased. Correction of volume depletion alone is usually sufficient to correct the alkalosis, since the kidney will then excrete the excess bicarbonate. HCl infusion is usually unnecessary and can be dangerous. Acetazolamide is unlikely to be effective in the face of distal Na^+ reabsorption (in exchange for H^+ secretion). Moreover, to the extent that acetazolamide causes natriuresis, it will exacerbate the volume depletion.

10. The answer is d. (*Greenfield, 2/e, pp 260–266.*) The patient presented in the question is in a state of metabolic acidosis as shown by a markedly increased anion gap of 28 meq unmeasured anions per liter of plasma. However, the respiratory response is greater than can be explained by a compensatory response, since the patient is mildly alkalemic. The disturbance cannot be pure respiratory alkalosis, since the serum bicarbonate does not drop below 15 meq/L as a result of renal compensation and the anion gap does not vary by more than 1–2 meq/L from its normal value of 12 in response to a respiratory disturbance. The renal response to hyperventilation involves wasting of bicarbonate and compensatory retention of chloride; it does not involve a change in the concentration of "unmeasured" anions, such as albumin and organic acids.

11. The answer is b. (*Anderson, Ann Intern Med 85:745–748, 1976.*) The acid-base disturbance in the patient described in the previous question demonstrates the value of extracting all available information from a small amount of rapidly retrievable data, e.g., arterial blood gases. Salicylates directly stimulate the respiratory center and produce respiratory alkalosis. By building up an accumulation of organic acids, salicylates also produce a concomitant metabolic acidosis. Characteristically both disturbances exist simultaneously following massive ingestion of salicylates. If sedative agents have been taken as well, the respiratory alkalosis (and even the respiratory compensation) may be absent. Phenformin and methanol overdoses also produce "high-anion-gap" metabolic acidosis, but without the simultaneous respiratory disturbance. In the case presented, the patient's history of tinnitus in conjunction with her mixed metabolic acidosis–respiratory alkalosis is essentially pathognomonic of salicylate intoxication.

12. The answer is c. (*Sabiston, 15/e, pp 131–133.*) Whenever significant bleeding is noted in the early postoperative period, the presumption should always be that it is due to an error in surgical control of blood vessels in the operative field. Hematologic disorders that are not apparent during the long operation are most unlikely to surface as problems postoperatively. Blood transfusion reactions can cause diffuse loss of clot integrity; the sudden appearance of diffuse bleeding during an operation may be the only evidence of an intraoperative transfusion reaction. In the postoperative period, transfusion reactions usually present as unexplained fever, apprehension, and headache—all symptoms difficult to interpret in the early postoperative period. Factor VIII deficiency (hemophilia) would almost certainly be known by history in a 65-year-old man, but if not, intraoperative bleeding would have been a problem earlier in this long operation. Severely hypothermic patients will not be able to form clots effectively, but clot dissolution does not occur. Care should be taken to prevent the development of hypothermia during long operations through the use of warmed intravenous fluid, gas humidifiers, and insulated skin barriers.

13. The answer is c. (*Goldman, J Cardiothorac Anesth 1:237, 1987.*) The work of Goldman and others has served to identify risk factors for perioperative myocardial infarction. The highest likelihood is associated with recent myocardial infarction: the more recent the event, the higher the risk up to 6 mo. It should be noted, however, that the risk never returns to normal. A non-Q-wave infarction may not have destroyed much myocardium, but it leaves the surrounding area with borderline perfusion; hence the particularly high risk of subsequent perioperative infarction. Evidence of congestive heart failure, such as jugular venous distention, or S_3 gallop also carries a high risk, as does the frequent occurrence of ectopic beats. Old age and emergency surgery are risk factors independent of these others. Coronary revascularization by coronary artery bypass graft (CABG) tends to protect against myocardial infarction. Smoking, diabetes, hypertension, and hyperlipidemia (all of which predispose to coronary artery disease) are surprisingly not independent risk factors, although they may increase the death rate should an infarct occur. The value of this information and data derived from further testing is that it identifies the patient who needs to be monitored invasively with a systemic arterial catheter and pulmonary arterial catheter. Most perioperative infarcts occur postoperatively when the "third-space" fluids return to the circulation, which increases the preload and the myocardial oxygen consumption. This generally occurs around the third postoperative day.

14. The answer is c. (*Schwartz, 7/e, pp 966–967.*) Acute mesenteric ischemia may be difficult to diagnose. The condition should be suspected in patients with either systemic manifestations of arteriosclerotic vascular disease or low cardiac output states associated with a sudden development of abdominal pain that is out of proportion to the physical findings. Lactic acidosis and an elevated hematocrit reflecting hemoconcentration are common laboratory findings. Abdominal films show a nonspecific ileus pattern. The cause may be embolic occlusion or thrombosis of the superior mesenteric artery, primary mesenteric venous occlusion, or nonocclusive mesenteric ischemia secondary to low cardiac output states. A mortality of 65–100% is reported. The majority of affected patients are at high operative risk, but since early diagnosis followed by revascularization or resectional surgery or both is the only hope for survival, celiotomy must be performed once the diagnosis of arterial occlusion or bowel infarction has been made. Initial treatment of nonocclusive mesenteric ischemia includes measures to increase cardiac output and blood pressure and the direct intraarterial infusion of vasodilators such as papaverine into the superior mesenteric system. The patient presented in the question is at risk for both occlusive and nonocclusive mesenteric ischemic disease. If his clinical status permits, angiographic studies should be performed before the operation to establish the diagnosis and to determine whether embolectomy, revascularization, or nonsurgical management is indicated as initial treatment.

15. The answer is b. (*Schwartz, 7/e, pp 1007–1014.*) This patient has a left iliofemoral vein thrombosis, as evidenced by sudden massive swelling of her entire left lower extremity. Noninvasive venous testing should be quite helpful as the venous obstruction extends above the knee; therefore, venography and x-ray exposure are unnecessary. Heparin is the preferred agent because it does not cross the placenta, while warfarin does. The vena caval filter is not indicated because there is no contraindication to heparin therapy and there has not been any evidence of pulmonary embolus.

16. The answer is e. (*Sabiston, 15/e, pp 134–135.*) von Willebrand disease has an autosomal dominant pattern of inheritance that affects both men and women. The deficiency of factor VIII activity is generally less severe than in classic hemophilia and tends to fluctuate even in an untreated patient. However, the bleeding tendency is compounded by abnormal platelet function. This is responsible for the common occurrence of epistaxis and menorrhagia. In 70% of patients, platelets fail to aggregate in response to the diagnostic reagent ristocetin. Transfusion of cryoprecipitate provides factor VIII R:WF (the von Willebrand factor), whereas infusions of high-purity concentrates of factor VIII:C are not effective. These patients do not generally require treatment unless they need surgery or are severely injured; therefore, they have not usually received the contaminated concentrates responsible for the 80% prevalence of HIV seropositivity among hemophiliacs.

17. The answer is b. (*Schwartz, 7/e, pp 85–87.*) Intraoperative and postoperative hemorrhage is a significant problem in the patient with polycythemia vera. Despite thrombocytosis, these patients have a hemorrhagic tendency generally ascribed to a qualitative deficiency of the platelets. Elective surgery should be postponed until the hematocrit and platelet count reach normal levels. Alkylating agents, such as busulfan or chlorambucil, are effective in this regard. In the emergency situation, phlebectomy should be performed prior to operation and also an especially careful hemostatic technique should be employed. Infection is also a problem in patients with polycythemia vera, but hemorrhagic problems are the more frequently encountered complications.

18. The answer is c. (*Schwartz, 7/e, p 96.*) When large amounts of banked blood are transfused, the recipient becomes deficient in factors V and VIII (the "labile" factors) and an acquired coagulopathy ensues. Since banked blood is also deficient in platelets, thrombocytopenia may also develop.

19. The answer is b. (*Schwartz, 7/e, p 467.*) The misconception that the entire bowel does not function in the early postoperative period is still widely held. Intestinal motility and absorption studies have clarified the patterns by which bowel activity resumes. The stomach remains uncoordinated in its muscular activity and does not empty efficiently for about 24 h after abdominal procedures. The small bowel functions normally within hours of surgery and is able to accept nutrients promptly, either by nasoduodenal or percutaneous jejunal feeding catheters or, after 24 h, by gastric emptying. The colon is stimulated in large measure by the gastrocolic reflex but ordinarily is relatively inactive for 3–4 days.

20. The answer is a. (*Greenfield, 2/e, pp 96–97.*) In a heparinized patient with significant life-threatening hemorrhage, immediate reversal of heparin anticoagulation is indicated. Protamine sulfate is a specific antidote to heparin and should be given as 1 mg for each 100 U heparin if hemorrhage begins shortly after a bolus of heparin. For a patient (such as this) in whom heparin therapy is ongoing, the dose should be based on the half-life of heparin (90 min). Since protamine is also an anticoagulant, only half the calculated circulating heparin should be reversed. The protaminization should be followed by placement of a percutaneous vena cava filter (Greenfield filter). In this critically ill patient, exploration of the retroperitoneal space would be surgically challenging and meddlesome.

21. The answer is d. (*Diettrich, Arch Surg 126:860–865, 1991.*) Patients who have AIDS frequently present with problems that potentially require surgical care. The involvement of surgeons with these patients will increase as more effective treatments are developed and the AIDS patient's survival is prolonged. AIDS patients not only suffer from common surgical illnesses, they also develop problems especially associated with their altered immune status, such as bleeding from gastrointestinal lymphomas or Kaposi's lesions, bowel ischemia, perforation from parasitic or viral infection, acalculous cholecystitis, and retroperitoneal and intraabdominal masses due to massive lymphadenitis. With the exception of tracheostomy, experience has demonstrated that surgery can be performed with acceptable morbidity and mortality and that it seems to provide comfort and prolong quality life. Though it may facilitate nursing care, tracheostomy does not reverse or slow the pulmonary failure once the patient has become ventilator dependent.

22. The answer is c. *(Schwartz, 7/e, pp 1639–1640.)* Acute adrenal insufficiency is classically manifested as changing mental status, increased temperature, cardiovascular collapse, hypoglycemia, and hyperkalemia. The diagnosis can be difficult to make and requires a high index of suspicion. Its clinical presentation is similar to that of sepsis; however, sepsis is generally associated with hyperglycemia and no significant change in potassium. The treatment for adrenal crisis is hydrocortisone 100 mg intravenously, volume resuscitation, and other supportive measures to treat any new or ongoing stress. Then, 200–400 hydrocortisone mg is administered over the next 24 h, followed by a taper of the steroid as tolerated.

23. The answer is c. *(Schwartz, 7/e, pp 95–96.)* Transfusions with fresh frozen plasma (FFP) are given to replenish clotting factors. The effectiveness of the transfusion in maintaining hemostasis is dependent on the quantity of each factor delivered and its half-life. The half-life of the most stable clotting factor, factor VII, is 4–6 h. A reasonable transfusion scheme would be to give FFP on call to the operating room. This way the transfusion is complete prior to the incision with circulating factors to cover the operative and immediate postoperative period.

24. The answer is c. *(Sabiston, 15/e, pp 344–345.)* Serosanguineous drainage is classically associated with fascial dehiscence. A reasonable approach to this problem is to remove several sutures and gently explore the wound to determine the extent of the dehiscence. A small fascial dehiscence (1–2 cm) can be treated conservatively with local wound care and an abdominal binder to support the fascia. A larger dehiscence requires reoperation for formal reclosure of the fascia. High-risk patients with a large fascial dehiscence may be treated with an abdominal binder and modified bed rest, which allows both intraabdominal adhesion formation and local granulation. Although fascial dehiscence can occur from local infection, it is usually not an infectious process and does not require parenteral antibiotic therapy.

25. The answer is d. *(Sabiston, 15/e, pp 344–345.)* The appearance of a gush of serosanguineous fluid from an abdominal incision is pathognomonic of a disruption of the deep fascia. The source of large amounts of serous fluid is the peritoneum. The temptation to avoid direct reclosure of these wounds when the fascial defect is larger than 1–2 cm should be resisted because delayed resumption of normal ambulation and activity with a late ventral hernia is the best outcome to be hoped for. Evisceration, wound infection, or protracted convalescence is far more likely. Recurrence of eviscerations following reclosure of these wounds is extremely rare, though 10–20% will later develop incisional hernias. The Scultetus binder is a corsetlike cloth wrap that was once a favored support to reduce likelihood of evisceration in those wounds in which the fascia was left unrepaired after dehiscence.

26. The answer is d. *(Sabiston, 15/e, p 124.)* Allergic and febrile reactions occur in about 1% of all transfusions. Hemolytic transfusion reactions are much less common (0.2%) with fatal reactions in 1:100,000 transfusions. Hemolytic transfusion reactions are due to the reaction of recipient antibodies against transfused antigens. These reactions can be both immediate and delayed. Symptoms of a hemolytic transfusion reaction include fever, chills, and pain and heat at the infusion site, as well as respiratory distress, anxiety, hypotension, and oliguria. During surgery a hemolytic transfusion reaction can manifest as abnormal bleeding.

27. The answer is e. *(Sabiston, 15/e, p 124.)* Hemolytic transfusion reactions lead to hypotension and oliguria. The increased hemoglobin in the plasma will be cleared via the kidneys, which leads to hemoglobinuria. Placement of an indwelling Foley catheter with subsequent demonstration of oliguria and hemoglobinuria not only confirms the diagnosis of a hemolytic transfusion reaction but is useful in monitoring corrective therapy. Treatment begins with discontinuation of the transfusion, followed by aggressive fluid resuscitation to support the hypotensive episode and increase urine output. Inducing a diuresis through aggressive fluid resuscitation and osmotic diuretics is important to clear the hemolyzed red cell membranes, which can otherwise collect in glomeruli and cause renal damage. Alkalinization of the urine (pH > 7) helps prevent hemoglobin clumping and renal damage. Steroids do not have a role in the treatment of hemolytic transfusion reactions.

28. The answer is d. (*Sabiston, 15/e, p 133.*) Platelet dysfunction, measured by bleeding time, has been associated with a long list of drugs. Among nonsteroidal anti-inflammatory and analgesic medications, aspirin, indomethacin, phenylbutazone, acetominophen, and phenacetin have been implicated, along with aminopyrine and codeine. Ibuprofen, however, has not. In addition, many antibiotics, anticonvulsants, and sedatives have been associated with thrombasthenia. Any time platelet abnormalities are suspected, a careful review of the drugs the patient is receiving should be undertaken, and a measurement should be made of the platelet count and bleeding time. Platelet dysfunction does not affect APTT, PT, reptilase, or thrombin times.

29. The answer is d. (*Sabiston, 15/e, pp 60–62.*) The metabolic response to surgery (and other trauma) is a result of neuroendocrine stimulation that sharply accelerates protein breakdown, stimulates gluconeogenesis, and produces glucose intolerance. The glycogen stores are rapidly depleted because of a fall in insulin and a rise in glucagon levels in the plasma. The peripheral effects of the neuroendocrine secretion result in an increase in plasma levels of amino acids, free fatty acids, lactate, glucose, and glycerol. In the liver, the cortisol and glucagon stimulate glycogenolysis, gluconeogenesis, and increased substrate uptake.

30. The answer is a. (*Berci, Am J Surg 161:332–335, 1991.*) The indications for diagnostic laparoscopic exploration are increasing rapidly as the tools and techniques for such intervention improve. In the stable trauma patient with a tangential gunshot wound or with a stab wound to the lower chest wall or abdomen, laparoscopy may show no actual peritoneal penetration and might make a laparotomy unnecessary. If the peritoneum or diaphragm is injured, subsequent laparotomy and exploration are generally indicated to exclude other possible injuries and to facilitate repair of the diaphragm. All unstable patients or those with signs of peritoneal irritation (e.g., rebound tenderness) should undergo prompt celiotomy.

Laparoscopic staging of malignancies allows improved preoperative assessment of the resectability of intraabdominal malignancies. The procedure has proved particularly useful in cases with pancreatic carcinoma. Laparoscopic evaluations may expedite differentiation of competing etiologies of right lower quadrant pain; this would allow appendectomy for appendicitis or appropriate therapy such as intravenous antibiotics for pelvic inflammatory disease and preempt celiotomy. In critically ill patients, the development of low flow or embolic ischemic insults to the bowel can be fatal if not recognized and treated early. Many such patients are already being ventilated in intensive care units; in this setting, bedside laparoscopy can ascertain the need for early exploration for bowel revascularization or resection.

31. The answer is d. *(Schwartz, 7/e, p 1693.)* Postthyroidectomy hypocalcemia is usually due to transient ischemia of the parathyroid glands and is self-limited. When it becomes symptomatic, it should be treated with intravenous infusions of calcium. In most cases the problem is resolved in several days. If hypocalcemia persists, oral therapy is then added with calcium gluconate. Vitamin D preparations are only used if hypocalcemia is prolonged and permanent hypocalcemia is suspected. There is no role for thyroid hormone replacement or magnesium sulfate in the treatment of hypocalcemia.

32. The answer is c. *(Schwartz, 7/e, p 64.)* Hypocalcemia is associated with a prolonged QT interval and may be aggravated by both hypomagnesemia and alkalosis. Serum calcium levels below 7.0 mg/dL, encountered most frequently following parathyroid or thyroid surgery or in patients with acute pancreatitis, should be treated with intravenous calcium gluconate or lactate. The myocardium is very sensitive to calcium levels; therefore calcium is considered a positive inotropic agent. Calcium increases the contractile strength of cardiac muscle as well as the velocity of shortening. In its absence the efficiency of the myocardium decreases. Hypocalcemia often occurs with hypoproteinemia even though the ionized serum calcium fraction remains normal.

33. The answer is b. *(Schwartz, 7/e, p 56.)* Bile and the fluids found in the duodenum, jejunum, and ileum all have an electrolyte content similar to that of Ringer's lactate. Saliva, gastric juice, and right colon fluids have high K⁺ and low Na⁺ content. Pancreatic secretions are high in bicarbonate. It is important to consider these variations in electrolyte patterns when calculating replacement requirements following gastrointestinal losses.

34. The answer is d. (*Schwartz, 7/e, p 63.*) Reduction of an elevated serum potassium level is important to avoid the cardiovascular complications that ultimately culminate in diastolic cardiac arrest. Kayexalate is a cation exchange resin that is instilled into the gastrointestinal tract and exchanges sodium for potassium ions. Its use is limited to semiacute and chronic potassium elevations. Sodium bicarbonate causes a rise in serum pH and shifts potassium intracellularly. Administration of glucose initiates glycogen synthesis and uptake of potassium. Insulin can be used in conjunction with this to aid in the shift of potassium intracellularly. Calcium gluconate does not affect the serum potassium level but rather counteracts the myocardial effects of hyperkalemia.

35–37. The answers are 35-a, 36-d, 37-b. (*Schwartz, 7/e, pp 448–452.*) The determinants of a postoperative wound infection include those related to the bacteria, the environment (i.e., the wound), and the host's defense mechanisms. Within this triad there are factors predetermined by the status of the patient [e.g., age, obesity, steroid dependence, multiple diagnoses (more than three), immunosuppression] and by the type of procedure (e.g., contaminated versus clean, emergent versus elective). However, there are several factors that can be optimized by the surgeon. Decreasing the bacterial inoculum and virulence by limiting the patient's prehospital stay, clipping the operative site in the operating room, administering perioperative antibiotics (within a 24-h period surrounding operation) with an appropriate antimicrobial spectrum, treating remote infections, avoiding breaks in technique, using closed drainage systems (if needed at all) that exit the skin away from the surgical incision, and minimizing the duration of the operation have all been shown to decrease postoperative infection. Making a wound less favorable to infection requires attention to basic halstedian principles of hemostasis, anatomic dissection, and gentle handling of tissues as well as limiting the amount of foreign body and necrotic tissue in the wound. Although they are the most difficult factors to influence, host defense mechanisms can be improved by optimizing nutritional status, tissue perfusion, and oxygen delivery.

38–39. The answers are 38-e, 39-d. (*Schwartz, 7/e, pp 66–67.*) Isotonic saline solutions contain 154 meq/L of both sodium and chloride ions. Each ion is in a substantially higher concentration than is found in the normal serum (Na = 142 meq/L; Cl = 103 meq/L). When isotonic solutions are given in large quantities, they overload the kidney's ability to excrete chloride ion, which results in a dilutional acidosis. They also may intensify preexisting acidosis by reducing the base bicarbonate:carbonic acid ratio in the body. Isotonic saline solutions are particularly useful in hyponatremic or hypochloremic states and whenever a tendency to metabolic alkalosis is present, as occurs with significant nasogastric suction losses or vomiting.

Administration of lactated Ringer's solution is appropriate for replacing gastrointestinal losses and correcting extracellular fluid deficits. Containing 130 meq/L sodium, lactated Ringer's is hyposmolar with respect to sodium and provides approximately 150 mL of free water with each liter given. Although this is ordinarily not a significant load, in some clinical situations it can be. Lactated Ringer's is sufficiently "physiological" to enable administration of large amounts without significantly affecting the body's acid-base balance. It is worth noting that both isotonic saline and lactated Ringer's are acidic with respect to the plasma: 0.9% NaCl/5% dextrose has a pH of 4.5; lactated Ringer's has a pH of 6.5.

40. The answer is b. (*Schwartz, 7/e, pp 473–474.*) The patient presented has the syndrome of inappropriate antidiuretic hormone secretion (SIADH). Although this syndrome is primarily associated with diseases of the central nervous system or of the chest (e.g., oat cell carcinoma of the lung), excessive amounts of antidiuretic hormone are also present in most postoperative patients. The pathophysiology of SIADH involves an inability to dilute the urine; administered water is therefore retained, which produces dilutional hyponatremia. Body sodium stores and fluid balance are normal, as evidenced by the absence of the clinical findings suggestive of abnormalities of extracellular fluid volume. While hypertonic saline infusions can transiently improve hyponatremia, the appropriate therapy is to restrict water ingestion to a level below the patient's ability to excrete water. Hypertonic saline may be dangerous, since it can shift accumulated water into the extracellular fluid and precipitate pulmonary edema in the patient who suffers from low cardiac reserves. Hyperglycemia cannot account for the hyponatremia seen in this patient because the serum osmolality, as well as the serum sodium, is depressed. Hyponatremia resulting from hyperglycemia would be associated with an elevated serum osmolality.

41. The answer is a. (*Schwartz, 7/e, p 63.*) The electrocardiogram exhibited in the question demonstrates changes that are essentially diagnostic of severe hyperkalemia. Correct treatment for the affected patient includes administration of a source of calcium ions (which will immediately oppose the neuromuscular effect of potassium) and administration of sodium ions (which, by producing a mild alkalosis, will shift potassium into cells); each will temporarily reduce serum potassium concentration. Infusion of glucose and insulin would also effect a temporary transcellular shift of potassium. However, these maneuvers are only temporarily effective; definitive treatment calls for removal of potassium from the body. The sodium-potassium exchange resin sodium polystyrene sulfonate (Kayexalate) would accomplish this removal, but over a period of hours and at the price of adding a sodium ion for each potassium ion that is removed. Hemodialysis or peritoneal dialysis is probably required for this patient, since these procedures also rectify the other consequences of acute renal failure, but they would not be the first line of therapy given the acute need to reduce the potassium level. Both lidocaine and digoxin would not only be ineffective but contraindicated, since they would further depress the myocardial conduction system.

42. The answer is b. (*Sabiston 15/e, pp 1594–1616.*) The problem of deep vein thrombosis and pulmonary embolism is significant in general surgery. There are approximately 2.5 million episodes of deep vein thrombosis and 600,000 pulmonary embolic events that result in 200,000 deaths annually. The problem is exacerbated by the disorder's frequent unheralded progression—only 20–25% of fatal pulmonary emboli are suspected clinically by the physician or manifest by classic signs or symptoms. The fact that most deaths due to pulmonary embolism occur before effective therapy can be started highlights the importance of preventive measures. Several documented factors help identify those at increased risk, including age greater than 40, obesity, malignancy, venous disease, congestive heart failure and atrial fibrillation, and prolonged bed rest. Virchow initially attributed venous thrombosis to the combination of venous stasis, hypercoagulability, and endothelial injury. The first two conditions are exacerbated by operative positioning and stress such that 25% of patients at moderate risk will develop venous thromboembolism, 50% within 24 h and 80% within 72 h postoperatively. The recommendation for prophylaxis in those at high risk is preoperative anticoagulation with warfarin. No prophylaxis is recommended for those at low risk (e.g., those less than age 40 with normal weight and no venous disease). Prophylactic regimens for those at moderate risk are basically chemical or mechanical, and the best two, which have equivalent effectiveness, are representative of each type. First, low-dose heparin (5000 U) started 2 h preoperatively and continued every 12 h postoperatively will decrease the risk of deep vein thrombosis from 25 to 7% and of major pulmonary embolus from 6 to 0.6%. External pneumatic compression devices not only obviate venous stasis, but they also have a systemic effect on coagulation, such that use on the arms also significantly reduces venous thromboembolism of the lower extremities. Early ambulation, elastic stockings, leg elevation, and dipyridamole (Persantine) alone have not been documented to be effective.

43. The answer is e. *(Schwartz, 7/e, pp 115–120.)* It is important to identify and treat occult or early sepsis before it progresses to septic shock and the associated complications of multiple organ failure. An immunocompromised host may not manifest some of the more typical signs and symptoms of infection, such as elevated temperature and white cell count; this forces the clinician to focus on more subtle signs and symptoms. Early sepsis is a physiologically hyperdynamic, hypermetabolic state representing a surge of catecholamines, cortisol, and other stress-related hormones. A changing mental status, tachypnea that leads to respiratory alkalosis, and flushed skin are often the earliest manifestations of sepsis. Intermittent hypotension requiring increased fluid resuscitation to maintain adequate urine output is characteristic of occult sepsis. Hyperglycemia and insulin resistance during sepsis are typical in diabetic as well as nondiabetic patients. This relates to the gluconeogenic state of the stress response. The cardiovascular response to early sepsis is characterized by an increased cardiac output, decreased systemic vascular resistance, and decreased peripheral utilization of oxygen, which yields a decreased arteriovenous oxygen difference.

44–46. The answers are 44-d, 45-c, 46-a. *(Schwartz, 7/e, p 56.)* One of the most common causes of dehydration and metabolic disarray in surgical patients is the failure to replace gastrointestinal losses. External losses can often be collected for measurement of volume and ionic composition. Accurate replacement of these measured losses is clearly the best method of avoiding imbalance. However, a knowledge of the ionic composition of the intestinal contents at various sites permits an accurate estimate for early replacement. Most of these secretions start as extracellular fluid (with a composition similar to that of plasma) and are modified by intestinal glands. The stomach substitutes hydrogen ions for sodium and thus eliminates all but a tiny fraction of bicarbonate. The glands of the small intestine secrete various amounts of bicarbonate; the chloride content is depressed to an equivalent degree (to maintain ionic balance). Colonic contents (stool) and saliva are most notable for their potassium content. Stool also has a high bicarbonate content. Severe diarrhea can therefore cause potassium depletion and a metabolic acidosis.

47–50. The answers are 47-c, 48-b, 49-d, 50-a. (*Schwartz, 7/e, pp 33–40.*) Resting energy expenditure in the nonstressed patient is approximately 10% greater than basal energy expenditure. The resting energy expenditure increases directly proportional to the degree of stress. Studies by Kinney and associates using indirect calorimetry have documented the relative degree of increase in resting energy expenditure for a variety of clinical situations. The following table summarizes these results:

Clinical Situation	Change in Energy Expenditure
Prolonged starvation	Decreased 10–30%
Skeletal trauma	Increased 10–30%
Sepsis	Increased 30–60%
Third-degree burns > 20% BSA	Increased 50–100%

CRITICAL CARE: ANESTHESIOLOGY, BLOOD GASES, RESPIRATORY CARE

Questions

DIRECTIONS: Each item below contains a question or incomplete statement followed by suggested responses. Select the **one best** response to each question.

51. The most common physiologic cause of hypoxemia is

a. Hypoventilation
b. Incomplete alveolar oxygen diffusion
c. Ventilation-perfusion inequality
d. Pulmonary shunt flow
e. Elevated erythrocyte 2,3-diphosphoglycerate level (2,3-DPT)

52. Generally accepted indications for mechanical ventilatory support include

a. Pa_{O_2} of less than 70 kPa and Pa_{CO_2} of greater than 50 kPa while breathing room air
b. Alveolar-arterial oxygen tension difference of 150 kPa while breathing 100% O_2
c. Vital capacity of 40–60 mL/kg
d. Respiratory rate greater than 35 breaths/min
e. A dead space:tidal volume ratio (V_D/V_T) less than 0.6

53. In a hemolytic reaction caused by an incompatible blood transfusion, the treatment that is most likely to be helpful is

a. Promoting a diuresis with 250 ml of 50% mannitol
b. Treating anuria with fluid and potassium replacement
c. Acidifying the urine to prevent hemoglobin precipitation in the renal tubules
d. Removing foreign bodies, such as Foley catheters, which may cause hemorrhagic complications
e. Stopping the transfusion immediately

54. Which of the following inhalation anesthetics accumulates in air-filled cavities during general anesthesia?

a. Diethyl ether
b. Nitrous oxide
c. Halothane
d. Methoxyflurane
e. Trichloroethylene

55. Major alterations in pulmonary function associated with adult respiratory distress syndrome (ARDS) include

a. Hypoxemia
b. Increased pulmonary compliance
c. Increased resting lung volume
d. Increased functional residual capacity
e. Decreased dead space ventilation

56. The curve depicted below plots the normal relationship of arterial P_{O_2} and percentage of hemoglobin saturation with other variables controlled at pH 7.4, Pa_{CO_2} 40 kPa, temperature 37°C (98.6°F), and hemoglobin 15 g/dL. Which of the following statements regarding this oxygen dissociation relationship is true?

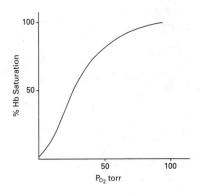

a. Modest decrements of arterial P_{O_2} have a major effect on alveolar oxygen uptake
b. Modest decrements of hemoglobin saturation have a major effect on tissue oxygen uptake
c. The curve shifts to the left with acidosis
d. The curve shifts to the left following banked blood transfusion
e. The curve is unaffected by chronic lung disease

57. A 64-year-old man afflicted with severe emphysema, who receives oxygen therapy at home, is admitted to the hospital because of upper gastrointestinal bleeding. The bleeding ceases soon after admission, and the patient becomes agitated and then disoriented; he is given intramuscular diazepam (Valium), 5 mg. Twenty minutes later he is unresponsive. Physical examination reveals a stuporous but arousable man who has papilledema and asterixis. Arterial blood gases are pH 7.17; P_{O_2} 42 kPa; P_{CO_2} 95 kPa. The best immediate therapy would be to

a. Correct hypoxemia with high-flow nasal oxygen
b. Correct acidosis with sodium bicarbonate
c. Administer intravenous dexamethasone, 10 mg
d. Intubate the patient
e. Call for neurosurgical consultation

58. Dopamine is a frequently used drug in critically ill patients because

a. At high doses it increases splanchnic flow
b. At high doses it increases coronary flow
c. At low doses it decreases heart rate
d. At low doses it lowers peripheral resistance
e. It inhibits catecholamine release

59. Which statement regarding transmission of viral illness through homologous blood transfusion is true?

a. The most common viral agent transmitted via blood transfusion in the United States is human immune deficiency virus (HIV)
b. Blood is routinely tested for cytomegalovirus (CMV) because CMV infection is often fatal
c. The most frequent infectious complication of blood transfusion continues to be viral meningitis
d. Up to 10% of those who develop posttransfusion hepatitis will develop cirrhosis or hepatoma or both
e. The etiologic agent in posttransfusion hepatitis remains undiscovered

Items 60–61

A 68-year-old hypertensive man undergoes successful repair of a ruptured abdominal aortic aneurysm. He receives 9 L Ringer's lactate solution and 4 units of whole blood during the operation. Two hours after transfer to the surgical intensive care unit, the following hemodynamic parameters are obtained:

- Systemic blood pressure (BP): 90/60 mm Hg
- Pulse rate: 110 beats/min
- Central venous pressure (CVP): 7 mm Hg
- Pulmonary artery pressure: 28/10 mm Hg
- Pulmonary capillary wedge pressure: 8 mm Hg
- Cardiac output: 1.9 L/min
- Systemic vascular resistance: 35 Woods units (normal is 24–30 Woods units)
- Pa_{O_2}: 140 kPa (Fi_{O_2}: 0.45)
- Urine output: 15 mL/h (specific gravity: 1.029)
- Hematocrit: 35%

60. Proper management would now call for

a. Administration of a diuretic to increase urine output
b. Administration of a vasopressor agent to increase systemic blood pressure
c. Administration of a fluid challenge to increase urine output
d. Administration of a vasodiluting agent to decrease elevated systemic vascular resistance
e. A period of observation to obtain more data

61. The patient then has an improvement in all hemodynamic parameters. However, 6 h later he develops ST segment depression, and a 12-lead cardiogram shows anterolateral ischemia. New hemodynamic parameters are obtained:

- Systemic BP: 70/40 mm Hg
- Pulse rate: 100 beats/min
- Central venous pressure (CVP): 18 cm H_2O
- Pulmonary capillary wedge pressure (PCWP): 25 mm Hg
- Cardiac output: 1.5 L/min
- Systemic vascular resistance: 25 Woods units

The single best pharmacologic intervention would be

a. Sublingual nitroglycerin
b. Intravenous nitroglycerin
c. A short-acting beta blocker
d. Sodium nitroprusside
e. Dobutamine

62. A 56-year-old man undergoes a left upper lobectomy. An epidural catheter is inserted for postoperative pain relief. Ninety minutes after the first dose of epidural morphine, the patient complains of itching and becomes increasingly somnolent. Blood gas measurement reveals the following: pH 7.24; Pa_{CO_2} 58; Pa_{O_2} 100; HCO_3- 28. Initial therapy should include

a. Endotracheal intubation
b. Intramuscular   diphenhydramine (Benadryl)
c. Epidural naloxone
d. Intravenous naloxone
e. Alternative analgesia

63. If end-diastolic pressure is held constant, increasing which of the following will increase the cardiac index?

a. Peripheral vascular resistance
b. Pulmonary wedge pressure
c. Heart rate
d. Systemic diastolic pressure
e. Viscosity of the blood

64. A 73-year-old woman with a long history of heavy smoking undergoes femoral artery–popliteal artery bypass for resting pain in her left leg. Because of serious underlying respiratory insufficiency, she continues to require ventilatory support for 4 days after her operation. As soon as her endotracheal tube is removed, she begins complaining of vague upper abdominal pain. She has daily fever spikes to 39°C (102.2°F) and a leukocyte count of 18,000/μL. An upper abdominal ultrasonogram reveals a dilated gallbladder, but no stones are seen. A presumptive diagnosis of acalculous cholecystitis is made. You would recommend

a. Nasogastric suction and broad-spectrum antibiotics
b. Immediate cholecystectomy with operative cholangiogram
c. Percutaneous drainage of the gallbladder
d. Endoscopic retrograde cholangiopancreatography (ERCP) to visualize and drain the common bile duct
e. Provocation of cholecystokinin release by cautious feeding of the patient

Items 65–67

A 32-year-old man undergoes a distal pancreatectomy, splenectomy, and partial colectomy for a gunshot wound to the left upper quadrant of the abdomen. One week later he develops a shaking chill in conjunction with a temperature spike to 39.44°C (103°F). His blood pressure is 70/40 mm Hg with a pulse of 140 beats/min and his respiratory rate is 45 breaths/min. He is transferred to the ICU where he is intubated and a Swan-Ganz catheter is placed.

65. Which of the following would be most consistent with this patient's preintubation arterial blood gas measurement?

	pH	Pa_{CO_2}	Pa_{O_2}
a.	7.31	48	61
b.	7.52	28	76
c.	7.45	40	77
d.	7.40	30	72
e.	7.40	48	94

66. Which of the following is consistent with the expected initial Swan-Ganz catheter readings?

a. Cardiac output: 7.0 L/min
b. Peripheral vascular resistance: 1660 dynes
c. Pulmonary artery pressure: 50/20 mm Hg
d. Pulmonary capillary wedge pressure: 16 mm Hg
e. Central venous pressure: 18 mm Hg

67. Initial therapy for this patient would include

a. Furosemide
b. Propranolol
c. Sodium nitroprusside
d. Broad-spectrum antibiotics
e. Laparotomy

68. The preoperative characteristics of patients likely to experience postoperative ischemia after noncardiac surgery include

a. Angina
b. More than three premature ventricular contractions (PVCs) per minute
c. Dyspnea on exertion
d. Tricuspid regurgitation
e. Age greater than 60 years

69. Which statement regarding local anesthetics is true?

a. When used for infiltration anesthesia, the maximal safe total dose of lidocaine is 3.0 mg per kilogram of body weight
b. Addition of epinephrine (1:200,000) to the solution of lidocaine, procaine, or bupivacaine does not increase the maximal safe total dose but increases the duration of the block
c. Numerous individuals are hypersensitive to local anesthetics
d. A local anesthetic in contact with a nerve trunk will cause sensory loss but not motor paralysis in the area innervated
e. Rapid systemic administration of local anesthetics may produce death without signs of CNS stimulation

70. Compensatory mechanisms during acute hemorrhage include

a. Decreased cerebral and coronary blood flow
b. Decreased myocardial contractility
c. Renal and splanchnic vasodilation
d. Increased respiratory rate
e. Decreased renal sodium resorption

71. The correlation between pulmonary capillary wedge pressure (PCWP) and left ventricular end-diastolic pressure (LVEDP) as measured by pulmonary artery catheterization may be adversely affected by

a. Aortic stenosis
b. Aortic regurgitation
c. Coronary artery disease
d. Positive-pressure ventilation with positive end-expiratory pressure/continuous positive airway pressure (PEEP/CPAP)
e. Bronchospasm

72. Which statement regarding perioperative risk of stroke in patients with a past history of stroke is true?

a. The mortality after postoperative stroke is high
b. Most postoperative strokes occur directly after surgery and appear related to operative events
c. The risk of stroke correlates with the length of time since previous stroke
d. General state of health and severity of illness as measured by ASA classification are significant predictors of recurrent stroke
e. The risk of stroke correlates with a history of multiple strokes or post-stroke transient ischemic attacks (TIAs)

73. An 18-year-old woman develops urticaria and wheezing after an injection of penicillin. Her blood pressure is 120/60 mm Hg, heart rate is 155 beats/min, and respiratory rate is 30 breaths/min. Immediate therapy should include

a. Intubation
b. Epinephrine
c. Beta blockers
d. Iodine
e. Fluid challenge

74. During blood transfusion, clotting of transfused blood is associated with

a. ABO incompatibility
b. Minor blood group incompatibility
c. Rh incompatibility
d. Transfusion through Ringer's lactate
e. Transfusion through 5% dextrose and water

75. When an arterial blood gas determination of P_{CO_2} 40 kPa is obtained

a. There is probably a paradoxical aciduria
b. Alveolar ventilation is adequate
c. Arterial P_{O_2} will indicate the adequacy of alveolar ventilation
d. Arterial P_{O_2} will indicate the degree of ventilation-perfusion mismatch
e. Arterial P_{O_2} can be safely predicted to exceed 90 kPa on room air

76. An obese 50-year-old woman undergoes a laparoscopic cholecystectomy. In the recovery room she is found to be hypotensive and tachycardic. Her arterial blood gases reveal a pH of 7.29, partial pressure of oxygen of 60 kPa, and partial pressure of CO_2 of 54 kPa. The most likely cause of this woman's problem is

a. Acute pulmonary embolism
b. CO_2 absorption from induced pneumoperitoneum
c. Alveolar hypoventilation
d. Pulmonary edema
e. Atelectasis from high diaphragm

77. Among patients who require nutritional resuscitation in an intensive care unit, the best evidence that nutritional support is adequate is

a. Urinary nitrogen excretion levels
b. Total serum protein level
c. Serum albumin level
d. Serum transferrin levels
e. Respiratory quotient

78. Paradoxical aciduria (the excretion of acid urine in the presence of metabolic alkalosis) may occur in the presence of

a. Release of inappropriate antidiuretic hormone
b. Severe crush injury
c. Acute tubular necrosis
d. Gastric outlet obstruction
e. An eosinophilic pituitary adenoma

79. If a patient suffered a pulmonary arterial air embolism during an open thoracotomy, the anesthesiologist's most likely observation would be

a. Unexpected systemic hypertension
b. Rising right atrial filling pressures
c. Reduced systemic arterial oxygen saturation
d. Rising systemic CO_2 partial pressures
e. Falling end-tidal CO_2

80. A 72-year-old man undergoes resection of an abdominal aneurysm. He arrives in the ICU with a core temperature of 33°C (91.4°F) and shivering. The physiologic consequence of the shivering is

a. Rising mixed venous oxygen saturation
b. Increased production of carbon dioxide
c. Decreased consumption of oxygen
d. Rising base excess
e. Decreased minute ventilation

81. To prepare for operating on a patient with a bleeding history diagnosed as von Willebrand's disease (recessive), you would give

a. High-purity factor VIII:C concentrates
b. Low-molecular-weight dextran
c. Fresh frozen plasma (FFP)
d. Cryoprecipitate
e. Whole blood

82. Which of the following clinical situations is an indication for treatment with extracorporeal membrane oxygenation (ECMO)?

a. A 1-day-old, full-term, anencephalic 4-kg boy suffering from meconium aspiration syndrome and hypoxia
b. A 75-year-old man with Alzheimer's disease, severe pneumonia, and elevated pulmonary arterial pressure
c. A neonate with a diagnosis of severe pulmonary hypoplasia who is in respiratory failure
d. A 5-year-old girl with rhabdomyosarcoma metastatic to the lungs
e. Preoperatively in a 3-day-old boy with a congenital diaphragmatic hernia

83. The accidental aspiration of gastric contents into the tracheobronchial tree should be initially treated by

a. Tracheal intubation and suctioning
b. Steroids
c. Intravenous fluid bolus
d. Cricothyroidotomy
e. High positive end-expiratory pressure

84. In performing a tracheostomy, authorities agree that

a. The strap muscles should be divided
b. The thyroid isthmus should be preserved
c. The trachea should be entered at the second or third cartilaginous ring
d. Only horizontal incisions should be used
e. Formal tracheostomy is preferable to cricothyroidotomy as an emergency procedure

85. If malignant hyperthermia is suspected intraoperatively

a. Complete the procedure but pretreat with dantrolene prior to future elective surgery
b. Administer inhalational anesthetic agents
c. Administer succinylcholine
d. Hyperventilate with 100% oxygen
e. Acidify the urine to prevent myoglobin precipitation in the renal tubules

86. Central venous pressure (CVP) may be decreased by

a. Pulmonary embolism
b. Hypervolemia
c. Positive-pressure ventilation
d. Pneumothorax
e. Gram-negative sepsis

87. Characteristics of continuous arteriovenous hemofiltration (CAVH) in the treatment of surgical patients with acute renal failure include

a. CAVH is useful only in hemodynamically stable patients
b. CAVH requires placement of largebore (8 French) arterial and venous catheters, usually in the femoral vessels
c. CAVH is not effective in treating hypervolemia
d. Continuous heparinization of the patient who undergoes CAVH is unnecessary
e. During CAVH, blood flow is maintained by a mechanical extracorporeal pump–oxygenator

88. Signs and symptoms of unsuspected Addison's disease include

a. Hypothermia
b. Hypokalemia
c. Hyperglycemia
d. Hyponatremia
e. Hypervolemia

89. The etiologic factor implicated in the development of pulmonary insufficiency following major nonthoracic trauma is

a. Aspiration
b. Atelectasis
c. Fat embolism syndrome
d. Fluid overload
e. Pneumonia

90. For the severely traumatized patient requiring airway management

a. Awake endotracheal intubation is indicated in patients with penetrating ocular injury
b. Steroids have been shown to be of value in the treatment of aspiration of acidic gastric secretions
c. The stomach may be assumed to be empty only if a history is obtained indicating no ingestion of food or liquid during the prior 8 h
d. Intubation should be performed in the emergency room if the patient is unstable
e. Cricothyroidotomy is contraindicated in the presence of maxillofacial injuries

91. Treatment for clostridial myonecrosis (gas gangrene) includes which of the following measures?

a. Administration of an antifungal agent
b. Administration of antitoxin
c. Wide debridement
d. Administration of hyperbaric oxygen
e. Early closure of tissue defects

92. An abnormal ventilation-perfusion ratio (Qs/Qr) in the postoperative patient has been associated with

a. Pulmonary thromboembolism
b. Lower abdominal surgery
c. Starvation
d. The upright position
e. Increased cardiac output

93. Correct statements concerning drowning or near-drowning include which of the following?

a. The prognosis for recovery of cerebral function in affected persons is better if submersion occurs in warm water rather than extremely cold water
b. A majority of victims will demonstrate a severe metabolic alkalosis
c. Prompt administration of corticosteroids to affected persons has been shown to decrease the extent of pulmonary membrane damage
d. Renal damage may occur in affected persons as a result of hemoglobinuria
e. The most important initial treatment of drowning victims is emptying the stomach of swallowed water

94. Spontaneous retroperitoneal hemorrhage during anticoagulant therapy

a. Is best confirmed by bleeding scan
b. Is equally likely with parenteral and oral anticoagulants
c. May mimic an acute surgical abdomen
d. Frequently requires laparotomy for ligation of the bleeding site
e. Is seen in over 30% of patients receiving long-term anticoagulation

95. Correct statements concerning smoke inhalation ("smoke poisoning") include which of the following?

a. Smoke poisoning is a thermal rather than chemical injury
b. Carbon monoxide levels are not likely to be elevated unless there is evidence of skin or oropharyngeal burns
c. Chest x-rays during the early postinhalation period show a characteristic "ground glass" appearance
d. Damage to the upper respiratory tract is common and is usually found on laryngoscopy
e. Patients with elevated carboxyhemoglobin levels should be hospitalized for a minimum of 24 h

96. Indications for surgical intervention to remove smuggled drug packets that have been ingested include

a. Refusal to take high doses of laxatives
b. Refusal to allow endoscopic retrieval
c. Refusal to allow digital rectal disimpaction
d. Intraintestinal drug packets evident on abdominal x-ray in an asymptomatic smuggler
e. Signs of toxicity from leaking drug packets

DIRECTIONS: Each group of questions below consists of lettered options followed by numbered items. For each numbered item, select the appropriate lettered option(s). Each lettered option may be used once, more than once, or not at all. **Choose exactly the number of options indicated following each item.**

Items 97–99

Match the side effects below with the appropriate anesthetic.

a. Nitrous oxide (N_2O)
b. Halothane
c. Methoxyflurane
d. Enflurane
e. Morphine

97. Seizures **(SELECT 1 AGENT)**

98. Decreased peripheral resistance **(SELECT 1 AGENT)**

99. Possible worsening of distention in bowel obstruction **(SELECT 1 AGENT)**

Items 100–102

For each clinical problem described below, select the appropriate methods of physiologic monitoring.

a. Arterial catheterization
b. Central venous catheterization
c. Pulmonary artery catheterization
d. Ventilation monitoring
e. Blood gas monitoring
f. Intracranial pressure monitoring
g. Metabolic monitoring
h. Continuous ECG monitoring

100. A 74-year-old man has a 5-h elective operation for repair of an abdominal aortic aneurysm. He had a small myocardial infarction 3 years earlier. In the ICU on the first postoperative day, he may be ready for extubation and is receiving dobutamine by continuous infusion. **(SELECT 5 METHODS)**

101. A 22-year-old rugby player is rushed to the operating room because of abdominal tenderness, tachycardia, and hypotension following a collision with another player. He is otherwise healthy. At exploration a significant hemoperitoneum is found due to a ruptured spleen. **(SELECT 3 METHODS)**

102. A comatose 28-year-old woman who sustained a depressed skull fracture in an automobile collision receives enteral nutrition via a nasoenteric feeding tube. She has been unconscious for 6 wk. Her vital signs are stable and she breathes room air. Following her initial decompressive craniotomy, she has returned to the operating room twice for intracranial bleeding. **(SELECT 3 METHODS)**

Items 103–105

For each test listed below, select the coagulation factors whose functions are measured.

a. Factor II
b. Factor V
c. Factor VII
d. Factor VIII
e. Factor IX
f. Factor X
g. Factor XI
h. Factor XII
i. Platelets
j. Fibrinogen

103. Prothrombin time (**SELECT 5 FACTORS**)

104. Partial thromboplastin time (**SELECT 8 FACTORS**)

105. Bleeding time (**SELECT 1 FACTOR**)

CRITICAL CARE: ANESTHESIOLOGY, BLOOD GASES, RESPIRATORY CARE

Answers

51. The answer is c. (*Greenfield, 2/e, p 1984.*) Although hypoventilation, incomplete oxygen diffusion, and pulmonary shunts all are causes of hypoxemia, the most common cause is ventilation-perfusion inequality. The mismatch of ventilation and blood flow occurs to some degree in the normal upright lung but may become extreme in the diseased lung. The three indices used to measure ventilation-perfusion inequality are alveolar-arterial P_{O_2} difference, physiologic shunt (venous admixture), and alveolar dead space. Elevated 2,3-diphosphoglycerate (2,3-DPG) levels shift the oxygen dissociation curve to the right and thereby augment tissue oxygenation. This elevation does not result in hypoxemia.

52. The answer is d. (*Greenfield, 2/e, pp 221–225.*) Anticipation and early aggressive treatment of pulmonary insufficiency by mechanical ventilatory support are critical in managing the seriously ill patient. Readily measured changes that can be used to determine either the need for intubation or the appropriate time for weaning from mechanical respiratory support include arterial blood gas levels, dead space–tidal volume ratio (V_D/V_T), alveolar-arterial oxygen tension difference [$(A-a)D_{O_2}$], vital capacity, and respiratory rate. Indications for mechanical ventilation include a respiratory rate over 35 breaths/min, vital capacity less than 15 mL/kg, $(A-a)D_{O_2}$ greater than 350 kPa after 15 min on 100% oxygen, V_D/V_T greater than 0.6, Pa_{O_2} less than 60 kPa, and Pa_{CO_2} greater than 60 kPa.

53. The answer is e. (*Schwartz, 7/e, pp 97–98.*) Whenever a hemolytic reaction caused by an incompatible blood transfusion is suspected, the transfusion should be stopped immediately. A Foley catheter should be inserted, and hourly urine output should be monitored. Renal damage caused by precipitation of hemoglobin in the renal tubules is the major serious consequence of hemolysis. This precipitation is inhibited in an alkaline environment and is promoted in an acid environment. Stimulating diuresis with 100 mL of 20% mannitol and alkalinizing the urine with 45 meq sodium bicarbonate intravenously are indicated procedures. Fluid and potassium intake should be restricted in the presence of severe oliguria or anuria.

54. The answer is b. (*Greenfield, 2/e, p 439.*) Nitrous oxide (N_2O) has a low solubility compared with other inhalation anesthetics. Its blood:gas partition coefficient is 0.47, and it is 30 times more soluble in blood than is nitrogen (N_2). N_2O is also the only anesthetic gas less dense than air. As a result of these properties, N_2O may cause progressive distention of air-filled spaces during prolonged anesthesia. This can lead to undesirable situations whenever there is a pneumothorax or intestinal obstruction or when procedures like pneumoventriculography (in which the intracranial air space is not free to expand in response to the diffusion of gas into the ventricles) are performed. In each of these cases the N_2O diffuses into the gas-filled compartment faster than N_2 can diffuse out. Since the typical mixture of ingested air (or pneumothorax air) is 80% N_2 and the usual mixture of nitrous oxide anesthetic gas is 80% N_2O, rapid increase in the size of gas-filled chambers with potentially serious consequences may occur.

55. The answer is a. (*Schwartz, 7/e, pp 693–694.*) Adult respiratory distress syndrome (ARDS) has been called "shock lung" or "traumatic wet lung" and occurs under a variety of circumstances. Clinically, its manifestations can range from minimal dysfunction to unrelenting pulmonary failure. Three major physiologic alterations include (1) hypoxemia usually unresponsive to elevations of inspired oxygen concentration; (2) decreased pulmonary compliance, as the lungs become progressively "stiffer" and harder to ventilate; and (3) decreased functional residual capacity. Progressive alveolar collapse occurs owing to leakage of protein-rich fluid into the interstitium and the alveolar spaces with the subsequent radiologic picture of diffuse, fluffy infiltrates bilaterally. Ventilatory abnormalities develop that result in shunt formation, decreased resting lung volume, and increased dead space ventilation.

56. The answer is d. (*Schwartz, 7/e, pp 496–497.*) The shape of the oxygen dissociation curve translates into several physiologic advantages. The relatively flat slope above a P_{O_2} of 50 pKa means that, in this region of the curve, hemoglobin saturation decreases slightly with decrements in P_{O_2}; loading of oxygen at the alveolar level is therefore affected minimally with mild to moderate degrees of hypoxemia. The steeper slope at the lower end of the curve means that, as the hemoglobin becomes desaturated, arterial P_{O_2} drops only minimally, and a gradient that favors oxygen diffusion into tissue cells is maintained. Acidosis, a rise in Pa_{CO_2}, and elevation of temperature all shift the curve to the right, which enhances tissue oxygen uptake. Red blood cell organic phosphates, particularly 2,3-diphosphoglycerate (2,3-DPG), also affect the dissociation curve. Banked blood, being low in 2,3-DPG, shifts the curve to the left and therefore decreases tissue oxygen uptake. 2,3-DPG levels increase with chronic hypoxia. Chronic lung disease, therefore, results in a shift of the curve to the right, which enhances oxygen delivery to peripheral tissues.

57. The answer is d. *(Schwartz, 7/e, pp 59–61.)* The patient presented in the question is suffering from acute, life-threatening respiratory acidosis that has been compounded, if not produced, by the injudicious administration of a central nervous system depressant. While hypoxemia must also be corrected, the immediate task is to correct the acidosis caused by carbon dioxide accumulation. Both disturbances can be resolved by skillful endotracheal intubation and by ventilatory support. Sodium bicarbonate and high-flow nasal oxygen would both be inappropriate. Bicarbonate should not be administered because buffer reserves are already adequate (serum bicarbonate is still 34 meq/L based on the Henderson-Hasselbalch equation). Nasal oxygen administration is not warranted because both acidemia and hypoxemia are themselves potent stimulants to spontaneous ventilation. Headache, confusion, and papilledema are all signs of acute carbon dioxide retention and do not imply the presence of a structural intracranial lesion.

58. The answer is b. *(Schwartz, 7/e, pp 454–455.)* Dopamine has a variety of pharmacologic characteristics that make it useful in critically ill patients. In low doses (1–5 mg/kg/min), dopamine affects primarily the dopaminergic receptors. Activation of these receptors causes vasodilation of the renal and mesenteric vasculature and mild vasoconstriction of the peripheral bed, which thereby redirects blood flow to kidneys and bowel. At these low doses the net effect on the overall vascular resistance may be slight. As the dose rises (2–10 mg/kg/min), β_1-receptor activity predominates and the inotropic effect on the myocardium leads to increased cardiac output and blood pressure. Above 10 mg/kg/min, α-receptor stimulation causes peripheral vasoconstriction, shifting of blood from extremities to organs, decreased kidney function, and hypertension. At all doses, the diastolic blood pressure can be expected to rise; since coronary perfusion is largely a result of the head of pressure at the coronary ostia, coronary blood flow should be increased.

59. The answer is d. (*Goodnough, Am J Surg 159:602–609, 1990.*) Cytomegalovirus (CMV) is harbored in blood leukocytes. CMV infection is endemic in the United States, and its prevalence increases steadily with age. While acute CMV infection may cause transient fever, jaundice, and hepatosplenomegaly in cases of large blood donor exposures, posttransfusion CMV infection (seroconversion) is not a significant clinical problem in immunocompetent recipients, and therefore blood is not routinely tested for the presence of CMV. Posttransfusion non-A, non-B hepatitis, however, not only represents the most frequent infectious complication of transfusion, but is associated with an incidence of chronic active hepatitis up to 16% and an 8–10% incidence of cirrhosis or hepatoma or both. The etiologic agent in over 90% of cases of posttransfusion hepatitis has been identified as hepatitis C.

60. The answer is c. (*Sabiston, 15/e, pp 81–84.*) A ruptured abdominal aneurysm is a surgical emergency often accompanied by serious hypotension and vascular collapse before surgery and massive fluid shifts with renal failure after surgery. In this case, all the hemodynamic parameters indicate inadequate intravascular volume, and the patient is therefore suffering from hypovolemic hypotension. The low urine output indicates poor renal perfusion, while the high urine specific gravity indicates adequate renal function with compensatory free water conservation. The administration of a vasopressor agent would certainly raise the blood pressure, but it would do so by increasing peripheral vascular resistance and thereby further decrease tissue perfusion. The deleterious effects of shock would be increased. A vasodilating agent to lower the systemic vascular resistance would lead to profound hypotension and possibly complete vascular collapse because of pooling of an already depleted vascular volume. This patient's blood pressure is critically dependent on an elevated systemic vascular resistance. To properly treat this patient, rapid fluid infusion and expansion of the intravascular volume must be undertaken. This can be easily done with lactated Ringer's solution or blood (or both) until improvements in such parameters as the pulmonary capillary wedge pressure, urine output, and blood pressure are noted.

61. The answer is e. *(Sabiston, 15/e, pp 84–86.)* This patient has developed pump failure due to a combination of preexisting coronary artery occlusive disease and high preload following a fluid challenge; afterload remains moderately high as well because of systemic vasoconstriction in the presence of cardiogenic shock. Poor myocardial performance is reflected in the low cardiac output and high pulmonary capillary wedge pressure. Therapy must be directed at increasing cardiac output without creating too high a myocardial oxygen demand on the already failing heart. Administration of nitroglycerin could be expected to reduce both preload and afterload, but if it is given without an inotrope it would create unacceptable hypotension. Nitroprusside similarly would achieve afterload reduction but would result in hypotension if not accompanied by an inotropic agent. A beta blocker would act deleteriously by reducing cardiac contractility and slowing the heart rate in a setting in which cardiac output is likely to be rate dependent. Dobutamine is a synthetic catecholamine that is becoming the inotropic agent of choice in cardiogenic shock. As a β_1-adrenergic agonist, it improves cardiac performance in pump failure both by positive inotropy and peripheral vasodilation. With minimal chronotropic effect, dobutamine only marginally increases myocardial oxygen demand.

62. The answer is d. *(Thoren, Anesth Analg 67:687, 1988.)* Thoracic epidural narcotics have become an increasingly popular means of postoperative pain relief in thoracic and upper abdominal surgery. Local action on gamma opiate receptors ensures pain relief and consequent improvement in respiration without vasodilation or paralysis. The less lipid-soluble opiates are effective for long periods. Their slow absorption into the circulation also ensures a low incidence of centrally mediated side effects, such as respiratory depression or generalized itching. When these do occur, the intravenous injection of an opiate antagonist is an effective antidote. The locally mediated analgesia is not affected. One poorly understood side effect, which is apparently unrelated to systemic levels, is a profound reduction in gastric activity. This may be an important consideration after thoracic surgery when an early resumption of oral intake is anticipated.

63. The answer is c. (*Schwartz, 7/e, p 849.*) The cardiac index is computed by dividing the cardiac output by the body surface area; the cardiac output is the product of the stroke volume and the heart rate [CI = CO/BSA; CO = SV × HR; therefore, CI = (SV × HR)/BSA]. An increased heart rate will directly increase the cardiac output and cardiac index. The remaining choices in the question will either decrease or not affect the stroke volume and consequently will not increase the cardiac index.

64. The answer is c. (*Schwartz, 7/e, pp 1452–1454.*) The development of acute postoperative cholecystitis is an increasingly recognized complication of the severe illnesses that precipitate admissions to the intensive care unit. The causes are obscure but probably lead to a common final pathway of gallbladder ischemia. The diagnosis is often extremely difficult because the signs and symptoms may be those of occult sepsis. Moreover, the patients are often intubated, sedated, or confused as a consequence of the other therapeutic or medical factors. Biochemical tests, though frequently revealing abnormal liver function, are nonspecific and nondiagnostic. Bedside ultrasonography is usually strongly suggestive of the diagnosis when a thickened gallbladder wall or pericholecystic fluid is present, but radiologic findings may also be nondiagnostic. If the diagnosis is delayed, mortality and morbidity are very high. Percutaneous drainage of the gallbladder is usually curative of acalculous cholecystitis and affords stabilizing palliation if calculous cholecystitis is present. Some authors have recommended prophylactic percutaneous drainage of the gallbladder under CT guidance in any ICU patient who is failing to thrive or has other signs of low-grade sepsis after appropriate therapy for the primary illness has been provided. The distractor items in the question are all either too aggressive to be safely done in critically ill patients or too cautious for a patient with a potentially fatal complication.

65–67. The answers are 65-b, 66-b, 67-d. (*Schwartz, 7/e, pp 115–120.*) The case presented is most consistent with septic shock from a postoperative intraabdominal abscess. In the early phase of septic shock the respiratory profile is characterized by mild hypoxia with a compensatory hyperventilation and respiratory alkalosis. Hemodynamically, a hyperdynamic state is seen with an increase in cardiac output and a decrease in peripheral vascular resistance in the face of relatively normal central pressures. Initial therapy is aimed at resuscitation and stabilization. This includes fluid replacement and vasopressors as well as antibiotic therapy aimed particularly at gram-negative rods and anaerobes for patients with presumed intraabdominal collections, especially after bowel surgery. Laparotomy and drainage of a collection is the definitive therapy but should await stabilization of the patient and confirmation of the presence and location of such a collection.

68. The answer is c. *(Charlson, Ann Surg 210:637–648, 1989.)* The landmark study by Goldman in 1978 identified cardiac risk factors in noncardiac surgical patients that included previous infarction (particularly infarction within 6 mo, but with increased risk continuing for life), functional impairment such as dyspnea on exertion, age over 70 years, mitral regurgitation, more than five premature ventricular contractions (PVCs) per minute, and a tortuous or calcified aorta. Angina alone was not a risk factor. Subsequent studies by others have differed regarding the importance of several of these factors, which probably reflects different comorbid characteristics in the study populations (e.g., diabetes and hypertension). Additional predictors of perioperative cardiac risk that achieved significance in some studies but not in others include cardiomegaly, upper abdominal or intrathoracic surgery, and intraoperative hypotension.

69. The answer is e. *(Schwartz, 7/e, p 681.)* The maximal safe total dose of lidocaine administered to a 70-kg man is 4.5 mg/kg, or approximately 30–35 mL of a 1% solution. The addition of epinephrine to lidocaine, procaine, or bupivacaine not only doubles the duration of infiltration anesthesia, but increases by one-third the maximal safe total dose by decreasing the rate of absorption of drug into the bloodstream. Epinephrine-containing solutions should not, however, be injected into tissues supplied by end arteries (e.g., fingers, toes, ears, nose, penis). Hypersensitivity to local anesthetics is uncommon and occurs most prominently with anesthetics of the ester type (procaine, tetracaine). While small nerve fibers seem to be most susceptible to the action of local anesthetics, these agents act on any part of the nervous system and on every type of nerve fiber. CNS toxicity usually appears as stimulation followed by depression, probably because of an early selective depression of inhibitory neurons; with a massive overdose, all neurons may be depressed simultaneously.

70. The answer is d. *(Schwartz, 7/e, pp 103–113.)* Acute hemorrhage triggers the potent vasopressor activity of both angiotensin and vasopressin to increase blood flow to the heart and brain via selective vasoconstriction of the skin, kidneys, and splanchnic organs. Adrenergic discharge also results in selective vasoconstriction of skin, renal, and splanchnic vessels. Myocardial contractility and heart rate are increased, with a resultant increased cardiac output. Hyperventilation is the typical response to the metabolic (lactic) acidosis associated with hemorrhagic shock and hypoperfusion. Aldosterone release, with subsequent increased renal sodium resorption, is mediated by angiotensin II and ACTH, which prevents further intravascular depletion.

71. The answer is e. *(Greenfield, 2/e, pp 195–197.)* When a Swan-Ganz pulmonary artery catheter is in the wedge position, i.e., isolating the pulmonary arterial system from the pulmonary capillaries, the measured pulmonary capillary wedge pressure (PCWP) is usually equivalent to both the left atrial pressure (LAP) and the left ventricular end-diastolic pressure (LVEDP). Pathologic processes in the pulmonary vasculature and heart valves, however, may alter this relationship. Pulmonary vasoocclusive disease may elevate the PCWP independently of the LAP or LVEDP. Bronchospasm affecting the airway but not the pulmonary vasculature should not affect the validity of Swan-Ganz catheter readings. Mitral stenosis and regurgitation cause increased LAP and PCWP, which result in an overestimated LVEDP. However, aortic stenosis and regurgitation elevate the PCWP, LAP, and LVEDP equally. Accurate measurement of PCWP by a Swan-Ganz catheter may not be possible in the presence of positive airway pressure with PEEP/CPAP; transmission of the positive airway pressure to the pulmonary microvasculature via the alveoli, especially in the upper lung zones, results in measurement of alveolar pressure rather than LAP or LVEDP. Coronary artery disease does not affect the relationship between PCWP, LAP, and LVEDP.

72. The answer is a. *(Landercasper, Arch Surg 125:986–989, 1990.)* In an 8-year, retrospective study of 173 consecutive patients with a documented medical history of stroke who underwent subsequent general anesthesia and surgery (excluding cardiac, cerebrovascular, and neurological surgery), 5 patients (2.9%) had documented postoperative strokes from 3 to 21 days (mean 12.2 days) after surgery. The risk of stroke did not correlate with age, sex, history of multiple strokes or poststroke transient ischemic attacks (TIAs), ASA classification, aspirin use, coronary artery disease, peripheral vascular disease, intraoperative blood pressure, time since previous stroke, or cause of previous stroke. The risk of recurrent stroke appears to be comparable with that of surgical patients who do not have a history of prior stroke and are undergoing cardiac and peripheral vascular surgery. Most recurrent strokes occur many hours to days following surgery and do not appear to be directly related to operative events. The mortality after postoperative stroke is high.

73. The answer is b. *(Schwartz, 7/e, pp 211–212.)* This patient is having an anaphylactoid reaction with destabilization of the cardiovascular and respiratory systems. Anaphylactoid reactions are most commonly caused by iodinated contrast media, β-lactam antibiotics (e.g., penicillin), and Hymenoptera stings. Manifestations of anaphylactoid reactions include both the lethal (bronchospasm, laryngospasm, hypotension, dysrhythmia) and the nonlethal (pruritus, urticaria, syncope, weakness, and seizure). Epinephrine is the initial treatment for laryngeal obstruction and bronchospasm, followed by histamine antagonists (H_1 and H_2 blockers), aminophylline, and hydrocortisone. Vasopressors and fluid challenges may be given for shock. Conscious patients are usually stabilized with injected or inhaled epinephrine, while unconscious patients and those with refractory hypotension or hypoxia should be intubated.

74. The answer is d. *(Schwartz, 7/e, pp 97–98.)* Most transfusion reactions are hemolytic and are due to clerical errors that result in administration of blood with major (ABO) and minor antigen incompatibility. Interestingly, Rh incompatibility is not associated with intravascular hemolysis. Administration of blood through hypotonic solutions such as 5% dextrose and water results in swelling of the erythrocytes and hemolysis. Calcium-containing solutions such as Ringer's lactate cause clotting within the intravenous line rather than hemolysis and may lead to pulmonary embolism. Delayed transfusion reactions, caused by a presumed anamnestic immune response that occurs 3–21 days after blood is infused, result in a hemolytic anemia.

75. The answer is b. (*Schwartz, 7/e, pp 494–496.*) Because of the highly efficient diffusion characteristics of the gas carbon dioxide, Pa_{CO_2} levels are reliable indicators of adequacy of alveolar ventilation. A Pa_{CO_2} of 40 kPa is the normal value. Paradoxical aciduria occurs when hypokalemic metabolic alkalosis is present as the kidney excretes hydrogen ion in an effort to conserve potassium ion. Though a Pa_{CO_2} of 40 kPa is not incompatible with metabolic alkalosis, it would ordinarily be higher as the patient tries to conserve carbolic acid by hypoventilating to compensate. Pa_{O_2} levels are influenced by so many other variables (e.g., age, concentration of inspired O_2, altitude) that no inferences can be made about adequacy of alveolar ventilation from Pa_{O_2} alone, nor can Pa_{O_2} be safely predicted by the presence of normocarbia. The ventilation-perfusion mismatch is a reflection of the gradient between alveolar and arterial oxygen tension in relationship to percentage of inspired O_2.

76. The answer is c. (*Schwartz, 7/e, pp 494–496.*) Because of the ease with which carbon dioxide diffuses across the alveolar membranes, the Pa_{CO_2} is a highly reliable indicator of alveolar ventilation. In this postoperative patient with respiratory acidosis and hypoxemia, the hypercarbia is diagnostic of alveolar hypoventilation. Acute hypoxemia can occur with pulmonary embolism, pulmonary edema, and significant atelectasis, but in all those situations the CO_2 partial pressures should be normal or reduced as the patient hyperventilates to improve oxygenation. The absorption of gas from the peritoneal cavity may affect transiently the Pa_{CO_2}, but should have no effect on oxygenation.

77. The answer is c. (*Schwartz, 7/e, pp 36–46.*) The serum albumin level provides a rough estimate of protein nutritional adequacy. The accuracy of this estimate is affected by the long half-life of albumin (3 wk) and vagaries of hemodilution. The acute-phase serum proteins have a very short half-life (hours) and may also provide good short-term indications of nutritional status. Transferrin is one of these acute-phase proteins, but unfortunately its levels too are influenced by changes in intravascular volume and, along with the other acute-phase reactants, rise nonspecifically during acute illness. All the listed responses provide some useful information about nutrition and adequacy of replacement.

78. The answer is d. (*Schwartz, 7/e, pp 60–62.*) The body has elaborate mechanisms to compensate for metabolic acidosis. Not only do most body functions work better in an acidotic state, the patient is able to move toward correction of the pH by excreting acid urine and by hyperventilating to "blow off" carbonic acid. On the other hand, we are poorly equipped to deal with metabolic alkalosis. We cannot hold our breath to save acid since the respiratory center overrides our efforts as the Pa_{CO_2} rises and the Pa_{O_2} falls. The kidney cannot make urine under any circumstance that is very far above normal pH. In the subtraction alkalosis that accompanies gastric outlet obstruction with loss of gastric acid by vomiting or suction, the potassium depletion and volume deficits provoke exchange of sodium for hydrogen ion in the distal tubule with resultant exacerbation of the metabolic alkalosis. All the other conditions listed would be expected to produce acidosis; consequently, acid urine would not be paradoxical.

79. The answer is e. *(Schwartz, 7/e, pp 159–161.)* Air carried into the pulmonary arterial vasculature creates an abnormal blood-air interface that leads to denaturing of plasma proteins and creates amorphous proteinaceous and cellular debris and endothelial injury. The ensuing increased capillary permeability results in alveolar flooding. The occlusion of pulmonary vessels increases the proportion of ventilated but underperfused alveoli. The increment in dead space results in a drop in end-tidal carbon dioxide.

80. The answer is b. *(Schwartz, 7/e, p 447.)* Shivering is the physiologic effort of the body to generate heat to maintain the core temperature. In healthy persons, shivering increases the metabolic rate by 3–5 times and results in increased oxygen consumption and carbon dioxide production. In critically ill patients these metabolic consequences are almost always counterproductive and should be prevented with other means employed to correct systemic hypothermia. In the presence of vigorous shivering, oxygen debt in the muscles and lactic acidemia develop.

81. The answer is d. *(Schwartz, 7/e, pp 78–84.)* von Willebrand disease is similar to true hemophilia in frequency of occurrence. It is being diagnosed more commonly today because of more reliable assays for factor VIII. This autosomal dominant disorder (recessive transmission can occur) is characterized by a diminution in factor VIII:C (procoagulant) activity. The reduction in activity is not as great as in classic hemophilia, and the clinical manifestations are more subtle. These manifestations are often overlooked until an episode of trauma or surgery makes them apparent. Treatment requires correcting the bleeding time and providing factor VIII R:WF (the von Willebrand factor). Only cryoprecipitate is reliably effective. High-purity factor VIII:C concentrates, effective in hemophilia, lack the von Willebrand factor and are, consequently, undependable.

82. The answer is e. *(Schwartz, 7/e, 1720–1721.)* Extracorporeal membrane oxygenation (ECMO) is a form of cardiopulmonary support that is useful in the setting of potentially reversible pulmonary or cardiac disease. Treatment of meconium aspiration syndrome, sepsis, pneumonia, and congenital diaphragmatic hernia (pre- or postoperatively) are thus appropriate uses. The technique is also applicable in some circumstances as a bridge to cardiac or lung transplantation since the outlook for survival is quite good if the child can be maintained in a good physiological state until donor organs are available. Hypoplastic lungs do not have enough surface area to perform adequate gas exchange and are unlikely to mature to a point where they can sustain life. Babies with hypoplastic lungs will be bypass dependent for life and consequently are not candidates for institution of ECMO therapy.

83. The answer is a. *(Schwartz, 7/e, p 458.)* Gastric aspiration is best treated by tracheal suctioning, oxygen, and positive-pressure ventilation. Bronchoscopy is helpful if particulate matter is causing bronchial obstruction or if the vomitus is found to contain particulate material. Bronchial lavage is no longer recommended, and steroids have not been shown to be of value. Fluids should be given sparingly because hypervolemia will worsen the risk of pulmonary edema following aspiration. Tracheostomy may be indicated for long-term airway management in obtunded or otherwise severely debilitated patients; however, initial control of the airway should be by orotracheal intubation whenever possible. High positive end-expiratory pressure is not required unless respiratory failure develops.

84. The answer is c. *(Schwartz, 7/e, p 156.)* Although tracheostomy is occasionally an emergency procedure, it can be more effectively performed in an operating room where hemostasis and antisepsis are readily achieved. Most authorities recommend a horizontal incision; however, limited direct midline incisions have the advantage of not opening any unnecessary tissue planes and perhaps reducing the incidence of bleeding complications. Both approaches have advocates. In either case, the skin incision is made just below the cricoid cartilage, the strap muscles are spared and retracted, the thyroid isthmus is divided if necessary, and the trachea is entered at the second tracheal ring. The second and third tracheal rings are incised vertically, allowing placement of the tracheostomy tube. The first tracheal ring and the cricoid cartilage must be left intact.

85. The answer is d. (*Schwartz, 7/e, pp 448, 499.*) The cause of malignant hyperthermia is unknown, but it is associated with inhalational anesthetic agents and succinylcholine. It may develop in an otherwise healthy person who has tolerated previous surgery without incident. It should be suspected in the presence of a history of unexplained fever, muscle or connective tissue disorder, or a positive family history (evidence suggests an autosomal dominant inheritance pattern). In addition to fever during anesthesia, the syndrome includes tachycardia, increased O_2 consumption, increased CO_2 production, increased serum K^+, myoglobinuria, and acidosis. Rigidity rather than relaxation following succinylcholine injection may be the first clue to its presence. Treatment of malignant hyperthermia should include prompt conclusion of the operative procedure and cessation of anesthesia, hyperventilation with 100% oxygen, and administration of intravenous dantrolene. The urine should be alkalinized to protect the kidneys from myoglobin precipitation. If reoperation is necessary, one should premedicate heavily, alkalinize the urine, and avoid depolarizing agents such as succinylcholine. Pretreatment for 24 h with dantrolene is helpful; it is thought to act directly on muscle fiber to attenuate calcium release.

86. The answer is e. (*Schwartz, 7/e, pp 487–493.*) Determination of CVP is an integral part of the overall hemodynamic assessment of the patient. This pressure can be affected by a variety of factors including those of cardiac, noncardiac, and artifactual origin. Venous tone, right ventricular compliance, intrathoracic pressure, and blood volume all influence CVP. Vasoconstrictor drugs, positive pressure, ventilation (with and without PEEP), mediastinal compression, and hypervolemia all increase CVP. Acute pulmonary embolism, when clinically significant, elevates CVP by causing right ventricular overload and increased right atrial pressure. Sepsis, on the other hand, decreases CVP through both the release of vasodilatory mediators and the loss of intravascular plasma volume due to increased capillary permeability.

87. The answer is b. (*Greenfield, 2/e, pp 238–239.*) Continuous arteriovenous hemofiltration (CAVH) is a relatively new method of therapy for acute renal failure in the intensive care unit. Continuous blood flow is maintained by the hydrostatic pressure gradient between an inflowing arterial cannula and the venous cannula that returns blood to the patient. The blood passes through an extracorporeal membrane, which clears an ultrafiltrate up to 12 L per day. This volume is replaced with an intravenous solution at a rate that achieves the desired fluid balance. CAVH in the surgical patient with acute renal failure allows a slow and continuous removal of fluid and is particularly advantageous in the volume-overloaded patient. Unlike traditional hemodialysis, it can be used over a wide range of blood pressures in the unstable patient. Solutes (such as urea nitrogen and potassium) that are not in the replacement intravenous fluid are also cleared. The main complications associated with CAVH relate to vascular access problems: arterial thrombosis, aneurysm, fistula formation, and infection. Anticoagulation, with the concomitant bleeding risks, must be maintained to prevent thrombosis of the filter and cannulae. The potential for electrolyte imbalance during long-term CAVH requires careful monitoring.

88. The answer is d. (*Greenfield, 2/e, pp 204–205.*) Clinical manifestations of adrenocortical insufficiency include hyperkalemia, hyponatremia, hypoglycemia, fever, weight loss, and dehydration. There is excessive sodium loss in the urine, contraction of the plasma volume, and perhaps hypotension or shock. Classic hyperpigmentation is present in chronic Addison's disease only. Addison's disease may present in newborns as a congenital atrophy, as an insidious chronic state often due to tuberculosis, as an acute dysfunction secondary to trauma or adrenal hemorrhage, or as a semiacute adrenal insufficiency seen during stress or surgery. In this last instance, signs and symptoms include nausea, lassitude, vomiting, fever, progressive salt wasting, hyperkalemia, and hypoglycemia. It may be confirmed by measurements of urinary Na^+ loss and absence of response to ACTH.

89. The answer is c. (*Schwartz, 7/e, pp 693–694.*) Posttraumatic pulmonary insufficiency in the absence of significant thoracic trauma has been attributed to a wide variety of etiologic agents, including aspiration, simple atelectasis, lung contusion, fat embolism, pneumonia, pneumothorax, pulmonary edema, and pulmonary thromboembolism. In a landmark monograph entitled *Respiratory Distress Syndrome of Shock and Trauma,* Blaisdell and Lewis identified fat embolism syndrome as the etiologic factor. The mechanism of this condition appears to be pulmonary alveolar injury due to the mobilization of free fatty acids in the blood as an adrenergic response to trauma, rather than pulmonary injury from embolization of fat globules from fractured bones, as was originally thought.

90. The answer is d. *(Sabiston, 15/e, p 296.)* Securing a stable airway is one of the most fundamental and important aspects of the management of the severely injured patient. The level of control required will vary from a simple oropharyngeal airway to tracheostomy, depending on the clinical situation. Full control of the airway should be secured in the emergency room if the patient is unstable. Endotracheal intubation will usually be the method chosen, but one should be prepared to do a tracheotomy if attempts at peroral or pernasal intubation are failing or are impractical because of maxillofacial injuries. The most dangerous period is just prior to and during the initial attempts to get control of the airway. Manipulation of the oronasopharynx may provoke combative behavior or vomiting in a patient already confused by drugs, alcohol, hypoxia, or cerebral trauma. The risk of aspiration is high during these initial attempts, and one should make no assumptions about the state of the contents of the patient's stomach. Antacids are recommended just prior to the intubation attempt, if feasible. Although steroids have been recommended in the past, they are no longer considered of value in the management of aspiration of acidic gastric juice. The best management requires prevention of the complication of aspiration. In a reasonably cooperative patient, awake intubation with topical anesthesia may help to avoid some of the risks of hypotension, arrhythmia, and aspiration associated with the induction of anesthesia. If awake intubation is inappropriate, then an alternative is rapid-sequence induction with a thiobarbiturate followed by muscle paralysis with succinylcholine. If elevated intracranial pressure is suspected, or if a penetrating eye injury exists, awake intubation is contraindicated.

91. The answer is c. *(Sabiston, 15/e, pp 269–270.)* Necrotizing skin and soft tissue infections may produce insoluble gases (hydrogen, nitrogen, methane) through anaerobic bacterial metabolism. While the term "gas gangrene" has come to imply clostridial infection, gas in tissues is more likely not to be due to *Clostridium* species but rather to other facultative and obligate anaerobes, particularly streptococci. Though fungi have also been implicated, they are less often associated with rapidly progressive infections. Treatment for necrotizing soft tissue infections includes repeated wide debridement, with wound reconstruction delayed until a stable, viable wound surface has been established. The use of hyperbaric oxygen in the treatment of gas gangrene remains controversial, due to lack of proven benefit, difficulty in transporting critically ill patients to hyperbaric facilities, and the risk of complications. Antitoxin has neither a prophylactic nor a therapeutic role in the treatment of myonecrosis.

92. The answer is a. (*Sabiston, 15/e, pp 1798–1799.*) Abnormalities of ventilation-perfusion ratio result from the shunting of blood to a hypoventilated lung or from the ventilation of hypoperfused regions of lung tissue. When this imbalance is extreme, as following massive pulmonary thromboembolism, the effect is life-threatening hypoxemia. Other common predisposing factors in the postoperative patient that contribute to this maldistribution include the assumption of a supine position, thoracic and upper abdominal incisions, obesity, atelectasis, and reduced cardiac output.

93. The answer is d. (*Shoemaker, 2/e, pp 39–41.*) The metabolic and physiologic effects of drowning and near-drowning depend upon variables that include fluid temperature, extent of aspiration, and whether the aspirate is fresh water or sea water. Cold-water submersion decreases oxygen consumption and results in preferential shunting of blood flow to the heart and brain. This shunting prolongs the period of submersion that can be endured without irreversible cerebral damage. Return of normal cerebral function after as long as 40 min of submersion in extremely cold water has been reported. One should also remember that cooling below 30°C (86°F) often causes cardiac arrhythmias. Ten percent of affected patients do not aspirate fluid but succumb to asphyxia because of breath holding or laryngospasm. Seventy percent have a significant metabolic acidosis requiring administration of sodium bicarbonate. Significant electrolyte and blood volume changes may or may not be present, depending on the degree of aspiration and toxicity of the fluid medium. Renal damage may occur as a result of hemoglobinuria (from hemolysis), acidosis, hypoxia, or changes in renal blood flow. The most important initial treatment of drowning victims is ventilation. Mouth-to-mouth or mouth-to-nose ventilation should be begun as soon as possible. Corticosteroids and prophylactic antibiotics are not recommended for the prevention of pulmonary complications. However, some workers feel that steroids may be of value in managing the complication of cerebral edema.

94. The answer is c. (*Greenfield, 2/e, pp 95–98.*) Major hemorrhage that requires the termination of anticoagulant therapy occurs in up to 15% of anticoagulated patients. Spontaneous retroperitoneal hemorrhage constitutes a small subset of such cases and can be a fatal complication. Heparin is much more frequently associated with spontaneous retroperitoneal hemorrhage than are oral agents. Advanced patient age and poor regulation of coagulation times also increase the likelihood of bleeding complications. Most cases of retroperitoneal hemorrhage present with flank pain and signs of peritoneal irritations suggestive of an acute intraabdominal process. CT scans are most useful in confirming the diagnosis and following the course of the bleeding. Successful management is usually nonoperative and consists of the discontinuation of anticoagulants, administration of vitamin K or protamine, possible transfusion of clotting factors, and repletion of intravascular volume with intravenous fluids.

95. The answer is e. (*Pruitt, J Trauma 30:363–368, 1990.*) Smoke inhalation injuries ("smoke poisoning") and asphyxia account for almost one-third of all fire fatalities. As opposed to respiratory burns, which are thermal injuries of the upper respiratory tract, smoke inhalation is a chemical injury to the distal tracheobronchial tree and alveoli. Most patients admitted for this injury have elevated carbon monoxide levels, but a minority will have physical evidence of skin burns (20%) or of oropharyngeal burns (25%). Visible damage to the respiratory tract is not a frequent finding. Chest films initially are often negative even in those patients who subsequently develop respiratory failure from pulmonary edema or pneumonitis. Patients with elevated carboxyhemoglobin levels or evidence of smoke inhalation should be hospitalized for a minimum of 24 h for observation regardless of normal arterial blood gases and chest x-ray.

96. The answer is e. (*Robinson, Surgery 113:709–711, 1993.*) Some drug smugglers, often called "body packers" or "mules," ingest cocaine- or heroin-filled packets and retrieve them at a later date from their stools. The drugs are usually contained in latex or plastic packets. Rupture or leakage of even one bag carries the risk of severe toxicity and death. Although conservative medical management with moderate doses of laxatives is usually safe in stable body packers, close physiologic monitoring is necessary until all packets are passed. High doses of laxatives, digital rectal disimpaction, or endoscopic removal create a high risk of rupture of the bags and therefore are generally discouraged. Emergency surgery is indicated when complications develop.

97–99. The answers are 97-d, 98-e, 99-a. (*Greenfield, 2/e, pp 438–443.*) Nitrous oxide (N_2O) is a frequently used inhalation analgesic. However, because the minimum alveolar anesthetic concentration (MAC) is so high (over 100), true anesthesia at 1 atm pressure cannot be obtained without compromising oxygen delivery to the patient. Since nitrous oxide is 30 times more soluble than nitrogen in blood, it enters a collection of trapped air at a rate faster than that at which nitrogen leaves the collection. Thus, the trapped air will increase in volume. If the trapped air is a result of bowel obstruction, intestinal distention will increase.

Halothane is a very potent anesthetic with an MAC of 0.75. Cardiovascular depression results from a number of different mechanisms. Hypotension and decreased cardiac output have been associated with a direct depression of myocardial muscle fibers and peripheral vascular smooth muscle fibers. An effect on the medullary vasomotor centers as well as on sympathetic ganglionic transmissions to the heart has been reported.

Enflurane is a halogenated inhalation anesthetic with an MAC of 1.2. It is similar to halothane in its anesthetic characteristics. However, in a small number of normal patients it may induce electroencephalographic changes similar to those seen in epilepsy.

Methoxyflurane is the most potent and least volatile halogenated inhalation anesthetic, with an MAC of 0.16. Its clinical use has been curtailed because of the high risk of nephrotoxicity of the free fluoride ions released during its biodegradation.

Morphine is a potent narcotic agent. Its use during general anesthesia can potentiate the analgesic effects of the inhalation agents. It causes histamine release with the risk of hypotension if given in a large bolus dose.

100–102. The answers are 100-a, c, d, e, h; 101-b, d, h; 102-f, g, h. (*Schwartz, 7/e, pp 485–507.*) The decision to extubate an elderly patient after major abdominal vascular surgery depends on accurate assessment of hemodynamic and respiratory factors. Adding to the complexity of this particular patient is his past history of cardiac disease and his need for inotropic support. Ventilatory and blood gas monitoring will determine whether the patient can be weaned from the respirator. Continuous blood pressure monitoring via arterial catheterization and pulmonary artery catheter readings will enable the responsible physicians to assess volume status and the ongoing need for inotropic support, both critical in the fluid management of a patient about to be extubated. Continuous ECG monitoring is essential for this patient because of the high incidence of perioperative cardiac arrhythmias, particularly atrial fibrillation, following surgery in which large fluid shifts are anticipated.

Conversely, an otherwise healthy young patient who is discovered to have a ruptured spleen during emergency laparotomy is unlikely to require prolonged intubation beyond the time of surgery. Nor is he likely to require hemodynamic support in the form of pressors or inotropes, since his problem is one of pure volume loss (blood), which can be met with rapid colloid and crystalloid administration in the operating room. Consequently, this patient may be managed with a central venous catheter (or even a large-bore peripheral catheter, if one can be placed quickly) and ECG and ventilatory monitoring during his operative procedure. If his hemorrhage is successfully controlled, early discontinuation of physiologic monitoring can be anticipated.

Chronically ill patients, such as brain-injured patients in vegetative states, require nutritional monitoring insofar as they are unable to articulate their nutritional needs. Caloric expenditure may be calculated to a modest degree of accuracy using noninvasive methods based on body surface area, age, and sex (Harris-Benedict equation). More accurate assessment, particularly appropriate in disease states where metabolic activity is accelerated, can be made using measurements of oxygen consumption and carbon dioxide production. A patient who has suffered blunt head trauma requiring repeated surgeries for intracranial bleeding will likely be monitored with an intracranial pressure device. Other indications for intracranial pressure monitoring include subarachnoid hemorrhage, hydrocephalus, postcraniotomy, and Reye syndrome. ECG monitoring may also be helpful in this setting, as increasing intracranial pressure may be presaged by bradycardia.

103–105. The answers are 103-a, b, c, f, j; 104-a, b, c, d, e, f, g, h; 105-i. (*Schwartz, 7/e, pp 88–90.*) Prothrombin time measures the speed of coagulation in the extrinsic pathway. A tissue source of procoagulant (thromboplastin) with calcium is added to plasma. The test will detect deficiencies in factors II, V, VII, X, and fibrinogen and is used to monitor patients receiving coumarin derivatives. However, even small amounts of heparin will artificially prolong the clotting time, so that accurate prothrombin times can only be obtained when the patient has not received heparin for at least 5 h.

The intrinsic pathway is measured by the partial thromboplastin time. This test is sensitive for defects in factors VIII, IX, XI, XII, and all the factors of the extrinsic pathway and is used to monitor the status of patients on heparin.

The bleeding time assesses the interaction of platelets and the formation of the platelet plug. Therefore it will pick up deficiencies in both qualitative and quantitative platelet function. Ingestion of aspirin within 1 wk of the test will alter the result.

The thrombin time assesses qualitative abnormalities in fibrinogen and the presence of inhibitors to fibrin polymerization. A standard amount of fibrin is added to a fixed volume of plasma and clotting time is measured.

Skin: Wounds, Infections, Burns; Hands; Plastic Surgery

Questions

DIRECTIONS: Each item below contains a question or incomplete statement followed by suggested responses. Select the **one best** response to each question.

106. Wasting of the intrinsic muscles of the hand can be expected to follow injury of the

a. Ulnar nerve
b. Radial nerve
c. Brachial nerve
d. Axillary nerve
e. Thenar and hypothenar nerves

107. Although wide surgical excision is the traditional treatment for malignant melanoma, narrow excision of thin (less than 1 mm deep) stage I melanomas has been found to be equally safe and effective when the margin of resection is as small as

a. 3 mm
b. 5 mm
c. 1 cm
d. 3 cm
e. 5 cm

108. With regard to wound healing, which one of the following statements is correct?

a. Collagen content reaches a maximum at approximately 1 wk after injury
b. Monocytes are essential for normal wound healing
c. Fibroblasts appear in the wound within 24–36 h after the injury
d. The function of the monocyte in wound healing is limited to phagocytosis of bacteria and debris
e. Early in wound healing, type I collagen is predominant

Items 109–110

109. While you are on duty in the emergency room, a 12-year-old boy arrives with pain and inflammation over the ball of his left foot and red streaks extending up the inner aspect of his leg. He remembers removing a wood splinter from the sole of his foot on the previous day. The most likely infecting organism is

a. *Clostridium perfingens*
b. *Clostridium tetani*
c. *Staphylococcus*
d. *Escherichia coli*
e. *Streptococcus*

110. The appropriate antibiotic to prescribe while awaiting specific culture verification is

a. Penicillin
b. Erythromycin
c. Tetracycline
d. Azathioprine
e. Cloxacillin

111. Proper treatment for frostbite consists of

a. Debridement of the affected part followed by silver sulfadiazine dressings
b. Administration of corticosteroids
c. Administration of vasodilators
d. Immersion of the affected part in water at 40–44°C (104–111.2°F)
e. Rewarming of the affected part at room temperature

112. The true statement regarding tendon injuries in the hand is

a. Flexor digitorum superficialis inserts on the distal phalanx
b. Flexor digitorum profundus inserts on the middle phalanx
c. The tendons of flexor digitorum superficialis arise from a common muscle belly
d. The best results for repair of a flexor tendon are obtained with injuries in the fibro-osseous tunnel (zone 2)
e. The process of healing a tendon injury involves formation of a tenoma

113. Which one of the following cases is considered a clean-contaminated wound?

a. Open cholecystectomy for cholelithiasis
b. Herniorrhaphy with mesh repair
c. Lumpectomy with axillary node dissection
d. Appendectomy with walled-off abscess
e. Gunshot wound to the abdomen with injuries to the small bowel and sigmoid colon

114. A 45-year-old woman undergoes an uneventful laparoscopic cholecystectomy for which she receives one dose of cephalosporin. One week later, she returns to the emergency room with fever, nausea, and copious diarrhea and is subsequently diagnosed with pseudomembranous colitis. With respect to this disease, which one of the following statements is correct?

a. Surgical intervention is frequently required
b. After appropriate antibiotic therapy, the relapse rate is less than 5%
c. Tissue culture assay for *Clostridium difficile* toxin B is neither sensitive nor specific; therefore diagnosis should be based on clinical findings
d. If surgery is performed, a left hemicolectomy is usually adequate to treat pseudo-membranous colitis
e. Indications for surgical treatment include intractable disease, failure of medical therapy, toxic megacolon, and colonic perforation

115. A 60-year-old woman presents with the skin lesion shown below, which had been present for 10 years. She reported a history of radiation treatments to that hand for "eczema." Correct statements concerning this lesion include

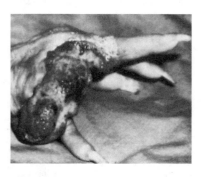

a. It is more malignant than basal cell carcinoma
b. It occurs more frequently in brunettes
c. It rarely metastasizes to regional lymph nodes
d. It should be treated by radiation therapy
e: It is rarely associated with chronic sun exposure

Items 116–117

116. A 25-year-old man is brought to the emergency room after sustaining burns during a fire in his apartment. He has blistering and erythema of his face, left upper extremity, and chest with frank charring of his right upper extremity. He is agitated, hypotensive, and tachycardiac. Which one of the following statements concerning this patient's initial wound management is correct?

a. Topical antibiotics should not be used, as they will encourage growth of resistant organisms
b. Early excision of facial and hand burns is especially important
c. Escharotomy should only be performed if neurologic impairment is imminent
d. Excision of areas of third-degree or of deep second-degree burns usually takes place 3–7 days after injury
e. Split-thickness skin grafts over the eschar of third-degree burns should be performed immediately in order to prevent fluid loss

117. Which one of the following statements regarding the above burn patient is correct?

a. High-dose penicillin should be administered prophylactically
b. Tetanus prophylaxis is not necessary if the patient has been immunized in the previous 3 years
c. This burn can be estimated at 60% total body surface area using the "rule of nines"
d. The most sensitive indicator of adequacy of fluid resuscitation is heart rate
e. This patient should undergo immediate intubation for airway protection and oxygen administration

118. True statements regarding squamous cell carcinoma of the lip include

a. The lesion often arises in areas of persistent hyperkeratosis
b. More than 90% of cases occur on the upper lip
c. The lesion constitutes 30% of all cancers of the oral cavity
d. Radiotherapy is considered inappropriate treatment for these lesions
e. Initially metastases are to the ipsilateral posterior cervical lymph nodes

119. Which of the following statements regarding carpal tunnel syndrome is correct?

a. It is rarely secondary to trauma
b. It may be associated with pregnancy
c. It most often causes dysesthesia during waking hours
d. It is often associated with vascular compromise
e. Surgical treatment involves release of the extensor retinaculum

120. Which of the following is true with regard to wound contraction?

a. It is the primary process affecting closure of a sutured or stapled surgical wound
b. Bacterial colonization significantly slows the process of contraction
c. It may account for a maximum of 50% decrease in the size of a wound
d. It is based on specialized fibroblasts that contain actin myofilaments
e. The percentage reduction of wound size is increased with increased adherency of skin to underlying tissue

121. Management of leukoplakia of the oral cavity includes

a. Excisional biopsy of all lesions
b. Application of topical antibiotics
c. Low-dose radiation therapy
d. Ascertaining that dentures fit properly
e. Application of topical chemotherapeutic agents

122. An 8-lb infant, born following uncomplicated labor and delivery, is noted to have a unilateral cleft lip and palate. The parents should be advised that

a. The child almost certainly has other congenital anomalies
b. Rehabilitation requires adjunctive speech therapy
c. Lip repair is indicated at 1 year of age
d. Palate repair is indicated prior to 6 mo of age
e. Cosmetic revisions to the nose should be performed at the same time as cleft lip repair

123. A 40-year-old woman undergoes wide excision of a pigmented lesion of her thigh. Pathologic examination reveals malignant melanoma that is Clark's level IV. Findings on examination of the groin are normal. The patient should be advised that

a. Radiotherapy will be an important part of subsequent therapy
b. The likelihood of groin node metastases is remote
c. Immunotherapy is an effective form of adjunctive treatment for metastatic malignant melanoma
d. Groin dissection is not indicated unless and until groin nodes become palpable
e. Intralesional bacille Calmette-Guérin (BCG) administration has been found to aid in local control in the majority of patients

DIRECTIONS: Each group of questions below consists of lettered options followed by numbered items. For each numbered item, select the appropriate lettered option(s). Each lettered option may be used once, more than once, or not at all. **Choose exactly the number of options indicated following each item.**

Items 124–127

Match each description with the correct skin or subcutaneous lesions.

a. Cystic hygroma
b. Basal cell carcinoma
c. Port-wine stain
d. Strawberry hemangioma
e. Malignant melanoma
f. Squamous cell carcinoma

124. A 56-year-old woman presents with a small, pigmented lesion on her forearm, which has been growing over the last 2 mo. She is a fair-complected woman with a history of sun exposure. **(SELECT 3 LESIONS)**

125. A 6-mo-old child presents with a red lesion on the face. **(SELECT 2 LESIONS)**

126. Surgical excision is the first line of therapy. **(SELECT 5 LESIONS)**

127. Radiation may be useful as adjuvant therapy. **(SELECT 3 LESIONS)**

Items 128–131

Match each description with the correct growth factors or cytokines.

a. Platelet-derived growth factor (PDGF)
b. Transforming growth factor
c. Tumor necrosis factor (TNF)
d. Fibroblast growth factor
e. Interleukin 1 (IL-1)
f. Thromboxane A_2

128. Platelets are the cell of origin. **(SELECT 3 CHOICES)**

129. Macrophages are the cell of origin. **(SELECT 5 CHOICES)**

130. They stimulate fibroblast proliferation. **(SELECT 4 CHOICES)**

131. They stimulate collagen synthesis. **(SELECT 3 CHOICES)**

SKIN: WOUNDS, INFECTIONS, BURNS; HANDS; PLASTIC SURGERY

Answers

106. The answer is a. (*Sabiston, 15/e, pp 1479–1485.*) The ulnar nerve innervates 15 of the 20 intrinsic muscles of the hand. The musculocutaneous, radial, ulnar, and median nerves are all important to hand function. The musculocutaneous and radial nerves allow forearm supination; the radial nerve alone innervates the extensor muscles. The median nerve is the "eye of the hand" because of its extensive contribution to sensory perception; it also maintains most of the long flexors, the pronators of the forearm, and the thenar muscles.

107. The answer is c. (*Schwartz, 7/e, pp 333, 523–527.*) Wide excision of melanomas, with margins of 3–5 cm beyond the lateral edges of tumor, has traditionally been considered mandatory. A 5-year prospective multicenter study of over 600 randomly assigned patients with thin stage I melanomas, however, showed that local recurrence rates, as well as the subsequent development of metastatic disease, were not different when margins of 1 cm or 3 cm were taken, provided that tumor thickness did not exceed 1 mm.

108. The answer is b. (*Greenfield 2/e, pp 67–83.*) Wound healing is an overlapping sequence of inflammation, proliferation, and remodeling. The inflammatory phase is characterized by a rapid influx of neutrophils, followed in about 2 days by an influx of mononuclear cells. These monocytes act not only by phagocytosing debris and bacteria, but also by secreting numerous growth factors including tumor necrosis factor (TNF), transforming growth factor, platelet-derived growth factor (PDGF), and fibroblast growth factor, which are essential to normal wound healing.

Angiogenesis and collagen formation take place during the proliferative phase of wound healing. Fibroblasts, which enter the wound at about day 3, continue to proliferate with increasing collagen deposition. Throughout the proliferative phase, type III collagen predominates. Collagen content is maximum at 2–3 wk, at which time the remodeling phase begins. Type III collagen, which is elastic fibrils, is gradually replaced by rigid fibrils, or type I collagen, at this time. During remodeling, collagen deposition and degradation reach a steady state, which may continue for up to 1 year.

109–110. The answers are 109-e, 110-a. (*Greenfield, 2/e, p 1970.*) The significant observation in this question is the description of lymphangitic inflammatory streaking up the inner aspect of the patient's leg. This is highly suggestive of a streptococcal infection and the presumptive therapy should be high doses of a bactericidal antibiotic. Penicillin remains the mainstay of therapy against presumed streptococcal infections. Most streptococcal cellulitis is adequately treated by penicillin, elevation of the infected extremity, and attention to the local wound to ascertain adequate local drainage and absence of any persisting foreign body. However, the clinician must be alert to the possibility of a more fulminant and life- or limb-threatening infection by clostridia, microaerophilic streptococcus, or other potentially synergistic organisms that can produce rapidly progressive deep infections in fascia of muscle. Smears and cultures of drainage fluid or aspirates should be taken. Close observation of the wound is essential, and aggressive debridement in the operating room is mandatory at the slightest suggestion that fasciitis or myonecrosis may be ensuing.

111. The answer is d. (*Greenfield, 2/e, pp 412–414.*) Many methods of treating frostbite have been tried throughout the years. These include massage, warm-water immersion, or covering the affected area. Rapid warming by immersion in water slightly above normal body temperature (40–448°C) is the most effective method; however, because the frostbitten region is numb and especially vulnerable, it should be protected from trauma or excessive heat during treatment. Further treatment may include elevation to minimize edema, administration of antibiotics and tetanus toxoid, and debridement of necrotic skin as needed.

112. The answer is e. (*Schwartz, 7/e, pp 2025–2056.*) Each digit has two long flexors, named *superficial* and *deep* according to the relative position of the muscle bellies. In the fingers each superficial flexor tendon divides around the corresponding deep tendon to reach its insertion on the base of the middle phalanx. The deep flexor tendon continues to its insertion on the base of the distal phalanx. Only the deep flexors can flex the distal interphalangeal joint. Since the tendons of the deep flexors share a common muscle belly, only the superficial flexors can move a finger when the adjacent fingers are immobilized. These tendons are prevented from bowstringing across the joints by the flexor retinaculum of the wrists and the fibroosseous tunnels, which extend from the distal palmar crease to the middle phalanx. They run within synovial sheaths and are nourished by vincula tendinum (short mesenteries). The process of healing a tendon injury involves the formation of a tenoma, which tends to become adherent to the surrounding sheath. A difficult balance has to be struck between the desire to prevent adhesions by early mobilization and the risk of rupturing an unhealed tendon. Verdan has divided the hand into six regions according to the anatomy surrounding the tendons. Zone 2, sometimes referred to as "no-man's land," refers to the fibroosseous tunnels. Repair in this region is fraught with difficulty.

113. The answer is a. (*Schwartz, 7/e, pp 130–131.*) Surgical wounds can be divided into three categories based on the amount of bacterial contamination. Clean wounds are those in which no part of the respiratory, gastrointestinal, or genitourinary tract is entered. Examples include herniorrhaphy and breast surgery. Clean-contaminated wounds encompass those cases in which the above systems are entered, but without evidence of active infection or gross spillage. Examples include elective cholecystectomy or elective colon resection with adequate bowel preparation. Contaminated wounds are those in which there is active infection (perforated appendicitis with abscess) or gross spillage (gunshot wound with large or small bowel injuries). While contaminated and clean-contaminated wounds require perioperative antibiotics, clean wounds need not be treated with prophylactic antibiotics.

114. The answer is e. (*Lipsett, Surgery 116:491–496, 1994.*) Pseudomembranous colitis is a common nosocomial infection most often caused by *Clostridium difficile* toxins A and B. Antibiotic use allows overgrowth of *C. difficile*, leading to abdominal pain, fever, diarrhea, and increased WBCs. Diagnosis is confirmed by isolation of *C. difficile* toxin B via tissue culture assay. Sensitivity and specificity are quite high (greater than 90%), but may require

24–48 h to complete. The vast majority of patients will respond to oral vancomycin or metronidazole, although 20–30% of patients may relapse. Because response to antibiotic therapy is high, surgical intervention is infrequently required (<1%). Indications for surgery include intractable or fulminant disease, failure of medical therapy, colonic perforation, and toxic megacolon. Pseudomembranous colitis often involves the entire colon, despite normal-appearing serosa. Therefore, the procedure of choice is a subtotal colectomy with ileostomy. Overall mortality of 35–40% is described, with <20% mortality for those patients undergoing subtotal colectomy.

115. The answer is a. *(Schwartz, 7/e, pp 257, 522, 527, 617–621.)* Squamous cell carcinoma occurs in people who have had chronic sun exposure, chronic ulcers or sinus tracts (draining osteomyelitis), and a history of radiation or thermal injury (Margolin's ulcer). It is more malignant than basal cell carcinoma, grows more rapidly, and metastasizes. It occurs more frequently in blondes and fair-skinned people. A radiation-induced carcinoma, or one arising in a burn scar, should not be treated with radiation therapy for fear of further damage.

116. The answer is d. *(Schwartz, 7/e, pp 242–244.)* Early wound management is characterized by early excision of areas of devitalized tissue, with the exception of deep wounds of the palms, soles, genitals, and face. Staged excision of deep partial-thickness or full-thickness burns occurs between 3 and 7 days after the injury. There are several proven advantages to early excision including decreased hospital stay and lower cost. This is especially true of burns encompassing >30–40% total body surface area. In conjunction with early excision, topical antimicrobials such as silver sulfadiazine are extremely important in delaying colonization of the newly excised or fresh burn wounds. Permanent coverage through split-thickness skin grafting usually occurs more than 1 wk after injury. Skin autograft requires a vascular bed and therefore cannot be placed over eschar. Meticulous attention to deep circumferential burns is crucial in the management of burn patients. Progressive tissue edema may lead to progressive vascular and neurologic compromise. Because the blood supply is the initial system affected, frequent assessment of flow is vital, with longitudinal escharotomy performed at the first sign of vascular compromise. A low threshold should be maintained in performing an escharotomy in the setting of severely burned limbs.

117. The answer is e. (*Schwartz, 7/e, pp 228–232, 234–238.*) Aggressive evaluation and treatment of burn victims has led to increased survival of the 2 million patients treated for burns each year in the United States. A systematic approach to the patient with attention to airway/vascular access and aggressive fluid resuscitation has proved essential. In the patient with obvious facial burns who is hemodynamically unstable, airway access is the first priority. Fluid resuscitation is initiated using the Parkland formula, with urine output of 0.5–1.0 mL/kg/h being the most sensitive indicator of the adequacy of resuscitation. The extent of the burn can be roughly estimated using the "rule of nines," in which the head and the upper extremities are each 9% of the total body surface area (TBSA) and the anterior trunk, posterior trunk, and the lower extremities are each 18% of the TBSA. The neck encompasses 1% of the TBSA. This patient has burns of roughly 40% TBSA (face 4.5%, upper extremities 18%, and anterior trunk 18%). Tetanus prophylaxis is indicated in all patients who have not been immunized within 1 year; prophylactic intravenous antibiotics are not indicated because they have not been shown to be of benefit in decreasing early cellulitic infections. Conversely, they have been shown to lead to increased complications secondary to resistant gram-negative organisms.

118. The answer is a. (*Schwartz, 7/e, pp 629, 631.*) Squamous cell carcinoma of the lip is the most common malignant tumor of the lip and constitutes 15% of all malignancies of the oral cavity. Basal cell carcinomas do occur on the lip, but much less frequently. There is a strong association between squamous cell tumors of the lip and sun exposure. Therefore, these lesions are more common in the southern United States and in occupational groups who work out of doors. Because of its greater sun exposure, the lower lip is the site of more than 90% of such lesions. Persistent hyperkeratosis precedes 35–40% of these lesions. The incidence of metastases increases with the size of the lesion, and spread is usually via lymphatics to the ipsilateral submental node. Contralateral nodal metastases are rare unless the lesion crosses the midline. Approximately 10–15% of all patients have metastases at the time of diagnosis. These lip tumors are very responsive to radiotherapy, which works well for small to medium-sized lesions. Large lesions treated with radiotherapy usually require surgical reconstruction. Radiotherapy should not be used in patients who will have ongoing sun exposure to the area because radiation therapy sensitizes the tissues to solar trauma.

119. The answer is b. (*Schwartz, 7/e, pp 2063–2070.*) Signs and symptoms of carpal tunnel syndrome are related to the distribution of the median nerve. This nerve, which passes through the carpal tunnel is the wrist with the finger flexor tendons, may suffer compression from fibrous scarring or malalignment following a fracture of the wrist. Nerve compression may also occur in patients with rheumatoid arthritis who develop flexor tenosynovitis. In women, the syndrome frequently first appears during pregnancy and recurs during the premenstrual phase of subsequent menstrual cycles. In these cases, symptoms are presumably the result of the effects of fluid retention and pressure on the median nerve owing to tissue swelling. In many instances, symptoms are limited to nocturnal pain and paresthesias. If conservative treatment of carpal tunnel syndrome is unsuccessful, surgical treatment may be required. Open and endoscopic techniques have been employed, both of which release adhesions of the median nerve and divide the transverse carpal ligament. The extensor retinaculum is located on the dorsal aspect of the wrist and contains the six compartments of extensor tendons.

120. The answer is d. (*Schwartz, 7/e, pp 270–277.*) While epithelialization is responsible for the healing of a closed incision, wound contraction is the primary method of closure in open wounds. During this process, the skin surrounding the wound is pulled over the wound surface and may account for up to a 90% reduction in the size of an open wound. In areas of greater adherence of skin to underlying tissue, the ability of contraction to close the wound is hindered due to the decreased mobility of the skin. Therefore, in areas of tight skin adherence such as the leg, contraction may only account for 30–40% reduction in wound size. Fibroblasts in the open wound, which predominate during the proliferative phase, contain increasing numbers of actin microfilaments, thereby becoming myofibroblasts. These specialized fibroblasts are felt to be responsible for wound contraction either through intrinsic cellular contraction or attachment to collagen strands. Bacterial colonization does not harm the process of wound contraction and surgical wound healing. While wound infection is often difficult to diagnose in open wounds, it is generally accepted that bacterial counts of 1 million bacteria per gram of tissue are deleterious to wound closure.

121. The answer is d. (*Schwartz, 7/e, pp 604, 610.*) White patches in the oral cavity (leukoplakia) sometimes are incorrectly interpreted as a premalignant condition. Microscopic examination of leukoplakia may in fact reveal hyperplasia, keratosis, or dyskeratosis, of which the last finding is the most serious because of its association with malignancy. Only about 5% of patients with leukoplakia develop cancer. A suggested treatment protocol for patients with thin lesions advocates a program of strict oral hygiene and avoidance of alcohol and tobacco. Biopsy is reserved only for those with thick lesions (since carcinoma in situ may be present). Radiation therapy is contraindicated. Approximately 50% of all oral cancers occur in patients who have associated areas of hyperkeratosis and dyskeratosis. Chronic irritation, as may occur with poorly fitting dentures, may result in leukoplakia.

122. The answer is b. (*Schwartz, 7/e, pp 2106–2110.*) Clefts of the lip and palate occur relatively frequently (1 in 750 live births); they may be unilateral or bilateral and can vary from a small notch to a complete cleft of the lip and palate. Most clefts occur as isolated anomalies, but occasionally they are associated with neurologic, orthopedic, or cardiac anomalies. A frequently recommended protocol for management is lip repair in the first 3 mo of life and palate repair at 12 to 18 mo. Other cosmetic procedures can be performed late in childhood and adolescence. Palate repair after 2 years of age is associated with a high incidence of speech impairment, often requiring speech therapy; repair in the early months of life can lead to a hazardous loss of blood that is poorly tolerated by the infant. Repair of the lip usually should be accomplished as soon as the infant is sufficiently stabilized to tolerate anesthesia with reasonable safety. Ten to twelve weeks is often recommended as the time for lip repair. At this age, the affected baby usually can be converted to dropper or cup feedings in the postoperative period, which thereby facilitates healing of the lip by reducing the need for suckling with the freshly wounded tissues.

123. The answer is d. (*Greenfield, 2/e, pp 2231–2242.*) The survival of patients with malignant melanoma correlates with the depth of invasion (Clark) and the thickness of the lesion (Breslow). It is widely held that patients with thin lesions (<0.76 mm) and Clark level I and II lesions are adequately managed by wide local excision. The incidence of nodal metastases rises with increasing Clark level of invasion such that a level IV lesion has a 30–50% incidence of nodal metastases. The assumption that removal of microscopic foci of disease is beneficial, in conjunction with retrospective data indicating improved survival in patients who have undergone removal of clinically negative but pathologically positive nodes, has led to the widely held belief that prophylactic node dissections are indicated for melanoma. Prospective data has challenged this concept. Veronesi and Sim have found that patients undergoing prophylactic node dissections survived no longer than those who were followed closely and underwent node dissections only after nodes became palpable. The subject remains controversial, and further study and follow-up are necessary. Immunotherapy has not been successful in controlling widespread metastatic melanoma even when added to chemotherapy. Intralesional administration of BCG has been demonstrated to control local skin lesions in only 20% of patients. Dinitrochlorobenzene (DNCB) can also be used.

124–127. The answers are 124-b, e, f; 125-c, d; 126-a, b, c, e, f; 127-b, e, f. (*Greenfield, 2/e, pp 2231–2245.*) Cutaneous neoplasms are extremely prevalent in the United States, with basal cell and squamous cell carcinoma being the most common. Patients who are at particular risk for malignant neoplasms are those with fair complexion and frequent sun exposure. Other risk factors for basal and squamous cell carcinomas include radiation damage, chronic wounds, and scar tissue. Surgical excision is the treatment of choice of all malignant cutaneous neoplasms. Radiation therapy may be useful for palliation of metastatic melanoma and may be considered as adjuvant therapy for squamous cell carcinoma and aggressive or invasive basal cell carcinoma. The pediatric population may suffer from multiple cutaneous lesions, including port-wine stains and strawberry hemangiomas. Both are capillary hemangiomas, but with very different clinical courses. Port-wine stains are present from birth and do not regress; therefore, surgical excision is a treatment option in small lesions. Other treatment options include laser cauterization or tattooing. Strawberry hemangiomas typically grow rapidly over 6–12 mo, but 90% regress spontaneously; therefore, commonly no intervention is required. For particularly large or rapidly growing lesions, excision, laser cauterization, or steroids may be considered. Cystic hygromas are masses of lymphatic vessels typically present in the head and neck region, usually apparent at birth. They are easily diagnosed with ultrasonography and are treated with surgical excision.

128–131. The answers are 128-a, b, f; 129-a, b, c, d, e; 130-b, c, d, e; 131-b, c, e. (*Greenfield, 2/e, pp 108–126.*) Numerous cytokines or growth factors are liberated from various cells at the time of injury. The process of wound healing requires that these factors act in an orchestrated manner. Platelets release ADP, thromboxane A_2, transforming growth factor, and platelet-derived growth factor within 1 h of injury. When macrophages become the predominant cell (at 2–3 days), numerous additional cytokines are released, including IL-1, fibroblast growth factor, TNF, transforming growth factor, and PDGF, among others. Integral to adequate wound healing is fibroblast proliferation and collagen synthesis. Stimulants of fibroblast proliferation include TNF, IL-1, fibroblast growth factor, transforming growth factor, epithelial growth factor, and plasminogen activator inhibitor. Collagen synthesis is then initiated and progresses during the proliferative phase of wound healing upon stimulation by IL-1, TNF, and transforming growth factor. Excessive or unopposed release of cytokines is thought to be responsible in various pathologic states of wound healing, such as pulmonary fibrosis or hepatic cirrhosis, and can lead to failure of multiple organ systems.

TRAUMA AND SHOCK

Questions

DIRECTIONS: Each item below contains a question or incomplete statement followed by suggested responses. Select the **one best** response to each question.

132. A teenage boy falls from his bicycle and is run over by a truck. On arrival in the emergency room, he is awake and alert and appears frightened but in no distress. The chest radiograph suggests an air-fluid level in the left lower lung field and the nasogastric tube seems to coil upward into the left chest. The next best step in management is

a. Placement of a left chest tube
b. Immediate thoracotomy
c. Immediate celiotomy
d. Esophagogastroscopy
e. Removal and replacement of the nasogastric tube; diagnostic peritoneal lavage

133. Which of the following conditions is most likely to follow a compression-type abdominal injury?

a. Renal vascular injury
b. Superior mesenteric thrombosis
c. Mesenteric vascular injury
d. Avulsion of the splenic pedicle
e. Diaphragmatic hernia

134. A 65-year-old man who smokes cigarettes and has chronic obstructive pulmonary disease falls and fractures the 7th, 8th, and 9th ribs in the left anterolateral chest. Chest x-ray is otherwise normal. Appropriate treatment might include

a. Strapping the chest with adhesive tape
b. Immobilization with sandbags
c. Tube thoracostomy
d. Peritoneal lavage
e. Surgical fixation of the fractured ribs

135. Blunt trauma to the abdomen most commonly injures which of the following organs?

a. Liver
b. Kidney
c. Spleen
d. Intestine
e. Pancreas

136. Ligation of injured major peripheral veins is rarely preferable to repair, but may be justified for which reason?

a. In severe popliteal vascular injuries, venous ligation leads to a decreased amputation rate following successful arterial reconstruction when compared with combined arterial and venous repair

b. Venous ligation leads to a decreased incidence of chronic venous insufficiency when compared with venous repair

c. Venous ligation leads to a decreased operative time in patients with multiple injuries or severe trauma when compared with venous repair

d. In the presence of extensive associated soft tissue injury, venous return is already sufficiently impaired to render venous repair pointless

e. Even though ligated veins thrombose, they often recanalize

137. A 27-year-old man sustains a single gunshot wound to the left thigh. In the emergency room he is noted to have a large hematoma of his medial thigh. He complains of paresthesias in his foot. On examination there are weak pulses palpable distal to the injury and the patient is unable to move his foot. The appropriate initial management of this patient would be

a. Angiography
b. Immediate exploration and repair
c. Fasciotomy of anterior compartment
d. Observation for resolution of spasm
e. Local wound exploration

Items 138–139

A 25-year-old woman arrives in the emergency room following an automobile accident. She is acutely dyspneic with a respiratory rate of 60 breaths/min. Breath sounds are markedly diminished on the right side.

138. The first step in managing the patient should be to

a. Take a chest x-ray
b. Draw arterial blood for blood gas determination
c. Decompress the right pleural space
d. Perform pericardiocentesis
e. Administer intravenous fluids

139. A chest x-ray of this woman before therapy would probably reveal

a. Air in the right pleural space
b. Shifting of the mediastinum toward the right
c. Shifting of the trachea toward the right
d. Dilation of the intrathoracic vena cava
e. Hyperinflation of the left lung

140. Among the physiologic responses to acute injury is

a. Increased secretion of insulin
b. Increased secretion of thyroxine
c. Decreased secretion of vasopressin (ADH)
d. Decreased secretion of glucagon
e. Decreased secretion of aldosterone

141. In a stable patient, the management of a complete transection of the common bile duct distal to the insertion of the cystic duct would be optimally performed with a

a. Choledochoduodenostomy
b. Loop choledochojejunostomy
c. Primary end-to-end anastomosis of the transected bile duct
d. Roux-en-Y choledochojejunostomy
e. Bridging of the injury with a T tube

142. Nonoperative management of penetrating neck injuries has been advocated as an alternative to mandatory exploration in asymptomatic patients. Which of the following findings would constitute a relative, rather than an absolute, indication for formal neck exploration?

a. Expanding hematoma
b. Dysphagia
c. Dysphonia
d. Pneumothorax
e. Hemoptysis

143. Following blunt abdominal trauma, a 12-year-old girl develops upper abdominal pain, nausea, and vomiting. An upper gastrointestinal series reveals a total obstruction of the duodenum with a "coiled spring" appearance in the second and third portions. Appropriate management is

a. Gastrojejunostomy
b. Nasogastric suction and observation
c. Duodenal resection
d. TPN to increase the size of the retroperitoneal fat pad
e. Duodenojejunostomy

144. Following traumatic peripheral nerve transection, regrowth usually occurs at which of the following rates?

a. 0.1 mm per day
b. 1 mm per day
c. 5 mm per day
d. 1 cm per day
e. None of the above

Items 145–147

A 28-year-old man is brought to the emergency room for a severe head injury after a fall. Initially lethargic, he becomes comatose and does not move his right side. His left pupil is dilated and responds only sluggishly.

145. The most common initial manifestation of increasing intracranial pressure in the victim of head trauma is

a. Change in level of consciousness
b. Ipsilateral (side of hemorrhage) pupillary dilation
c. Contralateral pupillary dilation
d. Hemiparesis
e. Hypertension

146. Initial emergency reduction of intracranial pressure is most rapidly accomplished by

a. Saline-furosemide (Lasix) infusion
b. Urea infusion
c. Mannitol infusion
d. Intravenous dexamethasone (Decadron)
e. Hyperventilation

147. In the patient described, compression of the affected nerve is produced by

a. Infection within the cavernous sinus
b. Herniation of the uncal process of the temporal lobe
c. Laceration of the corpus callosum by the falx cerebri
d. Occult damage to the superior cervical ganglion
e. Cerebellar hypoxia

148. A 31-year-old man is brought to the emergency room following an automobile accident in which his chest struck the steering wheel. Examination reveals stable vital signs, but the patient exhibits multiple palpable rib fractures and paradoxical movement of the right side of the chest. Chest x-ray shows no evidence of pneumothorax or hemothorax, but a large pulmonary contusion is developing. Proper treatment would consist of which of the following?

a. Tracheostomy, mechanical ventilation, and positive end-expiratory pressure
b. Stabilization of the chest wall with sandbags
c. Stabilization with towel clips
d. Immediate operative stabilization
e. No treatment unless signs of respiratory distress develop

149. A 30-year-old man is stabbed in the arm. There is no evidence of vascular injury, but he cannot flex his three radial digits. He has injured the

a. Flexor pollicis longus and flexor digitus medius tendons
b. Radial nerve
c. Median nerve
d. Thenar and digital nerves at the wrist
e. Ulnar nerve

150. Following a 2-h fire-fighting episode, a 36-year-old fireman begins complaining of a throbbing headache, nausea, dizziness, and visual disturbances. He is taken to the emergency room where his carboxyhemoglobin (COHb) level is found to be 31%. Appropriate treatment would be to

a. Begin an immediate exchange transfusion
b. Transfer the patient to a hyperbaric oxygen chamber
c. Begin bicarbonate infusion and give 250 mg acetazolamide (Diamox) intravenously
d. Administer 100% oxygen by mask
e. Perform flexible bronchoscopy with further therapy determined by findings

151. An elderly pedestrian collides with a bicycle-riding pizza delivery man and suffers a unilateral fracture of his pelvis through the obturator foramen. You would manage this injury by

a. External pelvic fixation
b. Angiographic visualization of the obturator artery with surgical exploration if the artery is injured or constricted
c. Direct surgical approach with internal fixation of the ischial ramus
d. Short-term bed rest with gradual ambulation as pain allows after 3 days
e. Hip spica

152. Regarding high-voltage electrical burns to an extremity

a. Injuries are generally more superficial than those of thermal burns
b. Intravenous fluid replacement is based on the percentage of body surface area burned
c. Antibiotic prophylaxis is not required
d. Evaluation for fracture of the other extremities and visceral injury is indicated
e. Cardiac conduction abnormalities are unlikely

153. Which of the following fractures or dislocations of the extremities induced by blunt trauma is associated with significant vascular injuries?

a. Knee dislocation
b. Closed posterior elbow dislocation
c. Midclavicular fracture
d. Supracondylar femur fracture
e. Tibial plateau fracture

154. A 23-year-old previously healthy man presents to the emergency room after sustaining a single gunshot wound to the left chest. The entrance wound is 3 cm inferior to the nipple and the exit wound is just below the scapula. A chest tube is placed that drains 400 mL of blood and continues to drain 50–75 mL/h during the initial resuscitation. Initial blood pressure of 70/0 mm Hg responds to 2 L crystalloid and is now 100/70 mm Hg. Abdominal examination is unremarkable. Chest x-ray reveals a reexpanded lung and no free air under the diaphragm. The next management step should be

a. Admission and observation
b. Peritoneal lavage
c. Exploratory thoracotomy
d. Exploratory celiotomy
e. Local wound exploration

155. A patient is brought to the emergency room after a motor vehicle accident. He is unconscious and has a deep scalp laceration and one dilated pupil. His heart rate is 120 beats/min, blood pressure is 80/40 mm Hg, and respiratory rate is 35 breaths/min. Despite rapid administration of 2 L normal saline, the patient's vital signs do not change significantly. The injury likely to explain this patient's hypotension is

a. Epidural hematoma
b. Subdural hematoma
c. Intraparenchymal brain hemorrhage
d. Basilar skull fracture
e. None of the above

156. When operating to repair civilian colon injuries

a. A colostomy should be performed for colonic injury in the presence of gross fecal contamination
b. The presence of shock on admission or more than two associated intraabdominal injuries is an absolute contraindication to primary colonic repair
c. Distal sigmoidal injuries should not be repaired primarily
d. Right-sided colonic wounds should not be repaired primarily
e. Administration of intravenous antibiotics with aerobic and anaerobic coverage has not been shown to decrease the incidence of wound infections after repair of colonic injuries

157. A 34-year-old prostitute with a history of long-term intravenous drug use is admitted with a 48-h history of pain in her left arm. Physical examination is remarkable for crepitus surrounding needle track marks in the antecubital space with a serous exudate. The plain x-ray of the arm is shown below. Which of the following organisms is most likely to be responsible for this condition?

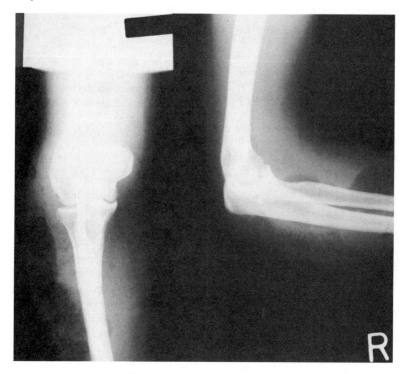

a. Anaerobic streptococcus
b. *Staphylococcus aureus*
c. *Pseudomonas aeruginosa*
d. *Clostridium perfringens*
e. *Escherichia coli*

158. Regarding myocardial contusion from blunt chest trauma, which of the following statements is correct?

a. Elevated cardiac isoenzyme levels sensitively identify patients at risk for life-threatening arrhythmias
b. The majority of patients have abnormalities on the initial ECG post injury
c. First-pass radionuclide angiography (RNA) and echocardiography are considered the "gold standard" for diagnosis
d. RNA and echocardiography are good predictors of subsequent cardiac complications such as arrhythmias and pump failure
e. All patients diagnosed with myocardial contusion should be monitored in an intensive care unit setting for 72 h

159. Protein metabolism after trauma is characterized by

a. Decreased liver gluconeogenesis
b. Inhibition of skeletal muscle breakdown by interleukin 1 and tumor necrosis factor (TNF, cachectin)
c. Decreased urinary nitrogen loss
d. Hepatic synthesis of acute-phase reactants
e. Decreased glutamine consumption by fibroblasts, lymphocytes, and intestinal epithelial cells

160. A 36-year-old man sustains a gunshot wound to the left buttock. He is hemodynamically stable. There is no exit wound, and an x-ray of the abdomen shows the bullet to be located in the right lower quadrant. Correct management of a suspected rectal injury would include

a. Barium studies of the colon and rectum
b. Barium studies of the bullet track
c. Endoscopy of the bullet track
d. Angiography
e. Sigmoidoscopy in the emergency room

161. Correct statements regarding blunt trauma to the liver include which of the following?

a. Hepatic artery ligation for control of bleeding is associated with decreased morbidity and mortality
b. The incidence of intraabdominal infections is significantly lower in patients with abdominal drains
c. Intracaval shunting has dramatically improved survival among patients with hepatic vein injuries
d. Nonanatomic hepatic debridement, with removal of the injured fragments only, is preferable to resection along anatomic planes
e. Major hepatic lacerations that are sutured closed will result in intrahepatic hematomas, hemobilia, and bile fistulas

162. If injury to a major artery in an extremity is suspected, surgical exploration should be carried out regardless of the presence of palpable pulses distal to the injury. The rationale is that the presence of palpable distal pulses does not reliably exclude

a. Significant arterial injury
b. Significant injury to adjacent motor nerve trunks
c. Significant injury to adjacent long bones
d. Significant injury to adjacent veins
e. Subsequent development of a compartment syndrome and the need for fasciotomy

163. The response to shock includes which of the following metabolic effects?

a. Increase in sodium and water excretion
b. Increase in renal perfusion
c. Decrease in cortisol levels
d. Hyperkalemia
e. Hypoglycemia

164. Appropriate treatment for an acute stable hematoma of the pinna of the ear includes which of the following measures?

a. Ice packs and prophylactic antibiotics
b. Excision of the hematoma
c. Needle aspiration
d. Incision, drainage, and pressure bandage
e. Observation alone

165. Animal and clinical studies have shown that administration of lactated Ringer's solution to patients with hypovolemic shock may

a. Increase serum lactate concentration
b. Impair liver function
c. Improve hemodynamics by alleviating the deficit in the interstitial fluid compartment
d. Increase metabolic acidosis
e. Increase the need for blood transfusion

Items 166–167

An 18-year-old high school football player is kicked in the left flank. Three hours later he develops hematuria. His vital signs are stable.

166. The diagnostic tests performed reveal extravasation of contrast into the renal parenchyma. Treatment should consist of

a. Resumption of normal daily activity excluding sports
b. Exploration and suture of the laceration
c. Exploration and wedge resection of the left kidney
d. Nephrostomy
e. Antibiotics and serial monitoring of blood count and vital signs

167. Initial diagnostic tests in the emergency room should include which of the following?

a. Retrograde urethrography
b. Retrograde cystography
c. Arteriography
d. Intravenous pyelogram
e. Diagnostic peritoneal lavage

168. True statements concerning penetrating pancreatic trauma include

a. Most injuries do not involve adjacent organs
b. Management of a ductal injury to the left of the mesenteric vessels is Roux-en-Y pancreaticojejunostomy
c. Management of a ductal injury in the head of the pancreas is pancreaticoduodenectomy
d. Small peripancreatic hematomas need not be explored to search for pancreatic injury
e. The major cause of death is exsanguination from associated vascular injuries

169. Rapid fluid resuscitation of the hypovolemic patient after abdominal trauma is significantly enhanced by which of the following?

a. Placement of long 18-gauge subclavian vein catheters
b. Placement of percutaneous femoral vein catheters
c. Bilateral saphenous vein cutdowns
d. Placement of short, large-bore percutaneous peripheral intravenous catheters
e. Infusion of cold whole blood

170. Use of the pneumatic antishock garment (PASG)

a. Elevates blood pressure by an "autotransfusion" effect, with augmentation of venous return and cardiac output
b. Is not recommended for control of persistent bleeding in the setting of severe pelvic fracture
c. Increases peripheral vascular resistance
d. Expedites assessment of lower body injuries in the trauma patient
e. Should be terminated by means of prompt deflation as soon as the trauma patient reaches the emergency department

171. Which of the following situations would be an indication for performance of a thoracotomy in the emergency room?

a. Massive hemothorax following blunt trauma to the chest
b. Blunt trauma to multiple organ systems with obtainable vital signs in the field but none on arrival in the emergency room
c. Rapidly deteriorating patient with cardiac tamponade from penetrating thoracic trauma
d. Penetrating thoracic trauma and no signs of life in the field
e. Penetrating abdominal trauma and no signs of life in the field

172. A 22-year-old man sustains a gunshot wound to the abdomen. At exploration, an apparently solitary distal small-bowel injury is treated with resection and primary anastomosis. On postoperative day 7, small-bowel fluid drains through the operative incision. The fascia remains intact. The fistula output is 300 mL/day and there is no evidence of intraabdominal sepsis. Correct treatment includes

a. Early reoperation to close the fistula tract
b. Broad-spectrum antibiotics
c. Total parenteral nutrition
d. Somatostatin to lower fistula output
e. Loperamide to inhibit gut motility

173. A 26-year-old man sustains a gunshot wound to the left thigh. Exploration reveals that a 5-cm portion of superficial femoral artery is destroyed. Appropriate management includes

a. Debridement and end-to-end anastomosis
b. Debridement and repair with an interposition prosthetic graft
c. Debridement and repair with an interposition arterial graft
d. Debridement and repair with an interposition vein graft
e. Ligation and observation

174. The patient illustrated on the chest x-ray film and contrast study on the following page was hospitalized after a car collision in which he suffered blunt trauma to the abdomen. He sustained several left rib fractures, but was hemodynamically stable. True statements about the injury demonstrated in the films include

a. The injury depicted is the most frequent organ injury in the setting of blunt trauma to the abdomen
b. Delayed operative repair is indicated after the patient's rib fractures are allowed to stabilize
c. Surgical treatment of this injury is indicated during this hospitalization
d. Early repair of this injury is preferably accomplished through a left posterolateral thoracotomy
e. If this injury is incidentally discovered during a surgical exploration, it should not be repaired

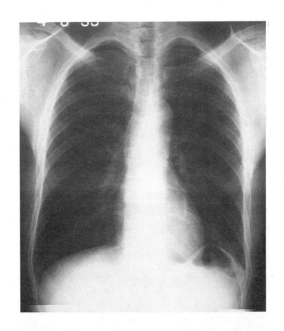

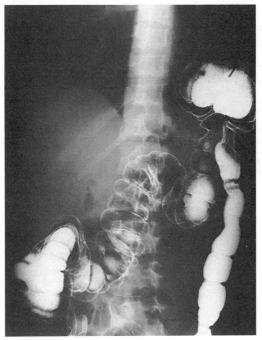

DIRECTIONS: Each group of questions below consists of lettered options followed by numbered items. For each numbered item, select the appropriate lettered option(s). Each lettered option may be used once, more than once, or not at all. **Choose exactly the number of options indicated following each item.**

Items 175–177

For each diagnostic technique listed below, select the injuries it reliably identifies.

a. Significant intraperitoneal bleeding
b. Injury of a retroperitoneal organ
c. Retroperitoneal (pelvic and visceral) vascular extravasation
d. Minor lacerations of liver and spleen
e. Subcapsular hematomas of liver and spleen
f. Injury of the small intestine
g. Diaphragmatic injury

175. Diagnostic peritoneal lavage **(SELECT 2 INJURIES)**

176. Abdominal computed tomography **(SELECT 3 INJURIES)**

177. Visceral angiography **(SELECT 1 INJURY)**

Items 178–180

For each scenario listed below, choose the abdominal organs most likely to be injured.

a. Diaphragm
b. Liver
c. Spleen
d. Small intestine
e. Large intestine
f. Kidneys
g. Stomach
h. Pancreas
i. Bladder
j. Great vessels (aorta/vena cava)

178. A motorist decelerates rapidly after striking a stalled vehicle. He is traveling at 55 mi/h at the time of impact. He is wearing a seat belt and his car is equipped with an air bag. **(SELECT 3 ORGANS)**

179. A man is shot with a high-velocity bullet that traverses his mid-abdomen at the level of the umbilicus. **(SELECT 3 ORGANS)**

180. An unsuspecting victim is struck forcefully in the upper abdomen by a mugger with a baseball bat. **(SELECT 4 ORGANS)**

Items 181–185

For each of the immediately life-threatening injuries of the chest listed below, select the proper intervention.

a. Endotracheal intubation
b. Cricothyroidotomy
c. Subxiphoid window
d. Tube thoracostomy
e. Occlusive dressing

181. Laryngeal obstruction (SELECT 1 INTERVENTION)

182. Open pneumothorax (SELECT 1 INTERVENTION)

183. Flail chest (SELECT 1 INTERVENTION)

184. Tension pneumothorax (SELECT 1 INTERVENTION)

185. Pericardial tamponade (SELECT 1 INTERVENTION)

TRAUMA AND SHOCK

Answers

132. The answer is c. (*Greenfield, 2/e, pp 284, 337.*) The finding of an air-fluid level in the left lower chest with a nasogastric tube entering it after blunt trauma to the abdomen is diagnostic of diaphragmatic rupture with gastric herniation into the chest. This lesion needs to be fixed immediately. With continuing negative pressure in the chest, each breath sucks more of the abdominal contents into the chest and increases the likelihood of vascular compromise of the herniated viscera. While the diaphragm is easily fixed from the left chest, this injury should be approached from the abdomen. The possibility of injury below the diaphragm after sufficient blunt injury to rupture the diaphragm mandates examination of the intraabdominal solid and hollow viscera; adequate exposure of the diaphragm to allow secure repair is possible from this approach.

133. The answer is e. (*Sabiston, 15/e, pp 308–312.*) In the rapid-deceleration injury associated with automobile crashes, the abdominal viscera tend to continue moving anteriorly after the body wall has been stopped. These organs exert great stress upon the structures anchoring them to the retroperitoneum. Intestinal loops stretch and may tear their mesenteric attachments, injuring and thrombosing the superior mesenteric artery; kidneys and spleen may similarly shear their vascular pedicles. In these injuries, however, ordinarily the intraabdominal pressure does not rise excessively and diaphragmatic hernia is not likely. Diaphragmatic hernia is primarily associated with compression-type abdominal or thoracic injuries that increase intraabdominal or intrathoracic pressure sufficiently to tear the central portion of the diaphragm.

134. The answer is d. (*Sabiston, 15/e, pp 307–309.*) The preeminent concern in treatment of rib fractures is the prevention of pulmonary complications (atelectasis and pneumonia), particularly for patients with preexisting pulmonary disease, who are in danger of progressing to respiratory failure. Attempts to relieve pain by immobilization or splinting, such as strapping the chest, merely compound the problem of inadequate ventilation. Tube thoracostomy is indicated only if pneumothorax is diagnosed. Mild pain may be controlled with oral analgesics, and patients with minor fracture injuries, if they can be closely monitored, may be managed at home with appropriate instructions for coughing and deep breathing. Patients with significant fractures or severe pain should be hospitalized. Rib fractures in the elderly are particularly treacherous. Intercostal nerve blocks often provide prolonged periods of pain relief and, together with appropriate pulmonary physiotherapy, will inhibit development of respiratory complications. Rib fractures are often associated with either intrathoracic or intraabdominal injuries. In particular, fractures of the left chest wall should arouse suspicion of splenic trauma. In equivocal cases, peritoneal lavage will often be diagnostic. Rib fractures heal spontaneously, without need for surgical fixation.

135. The answer is c. *(Sabiston, 15/e, pp 312–325.)* The diagnosis of injuries resulting from blunt abdominal trauma is difficult; injuries are often masked by associated injuries. Thus, trauma to the head or chest, together with fractures, frequently conceals intraabdominal injury. Apparently trivial injuries may rupture abdominal viscera in spite of the protection offered by the rib cage. The structures most likely to be damaged in blunt abdominal trauma are, in order of frequency, the spleen, kidney, intestine, liver, abdominal wall, mesentery, pancreas, and diaphragm. Abdominal paracentesis is a rapid, sensitive diagnostic test for patients with suspected intraabdominal injury and may be extremely helpful in the management of patients with associated head, thoracic, or pelvic trauma in whom signs and symptoms of the abdominal injuries may be masked or overlooked. Abdominal CT scans, which should be done promptly and rapidly, are being used more frequently to evaluate these injuries.

136. The answer is c. *(Sabiston, 15/e, p 333.)* In the past, ligation rather than repair of large veins in the extremities has been advocated in patients with multiple injuries or severe trauma. Venous repair adds to the operative time, often results in thrombosis and occlusion, and was thought to lead to an increased incidence of pulmonary embolization. Recent studies, including reviews of the Viet Nam Vascular Registry, indicate that the risk of pulmonary embolization is not increased with repair and that vein repair, in conjunction with arterial repair, increases limb salvage, particularly in popliteal injuries. Venous repair may also be necessary in the presence of extensive soft tissue trauma and an already severely compromised venous return. Long-term follow-up reveals that the sequelae of chronic venous insufficiency develop with increasing frequency in those patients who have had ligations of lower-extremity veins. Morbidity from chronic deep venous occlusion may be diminished even in those patients who develop thrombosis following repair, because recanalization often occurs. Ligated veins do not recanalize. For these reasons, it is currently recommended that large veins be repaired whenever clinically feasible.

137. The answer is b. *(Sabiston, 15/e, pp 332–333.)* The **five P's** of arterial injury include **P**ain, **P**aresthesias, **P**allor, **P**ulselessness, and **P**aralysis. In the extremities the tissues most sensitive to anoxia are the peripheral nerves and striated muscle. The early developments of paresthesias and paralysis are signals that there is significant ischemia present and immediate exploration and repair are warranted. The presence of palpable pulses does not exclude an arterial injury because this presence may represent a transmitted pulsation through a blood clot. When severe ischemia is present, the repair must be completed within 6–8 h to prevent irreversible muscle ischemia and loss of limb function. Delay to obtain an angiogram or to observe for change needlessly prolongs the ischemic time. Fasciotomy may be required but should be done in conjunction with and after reestablishment of arterial flow. Local wound exploration is not recommended because brisk hemorrhage may be encountered without the securing of prior vascular control.

138–139. The answers are 138-c, 139-a. *(Sabiston, 15/e, p 308.)* Tension pneumothorax is a life-threatening problem requiring immediate treatment. A lung wound that behaves as a ball or flap valve allows escaped air to build up pressure in the intrapleural space. This causes collapse of the ipsilateral lung and shifting of the mediastinum and trachea to the contralateral side, in addition to compression of the vena cava and contralateral lung. Sudden death may ensue because of a decrease in cardiac output; hypoxemia; and ventricular arrhythmias. To accomplish rapid decompression of the pleural space, a large-gauge needle should be passed into the intrapleural cavity through the second intercostal space at the midclavicular line. This may be attached temporarily to an underwater seal with subsequent insertion of a chest tube after the life-threatening urgency has been relieved.

Tension pneumothorax produces characteristic x-ray findings of ipsilateral lung collapse, mediastinal and tracheal shift, and compression of the contralateral lung. Occasionally, adhesions prevent complete lung collapse, but the tension pneumothorax is evident because of the mediastinal displacement. A pleural effusion would not be expected acutely in the absence of associated intrapleural blood.

140. The answer is a. *(Schwartz, 7/e, pp 103–105.)* Though the immediate release of catecholamines causes a transient drop in the insulin levels, shortly thereafter there is a significant rise in plasma insulin levels in injured humans. Since injured patients are highly hypermetabolic, it might be expected that the activity of the thyroid hormones would be increased following injury. This is not the case, however, and increased levels of the thyroid hormones are not seen. Vasopressin (ADH) is regulated by the serum osmolality. In the postinjury period many factors are at play that provoke the excretion of vasopressin. Glucagon secretion is normal or increased after injury; not only are aldosterone levels elevated, but the diurnal fluctuations ordinarily seen are lost.

141. The answer is d. *(Schwartz, 7/e, pp 192–193.)* Traumatic injury to the common bile duct must be considered in two separate categories. Complete transection of the common bile duct can be handled in many ways. If the patient is unstable and time is limited, simply placing a T tube in either end of the open common bile duct and staging the repair is the treatment of choice. In a stable patient a biliary enteric bypass is preferred. This can be accomplished by Roux-en-Y choledochojejunostomy or cholecystojejunostomy. The jejunum is favored over the duodenum because if the anastomosis leaks, a lateral duodenal fistula is avoided. For similar reasons the defunctionalizing of the jejunal limb is also preferable. This can be accomplished by creating a Roux-en-Y limb of jejunum. Primary end-to-end repair of a completely transected common bile duct is not recommended because of the high incidence of stricture and need for reoperation and creation of a biliary enteric bypass. However, primary repair is the procedure of choice if the common bile duct is lacerated or only partially transected.

142. The answer is d. *(Schwartz, 7/e, pp 163–166.)* Reports of a more than 50% incidence of negative explorations of the neck, iatrogenic complications, and serious injuries overlooked at operation have caused a reassessment of the dictum that all penetrating neck wounds that violate the platysma must be explored. Stable patients with zone III (between the angle of the mandible and the skull) or zone I (inferior to the cricoid cartilage) injuries, or multiple neck wounds, should undergo initial angiography irrespective of the ultimate treatment plan. Algorithms exist for nonoperative management of asymptomatic patients that employ observation alone or combinations of vascular and aerodigestive contrast studies and endoscopy. Nevertheless, recognition of acute signs of airway distress (stridor, hoarseness, dysphonia), visceral injury (subcutaneous air, hemoptysis, dysphagia), hemorrhage (expanding hematoma, unchecked external bleeding), or neurologic symptoms referable to carotid injury (stroke or altered mental status) or lower cranial nerve or brachial plexus injury requires formal neck exploration. Pneumothorax would mandate a chest tube; the necessity for exploration would depend on clinical judgment and institutional policy.

143. The answer is b. (*Schwartz, 7/e, pp 194–195.*) Duodenal hematomas result from blunt abdominal trauma. They present as a high bowel obstruction with abdominal pain and occasionally a palpable right upper quadrant mass. An upper gastrointestinal series is almost always diagnostic with the classic coiled spring appearance of the second and third portions of the duodenum secondary to the crowding of the valvulae conniventes (circular folds) by the hematoma. Nonsurgical management is the mainstay of therapy because the vast majority of duodenal hematomas resolve spontaneously. Simple evacuation of the hematoma is the operative procedure of choice. However, bypass procedures and duodenal resection have been performed for this problem. In patients with duodenal obstruction from the superior mesenteric artery syndrome, the obstruction is usually the result of a marked weight loss and, in conjunction with this, loss of the retroperitoneal fat pad that elevates the superior mesenteric artery from the third and fourth portions of the duodenum. Nutritional repletion and replenishment of this fat pad will elevate the artery off the duodenum and relieve the obstruction.

144. The answer is b. (*Schwartz, 7/e, pp 1884–1885.*) Transection of a peripheral nerve results in hemorrhage and in retraction of the severed nerve ends. Almost immediately, degeneration of the axon distal to the injury begins. Degeneration also occurs in the proximal fragment back to the fist node of Ranvier. Phagocytosis of the degenerated axonal fragments leaves a neurilemmal sheath with empty cylindrical spaces where the axons were. Several days following the injury, axons from the proximal fragment begin to regrow. If they make contact with the distal neurilemmal sheath, regrowth occurs at about the rate of 1 mm per day. However, if associated trauma, fracture, infection, or separation of neurilemmal sheath ends precludes contact between axons, growth is haphazard and a traumatic neuroma is formed. When neural transection is associated with widespread soft tissue damage and hemorrhage (with increased probability of infection), many surgeons choose to delay reapproximation of the severed nerve end for 3–4 wk.

145–147. The answers are 145-a, 146-e, 147-b. *(Schwartz, 7/e, pp 179–180.)* Closed head injuries may result in cerebral concussion from depression of the reticular formation of the brainstem. This type of injury is usually reversible.

Local bleeding and swelling (intracranial or extracranial) produce an increase in the intracranial pressure. A characteristic symptom pattern occurs initiated by progressive depression of mental status. Increasing intracranial pressure tends to displace brain tissue away from the source of the pressure; if the pressure is sufficient, herniation of the uncal process through the tentorium cerebri occurs.

Pupillary dilation is caused by compression of the ipsilateral oculomotor nerve and its parasympathetic fibers. If the pressure is not relieved, the contralateral oculomotor nerve will become involved and, ultimately, the brainstem will herniate through the foramen magnum and cause death. Hypertension and bradycardia are preterminal events.

Emergency measures to reduce intracranial pressure while preparing for localization of the clot or for a craniotomy or both include hyperventilation, dexamethasone (Decadron), and mannitol infusion. Of these, hyperventilation produces the most rapid decrease in brain swelling.

148. The answer is a. *(Schwartz, 7/e, pp 688–689.)* Flail chest is diagnosed in the presence of paradoxical respiratory movement in a portion of the chest wall. At least two fractures in each of three adjacent rib or costal cartilages are required to produce this condition. Complications of flail chest include segmental pulmonary hypoventilation with subsequent infection and ultimately respiratory failure. Management of flail chest should be individualized. If adequate pain control and pulmonary toilet can be provided, patients may be managed without stabilization of the flail. Often, intercostal nerve blocks and tracheostomy aid in this form of management. If stabilization is required, external methods such as sandbags or towel clips are no longer used. Surgical stabilization with wires is used if thoracotomy is to be performed for another indication. If this is not the case, "internal" stabilization is performed by placing the patient on mechanical ventilation with positive end-expiratory pressure. Tracheostomy is recommended because these patients usually require 10–14 days to stabilize their flail segment and postventilation pulmonary toilet is simplified by tracheostomy. Indications for mechanical ventilation include significant impedance to ventilation by the flail segment, large pulmonary contusion, an uncooperative patient (e.g., owing to head injury), general anesthesia for another indication, more than five ribs fractured, and the development of respiratory failure.

149. The answer is c. (*Schwartz, 7/e, pp 2048–2050.*) The motor components of the median nerve maintain the muscular function of most of the long flexors of the hand as well as the pronators of the forearm and the thenar muscles. The median nerve is also an extremely important sensory innervator of the hand and is commonly described as the "eye of the hand" because the palm, the thumb, and the index and middle fingers all receive their sensation via the median nerve.

150. The answer is d. (*Schwartz, 7/e, pp 238–239.*) Carbon monoxide (CO) is the leading cause of toxin-related death in the United States. It is produced by the incomplete combustion of fossil fuels and is emitted by virtually all gas-powered engines and appliances that burn fossil fuel, e.g., home furnaces, water heaters, stoves, pool heaters, kerosene heaters, and charcoal fires. Tobacco smoke—particularly smoke released from the tip of the cigarette, which has 2.5 times more CO than inhaled smoke—produces a significant amount of the gas; nonsmokers working in closed quarters with smokers may have carboxyhemoglobin (COHb) levels as high as 15%, easily enough to cause headache and some impairment of judgment. Fire fighters are at particularly high risk for CO intoxication. The pathophysiology of CO poisoning is unclear. It is known to cause an adverse shift in the oxygen-hemoglobin dissociation curve, to cause direct cardiovascular depression, and to inhibit cytochrome A_3. Tissue hypoxia is the result.

Treatment is directed toward increasing the partial pressures of O_2 to which the transalveolar hemoglobin is exposed. In most cases, administering 100% oxygen through a tightly fitted face mask will result in a serum elimination half-life of COHb of 80 min (compared with 520 min when one breathes room air). In severe cases, where coma, seizures, or respiratory failure are present, the partial pressure of O_2 is increased by administering it in a hyperbaric chamber with an atmospheric pressure of 2.8. In this situation the serum elimination half-life is reduced to 23 min. In any case, the oxygen therapy should continue until the COHb levels reach 10%.

151. The answer is d. (*Schwartz, 7/e, pp 169, 204.*) Most pelvic fractures are the result of automobile-pedestrian accidents and these fractures are a frequent cause of death. The pelvis is extremely vascular with a diffuse blood supply that makes hemorrhage common and surgical control of bleeding difficult. This patient has a type II fracture (single break in pelvic ring) through a non-weight-bearing portion of the pelvis. These fractures are best treated by bed rest until hemodynamic stability is assured and thereafter by gentle ambulation as pain permits. The clinician must watch carefully for associated injuries to bladder, urethra, and colon and be alert to the many other possible concurrent injuries to an elderly patient who has suffered a collision, even a low-velocity attack from a pizza man.

152. The answer is d. (*Schwartz, 7/e, pp 250–252.*) The treatment of electrical injury should be modified from that of thermal burns because tissue damage is much deeper than is apparent at first inspection. The heat generated is proportional to the resistance to the flow of current. Bone, fat, and tendons offer the greatest resistance. Therefore, the tissue deep within the center of an extremity may be injured while more superficial tissues are spared. For this reason, the quantification of fluid requirements cannot be based on the percentage of body surface area involved, as in the Parkland, Brooke, or Baxter formulas, which are used to calculate fluid replacement after thermal burns. Massive fluid replacement is usually essential. A brisk urine output is desirable because of the likelihood of myonecrosis with consequent myoglobinuria and renal damage. As with deep thermal burns, debridement, skin grafting, and amputation of extremities may be required following electrical injury. However, fasciotomy is more frequently required than escharotomy with electrical injury because deep myonecrosis results in increased intracompartmental pressures and compromised limb perfusion. In addition, distant fractures may result owing to vigorous muscle contraction during the accident or if subsequent falls occur. Cardiac or respiratory arrest may occur if the pathway of the current includes the heart or brain. An electrical current can also damage the pulmonary alveoli and capillaries and lead to respiratory infections, a major cause of death in these victims. Owing to the deep myonecrosis that often accompanies high-voltage injury, prophylaxis for clostridia with high-dose penicillin may be considered. Mafenide acetate is preferred over other topical antimicrobials because of its deeper penetration of eschar.

153. The answer is a. *(Bunt, Am J Surg 160:226–228, 1990.)* In a 4-year retrospective study of 569 at-risk parajoint fractures or dislocations resulting from blunt trauma, there was only a 1.5% incidence of associated vascular injury. Angiograms and vascular surgical consultations were obtained when vascular compromise was suspected owing to clinical examination or Doppler confirmation of flow abnormalities. While vascular injuries due to fractures on either side of a joint (e.g., supracondylar femur fracture or tibial plateau fracture) were uncommon, major joint dislocations were more commonly associated with vascular injury. An exception to this rule is the type III supracondylar humerus fracture, where displacement of bone may injure or entrap the tethered brachial artery. Clavicular fractures are rarely associated with significant vascular injury. The highest rate of vascular injury occurs with knee dislocations because of the extreme force required to dislocate the joint. In open elbow dislocations, the brachial artery is often disrupted by forcible hyperextension of the joint; closed elbow dislocations are rarely associated with vascular injury unless the dislocation is anterior.

154. The answer is d. *(Greenfield, 2/e, pp 317–331.)* Gunshot wounds to the lower chest are often associated with intraabdominal injuries. The diaphragm can rise to the level of T4 during maximal expiration. Therefore, any patient with a gunshot wound below the level of T4 should be subjected to abdominal exploration. Exploratory thoracotomy is not indicated because most parenchymal lung injuries will stop bleeding and heal spontaneously with the use of tube thoracostomy alone. Indication for thoracic exploration for bleeding is usually in the range of 100–150 mL/h over several hours. Peritoneal lavage is not indicated even though the abdominal examination is unremarkable. As many as 25% of patients with negative physical findings and negative peritoneal lavage will have significant intraabdominal injuries in this setting. These injuries include damage to the colon, kidney, pancreas, aorta, and diaphragm. Local wound exploration is not recommended because the determination of diaphragmatic injury with this technique is unreliable.

155. The answer is e. *(Sabiston, 15/e, pp 297–298.)* Loss of consciousness following head trauma should be assumed to be due to intracranial hemorrhage until proved otherwise. However, a thorough evaluation of the head-injured patient includes assessment for other potentially life-threatening injuries. Rarely, a patient may have sufficient hemorrhage from a scalp laceration to cause hypotension. In the patient described, hypotension and tachycardia should not be uncritically attributed to the head injury, since these findings in the setting of blunt trauma are suggestive of serious thoracic, abdominal, or pelvic hemorrhage. When cardiovascular collapse occurs as a result of rising intracranial pressure, it is generally accompanied by hypertension, bradycardia, and respiratory depression.

156. The answer is b. *(Sabiston, 15/e, pp 324–325.)* Because of the colon's poor blood supply and its fecal content, colon injuries are more difficult to manage than small-bowel injuries. Recently the necessity of mandatory colostomy for civilian colon injuries has been questioned. About 85% of civilian colon injuries are small wounds from low- or medium-velocity gunshots or stab wounds, which are less likely to produce gross fecal spillage. These injuries can be repaired primarily in the absence of gross contamination, regardless of the right- or left-sided location of injury. Shock on admission and multiple associated injuries are not universally viewed as absolute contraindications to primary repair in such cases. Gross contamination or large amounts of hard intraluminal feces remain generally accepted contraindications to primary repair. Alternatives include end colostomy with mucous fistula or Hartmann's pouch, exteriorization of a primary repair, and protection of a primary repair in the distal colon by formation of a proximal colostomy. In all cases in which traumatic colon injury is suspected, the early administration of broad-spectrum intravenous antibiotics seems to reduce the incidence of postoperative infectious complications.

157. The answer is d. *(Sabiston, 15/e, pp 269–270.)* Because they are so often malnourished and at high risk for other conditions that alter their immunocompetence, drug addicts have an extraordinary susceptibility to infections of the type that can quickly progress to threaten life and limb. Among the most virulent are those that give rise to anaerobic cellulitis. Terms sometimes used for these infections are *gas abscess, gangrenous cellulitis, localized gas gangrene,* and *epifascial gangrene.* Suppuration and extensive gas formation are common and usually localized, unlike the infections associated with myonecrosis. These lesions may be clostridial or nonclostridial. *Clostridium perfringens* is the most common culprit, but anaerobic cellulitis and gas formation have been associated with a variety of obligate anaerobes including *Bacteroides* species, *Peptostreptococcus,* and *Peptococcus,* and the gram-negative enteric bacilli (*E. coli, Klebsiella*), staphylococci, and streptococci. *Pseudomonas aeruginosa* is not implicated in these aggressive infections. Since the progressive injury results from liberation of bacterial exotoxins, antitoxin administration at this stage is futile. Treatment is determined by immediate inspection of a Gram stain of the thin, dark, malodorous wound drainage or a needle aspirate of the crepitant area: if large, "boxcar-shaped" gram-positive bacilli are present, it is a clostridial infection and high doses of parenteral penicillin G (20 million U/day) are indicated; if a polymicrobial Gram stain is seen, clindamycin-aminoglycoside should be added until specific sensitivities are known. Aggressive debridement is always indicated.

158. The answer is c. (*Dubrow, Surgery 106:267–273, 1989. Miller, Arch Surg 124:805–807, 1989.*) The spectrum of blunt cardiac injuries includes myocardial contusion, rupture, and internal (chamber and septal) disruptions such as traumatic septal defects, papillary muscle tears, and valvular tears. Myocardial contusions are by far the most common of these injuries. They usually occur in persons who sustain a direct blow to the sternum, as seen in a driver whose sternum is forcibly compressed by the steering column in a deceleration injury. Over 50% of patients with myocardial contusion demonstrate external signs of thoracic trauma, including sternal tenderness, abrasions, ecchymosis, palpable crepitus, rib fractures, or flail segments. Overall, fewer than 10% of patients have conduction abnormalities, dysrhythmias, or ischemic patterns on initial ECG. Elevated cardiac isoenzyme levels are specific for myocardial injury, but they lack clinical significance in patients without ECG abnormalities or hemodynamic instability. First-pass radionuclide angiography (RNA) and echocardiography provide sensitive assessment of ventricular wall motion and ejection fraction after blunt chest trauma and are currently viewed as the "gold standard" for the diagnosis of myocardial contusion. But while RNA and echocardiography sensitively detect small abnormalities in myocardial function, they are poor predictors of the significant cardiac complications of pump failure and arrhythmia. Traditionally, management of patients with myocardial contusion has included continuous ECG monitoring in an intensive care unit for 48–72 h, even in hemodynamically stable patients without other injuries. Because of the large number of patients with blunt chest trauma from automobile accidents, however, this policy has been scrutinized. Virtually all patients who develop cardiac complications display ECG abnormalities on arrival in the emergency room or within the first 24 h. Since an abnormal ECG is a good predictor of subsequent complications, stable patients with possible myocardial contusions but with a normal ECG tracing may be placed on telemetry for 24 h, rather than monitored in an ICU.

159. The answer is d. (*Weissman, Anesthesiology 73:308–327, 1990.*) Injury and sepsis result in accelerated protein breakdown with increased urinary nitrogen loss and increased peripheral release of amino acids. The negative nitrogen balance represents the net result of breakdown and synthesis (with breakdown increased and synthesis increased or diminished). Amino acids such as alanine are released by muscle and transported to the liver for incorporation into acute-phase proteins including fibrinogen, complement, haptoglobin, and ferritin. The amino acids also undergo gluconeogenesis to glucose, which is utilized primarily by the brain and other glycolytic tissues such as peripheral nerves, erythrocytes, and bone marrow. Other tissues receive energy from fat in the form of fatty acids or ketone bodies during starvation following major trauma; this helps to conserve body protein. Glutamine is the most abundant amino acid in the blood, and its levels in muscle and blood decrease following injury and sepsis as it is consumed rapidly by replicating fibroblasts, lymphocytes, and intestinal endothelial cells. The use of glutamine may decrease protein catabolism in the intestine and may help prevent atrophy of the gastrointestinal tract in starved and parenterally nourished patients. Along with the counterregulatory hormones (glucagon, epinephrine, cortisol), interleukin 1 appears to mediate muscle breakdown. Recent studies have indicated that TNF (also called cachectin because of the role it plays in muscle wasting in septic or oncologic patients) also may be a principal catabolic cytokine in the traumatized patient. This protein is secreted by macrophages and further affects metabolism by inducing secretion of inter-leukin 1 and inhibiting synthesis and activity of lipogenic enzymes.

160. The answer is e. *(Sabiston, 15/e, pp 324–325. Schwartz, 7/e, pp 199–200.)* Penetrating injury to the intraperitoneal or extraperitoneal rectum should be diagnosed by immediate sigmoidoscopy. Contrast studies of the rectum, when sigmoidoscopy is inconclusive, should use a water-soluble radiopaque medium such as Gastrografin. The use of barium is contraindicated because its spillage in the peritoneal cavity mixed with feces would increase the likelihood of subsequent intraabdominal abscesses. Instrumentation of the bullet track is also contraindicated because of the risk of injury to adjacent structures (e.g., bladder, ureters, iliac vessels). Angiography is not a sensitive method for demonstrating injury of the intestinal wall.

161. The answer is d. *(Schwartz, 7/e, pp 188–192.)* The overwhelming majority of patients explored for blunt trauma to the liver sustain their injuries in motor vehicle accidents. In a large consecutive series of 323 patients with blunt hepatic trauma who were explored for the finding of hemoperitoneum on peritoneal lavage, the mortality was 31%. Forty-two percent of the deaths, due primarily to liver injury, occurred intraopera-tively during the initial operation following admission. All operations were performed at a regional trauma center by staff trauma surgeons. Their find-ings included the following observations: (1) intraoperative deaths were due to uncontrolled hemorrhage; (2) patients with major hepatic injuries who survived operation but nevertheless died appeared to succumb either to sepsis or to associated injuries, usually involving the head or chest; (3) hepatic artery ligation for control of bleeding yielded dismal results—of the 3 surviving patients who underwent hepatic artery ligation (an additional 11 died), 2 required reoperation for continued bleeding; (4) the use of drains (passive and active) was associated with a significantly greater inci-dence of intraabdominal infectious complications; (5) intracaval shunting was used in 7 severely injured patients without a survivor; (6) while minor hepatic injuries required little or no treatment, major lacerations could usually be controlled with simple absorbable sutures placed 2–3 cm from the fracture edge, without occurrence of subsequent intrahepatic hematoma, hemobilia, or bile fistulae; (7) hepatic fragmentation may be treated by nonanatomic debridement, with suture ligation of individual bleeding points—of nine attempts at formal anatomic resection in stable patients, all ended in uncontrollable hemorrhage and death.

162. The answer is a. (*Schwartz, 7/e, pp 172–175, 204–206.*) The presence of ischemic changes following vascular trauma is an indication for emergency exploration and repair. Nonsurgical management of arterial trauma when distal pulses are palpable may lead to delayed sequelae of embolization, occlusion, secondary hemorrhage, false aneurysm, and traumatic arteriovenous fistula. The presence of palpable pulses does not reliably exclude significant arterial injury. Injuries that may be missed if exploration is not performed include lacerations and partial transections containing hematomas, intramural or intraluminal thromboses, and intimal disruptions or tears. Injury to motor nerves would be apparent on neurologic examination. Injury to bone would be diagnosed by x-ray. Adjacent venous injury, in the absence of an expanding hematoma, would not by itself mandate exploration because there are numerous collateral venous channels in the extremities. Prophylactic fasciotomy is not routinely performed for all arterial injuries but is indicated in the presence of an ischemic period exceeding 4–6 h, combined arterial and major venous injury, prolonged periods of hypotension, massive associated soft tissue trauma, and massive edema.

163. The answer is d. (*Schwartz, 7/e, pp 102–105.*) The biochemical changes associated with shock result from tissue hypoperfusion, endocrine response to stress, and specific organ system failure. During shock, the sympathetic nervous system and adrenal medulla are stimulated to release catecholamines. Renin, angiotensin, antidiuretic hormone, adrenocorticotropin, and cortisol levels increase. Resultant changes include sodium and water retention and an increase in potassium excretion, protein catabolism, and gluconeogenesis. Potassium levels rise as a result of increased tissue release, anaerobic metabolism, and decreased renal perfusion. If renal function is maintained, potassium excretion is high and normal plasma potassium levels are restored.

164. The answer is d. (*Sabiston, 15/e, pp 1277–1278.*) A subperichondrial hematoma in the pinna of the ear may lead to avascular necrosis of the cartilage with shriveling of the pinna and fibrosis and calcification of the hematoma. The result is the deformity known as "cauliflower ear." Appropriate treatment consists of evacuation of the hematoma by incision and tight packing of the skin and perichondrium onto the cartilage with a pressure dressing. Needle aspiration does not effect adequate drainage. Ice packs may be helpful early, but are not sufficient to prevent the deformity; antibiotics are not indicated for this lesion. Since the hematoma is subperichondrial, excision of the hematoma would remove the perichondrium and lead to cartilage deformities.

165. The answer is c. *(Sabiston, 15/e, pp 83–84, 123.)* Infusion of lactated Ringer's solution is an effective immediate step, both clinically and experimentally, in managing hypovolemic shock. Use of this balanced salt solution helps correct the fluid deficit (in the extracellular, extravascular compartment) resulting from hypovolemic shock. This procedure may decrease requirements for whole blood in patients with hemorrhagic shock. If blood loss has been minimal and is controlled, whole blood transfusion may be avoided entirely. The theoretical objection to infusion of lactated Ringer's solution is that it will increase lactate levels and compound the problem of lactic acidosis. This has not been borne out in animal or clinical studies. Along with the hemodynamic improvement that follows volume restitution, liver function improves, lactate metabolism is improved, excess lactate levels drop, and metabolic acidosis improves.

166–167. The answers are 166-e, 167-d. *(Cass, Urol Clin North Am 16:213–220, 1989.)* In stable patients with suspected genitourinary tract injury, the first urologic study other than urinalysis should be the intravenous urogram. The technique of high-dose drip infusion is desirable because the high concentration of contrast achieved greatly facilitates interpretation in an unprepared patient. Intravenous pyelography should be performed before retrograde cystography to avoid obscuring visualization of the lower ureteral tract. The study also may preclude the need for retrograde urethrography in cases where, unlike the case presented, there is a suspicion of urethral injury. Renal arteriography is not indicated routinely but should be performed to rule out renal pedicle injury when no kidney function is demonstrated by drip infusion urography. Peritoneal lavage is not useful in the diagnosis of genitourinary injuries because the structures are retroperitoneal. Seventy to eighty percent of patients with blunt renal trauma are successfully treated nonsurgically. Bed rest may reduce the likelihood of secondary hemorrhage; antibiotics may reduce the chance of infection's developing in a perirenal hematoma. Failure of conservative treatment is indicated by rising fever, increasing leukocytosis, evidence of secondary hemorrhage, and persistent or increasing pain and tenderness in the region of the kidney.

168. The answer is e. *(Sabiston, 15/e, pp 315–317.)* The majority of penetrating pancreatic injuries can be managed with simple drainage. Injury to the major pancreatic duct to the left of the mesenteric vessels is effectively treated with a distal pancreatectomy. The high morbidity and mortality of a pancreaticoduodenectomy for trauma limit its use to extensive blunt injuries to both pancreatic head and duodenum. For ductal injury in the region of the head of the pancreas, a Roux-en-Y limb of jejunum should be brought up and used to drain the transected duct. The proximity of the pancreas to many other major structures makes combined injuries frequent (90%). Complications of pancreatic injury include fistula, pseudocyst, and abscess, but the cause of death in patients with pancreatic injury is most frequently exsanguination from associated injury to major vascular structures such as the splenic vessels, mesenteric vessels, aorta, or inferior vena cava. Finally, however small, all peripancreatic hematomas should be explored to search for pancreatic injury. Simple drainage is usually adequate treatment in such cases, but failure to recognize a pancreatic injury can have catastrophic sequelae.

169. The answer is d. *(Dutky, J Trauma 29:856–860, 1989.)* Rapid fluid administration is often the key to successful trauma resuscitation. Some of the important factors affecting the rate of fluid resuscitation include the diameter of the intravenous tubing, the size and length of the venous cannulae, the fluid viscosity, and the site of administration. According to Poiseuille's law, flow is proportional to the fourth power of the radius of a catheter and inversely proportional to its length. Therefore, the shorter a catheter and the larger its diameter, the faster one can infuse a solution through it. Central venous placement alone does not assure rapid flow. Importantly, the diameter of the intravenous tubing employed may be the rate-determining factor in fluid delivery: blood-infusion tubing allows twice the flow of standard intravenous tubing and should be used when rapid fluid resuscitation is needed. Any patient who is suspected of having a major abdominal injury should immediately have at least two short, large-bore (16-gauge or larger) intravenous cannulae placed in peripheral veins. Longer, smaller catheters, such as standard 18-gauge central venous catheters, may take more time to place and will have lower flow rates. Once fluid resuscitation is under way, one may elect to place an 8- or 9-French pulmonary artery catheter-introducer via a central venous approach for further volume administration, as well as for measurement of central venous pressure or for Swan-Ganz catheter insertion. Lower-extremity venous cannulae, placed by saphenous vein cutdown or percutaneously into the femoral veins, are no longer advised as primary access for patients with abdominal trauma, since possible disruption of iliac veins or the inferior vena cava will render volume infusion ineffective. Studies have demonstrated that the flow rate of cold whole blood is roughly two-thirds that of whole blood at room temperature. Diluting and warming the blood by "piggybacking" it into infusion lines that are delivering crystalloid will decrease the blood's viscosity, enhance flow, and minimize hypothermia.

170. The answer is c. *(Flint, Ann Surg 211:703–707, 1990. Trunkey, Can J Surg 27:479–486, 1984.)* The pneumatic antishock garment (PASG) is composed of inflatable overalls with three compartments, two for the legs and one for the abdomen. It has now been convincingly demonstrated that the PASG elevates blood pressure by increasing peripheral vascular resistance rather than by an "autotransfusion" effect on venous return and increased cardiac output. The PASG is beneficial for controlling bleeding from pelvic fractures by reduction of pelvic volume and immobilization to restrict fracture movement. The suit pressure must be released very slowly because rapid deflation can lead to sudden, irreversible hypotension. This is probably due to a sudden decrease in peripheral vascular resistance and to the effects of vasodilation and wash-out of accumulated metabolites of capillary beds under the suit. Upon reperfusion of the lower body, a systemic metabolic acidemia with hyperkalemia may result and must be closely monitored. For these reasons satisfactory intravenous volume must be attained prior to decompression of the PASG, a delay that may prevent adequate early evaluation of concealed injuries to the lower body.

171. The answer is c. *(Schwartz, 6/e, p 675.)* Although indications for thoracotomy in the emergency room are controversial, the procedure appears to be most beneficial when it is employed to (1) release cardiac tamponade in patients with penetrating thoracic trauma who are deteriorating too rapidly for a subxiphoid pericardial window to be created; (2) allow cross-clamping of the descending aorta in patients with intraabdominal bleeding for whom other measures are not effective in maintaining blood pressure; and (3) allow effective internal cardiac massage in patients who arrive in the emergency room with faint or absent pulses and distant heart sounds, and for whom other resuscitative efforts are unsuccessful. By contrast, existing evidence suggests that patients who are unsalvageable and do not benefit from emergency room thoracotomy include (1) those with no vital signs (pulse, pupillary reaction, spontaneous respiration) in the field and (2) those with blunt trauma to multiple organ systems and absent vital signs upon arrival in the emergency room.

172. The answer is c. *(Schwartz, 6/e, pp 1181–1182.)* Most enterocutaneous fistulas result from trauma sustained during surgical procedures. Irradiated, obstructed, and inflamed intestine is prone to fistulization. Complications of fistulas include fluid and electrolyte depletion, skin necrosis, and malnutrition. Fistulas are classified according to their location and the volume of output, because these factors influence prognosis and treatment. When the patient is stable, a barium swallow is obtained to determine (1) the location of the fistula, (2) the relation of the fistula to other hollow intraabdominal organs, and (3) whether there is distal obstruction. Proximal small-bowel fistulas tend to produce a high output of intestinal fluid and are less likely to close with conservative management than are distal, low-output fistulas. Small-bowel fistulas that communicate with other organs, particularly the ureter and bladder, may need aggressive surgical repair because of the risk of associated infections. The presence of obstruction distal to the fistula (e.g., an anastomotic stricture) can be diagnosed by barium contrast study and mandates correction of the obstruction. When these poor prognostic factors for stabilization and spontaneous closure are observed, early surgical intervention must be undertaken. The patient in the question, however, appears to have a low-output, distal enterocutaneous fistula. Control of the fistulous drainage should be provided by percutaneous intubation of the tract with a soft catheter. This is usually accomplished under fluoroscopic guidance. Antispasmodic drugs have not been proved effective; somatostatin has been used with mixed success in the setting of high-output (greater than 500 mL/day) fistulas. There is no indication for antibiotics in the absence of sepsis. Total parenteral nutrition (TPN) is given to maintain or restore the patient's nutritional balance while minimizing the quantity of dietary fluids and endogenous secretions in the gastrointestinal tract. A period of 4–6 wk of TPN therapy is warranted to allow for spontaneous closure of a low-output, distal fistula. Should conservative management fail, surgical closure of the fistula is performed.

173. The answer is d. *(Schwartz, 6/e, pp 981–982.)* Traumatic arterial injuries can be handled with several techniques. The basic principles of debridement of injured tissue and reestablishment of flow should be observed. Primary end-to-end anastomosis is preferable if this can be accomplished without tension. When 5 cm of artery has been destroyed, it is impossible to perform a tension-free primary anastomosis, and a reversed saphenous vein graft is the repair of choice. Ligation of the artery is to be avoided in order to prevent gangrene and limb loss. The use of prosthetic material (Gore-Tex) in a potentially infected field is also to be avoided as infection at the suture line often leads to delayed hemorrhage. Harvesting an arterial graft of similar diameter from elsewhere in the body is hazardous and unnecessary when vein is available.

174. The answer is c. *(Cameron, 4/e, pp 820–824.)* Traumatic injuries to the diaphragm are associated with both blunt and penetrating trauma. The spleen, kidneys, intestines, and liver are the most frequently injured abdominal organs in blunt trauma; the diaphragm is the least. Missed injuries lead to problems with herniation and bowel strangulation with sufficient frequency that repair should not be delayed. All such injuries require repair once the diagnosis is made and the patient has been stabilized. Most acute defects in the diaphragm can be repaired via an abdominal approach, which allows exploration for coexisting injuries.

175–177. The answers are 175-a, d; 176-a, b, e; 177-c. *(Davis, pp 2789–2790. Walters, Surg Gynecol Obstet 165:496–502, 1988.)* Peritoneal lavage is a diagnostic technique used to identify occult intraperitoneal injury in patients with abdominal trauma. An abnormal lavage is obtained when the lavage effluent exceeds allowable levels of blood, bile, or amylase; the presence of vegetable matter also constitutes an abnormal result. Lavage has been used most widely in the triage of hemodynamically stable victims of abdominal trauma who are suspected of having significant injuries but who manifest equivocal physical findings. Further indications for lavage are the suspicion of abdominal injury in patients with altered sensoria, patients with unexplained blood loss, and patients who require general anesthesia to treat other injuries. The technique is exquisitely sensitive to intraabdominal bleeding and will detect as little as 20 mL of free blood in the peritoneal cavity. Because stable retroperitoneal hematomas and minor lacerations of the liver and spleen often shed sufficient blood to produce a positive lavage, some authors have advocated abdominal CT as the preferred method of identifying occult operable injuries of the abdomen. Also, CT with oral and intravenous contrast can provide accurate images of the injured retroperitoneum and the solid intraabdominal viscera (as lavage cannot). Neither CT nor lavage has been a reliable indicator of small intestinal and diaphragmatic injuries, and neither has been useful in obtaining hemostasis nonoperatively. Angiography, however, may be employed to demonstrate visceral or pelvic arterial extravasation and to control hemorrhage by selective embolization.

178–180. The answers are 178-d, e, f; 179-d, e, j; 180-b, c, f, h. (*Schwartz, 6/e, pp 193–219.*) Deceleration injuries commonly result from high-speed motor vehicle accidents and falls from considerable heights. The mechanism of injury is the shearing of pedicled organs from their points of attachment to the retroperitoneum. Because these pedicles are usually vascular, the injury results in bleeding and ischemia of the affected organ. Pedicled organs in the abdomen include the intestines (small and large) and the kidneys. Deceleration injuries to the aorta occur in the mediastinum and are usually fatal.

The small intestine and its mesentery is by far the most commonly injured abdominal organ in penetrating trauma because of its sheer mass and central location. A midline bullet at the level of the umbilicus is most likely to strike small intestine, the transverse colon, and perhaps the aorta or vena cava. The great vessels bifurcate just at the level of the umbilicus. The diaphragm, stomach, and pancreas would be superior to this injury; the bladder below; and the liver, spleen, and kidneys lateral.

The relative incidence of organ injury in blunt trauma is highest for solid organs (spleen, liver, and kidneys). Although hollow viscera are less likely to be injured by blunt trauma, this rule does not apply when the hollow viscus is full; for example, rupture of a full urinary bladder is frequently described when blunt force is applied to the lower abdomen. In addition to the spleen, liver, and kidneys, extreme blunt force to the upper abdomen may fracture the pancreas, which is susceptible to injury because of its position overlying the rigid spinal column.

181–185. The answers are 181-b, 182-e, 183-a, 184-d, 185-c.
(Schwartz, 6/e, pp 672–684.) Flail chest describes the paradoxical motion of the chest wall that occurs when consecutive ribs are broken in more than one place, usually following blunt trauma to the thorax. Respiratory distress may ensue when the noncompliant flail segment interferes with generation of adequate positive and negative intrathoracic pressure needed to move air through the trachea. In addition, a blow sufficiently violent to cause a flail chest may also contuse the underlying pulmonary parenchyma, which compounds the respiratory distress. Treatment consists of stabilizing the chest wall. Although some temporary benefit may be gained by external buttressing of the chest (e.g., with sandbags, or by turning the patient onto the affected side), endotracheal intubation provides rapid and safe control of the airway, as well as stabilization of the chest internally by positive pressure ventilation.

Airway obstruction denotes partial or complete occlusion of the tracheobronchial tree by foreign bodies, secretions, or crush injuries of the upper respiratory tract. Patients may present with symptoms ranging from cough and mild dyspnea to stridor and hypoxic cardiac arrest. An initial effort should be made to digitally clear the airway and to suction visible secretions; in selected, stable patients, fiberoptic endoscopy may be employed to determine the cause of obstruction and to retrieve foreign objects. Unstable patients whose airways cannot be quickly reestablished by clearing the oropharynx must be intubated. An endotracheal intubation may be attempted, but cricothyroidotomy is indicated in the presence of proximal obstruction or severe maxillofacial trauma.

Blunt or penetrating trauma to the pericardium and heart will result in pericardial tamponade when fluid pressure in the pericardial space exceeds central venous pressure and thus prevents venous return to the heart. The result is shock, despite adequate volume and myocardial function. The treatment is pericardial decompression. A subxiphoid, supradiaphragmatic incision and creation of a pericardial "window," ideally performed in the operating room, provides a rapid, safe means of confirming the diagnosis of tamponade and of relieving venous obstruction. If heavy bleeding is encountered on opening the pericardial window, a sternotomy may be performed.

Tension pneumothorax occurs when a laceration of the visceral pulmonary pleura acts as a one-way valve that allows air to enter the pleural space from an underlying parenchymal injury but not to escape. Increasing intrapleural pressure causes collapse of the ipsilateral lung, compression of the contralateral lung due to mediastinal shift toward the opposite hemithorax, and diminished venous return. Treatment consists of relieving the pneumothorax. This is best accomplished by tube thoracostomy. Open pneumothorax occurs when a traumatic defect in the chest wall permits free communication of the pleural space with atmospheric pressure. If the defect is larger than two-thirds of the tracheal diameter, respiratory efforts will move air in and out through the defect in the chest wall rather than through the trachea. The immediate treatment is placement of an occlusive dressing over the defect; subsequent interventions include placement of a thoracostomy tube (preferably through a separate incision), formal closure of the chest wall, and ventilatory assistance if needed.

TRANSPLANTS, IMMUNOLOGY, AND ONCOLOGY

Questions

DIRECTIONS: Each item below contains a question or incomplete statement followed by suggested responses. Select the **one best** response to each question.

186. Tissue injury or infection results in the release of tumor necrosis factor (TNF) by which of the following cells?

a. Fibroblasts
b. Damaged vascular endothelial cells
c. Monocytes/macrophages
d. Activated T lymphocytes
e. Activated killer lymphocytes

187. A cross-match is performed by incubating

a. Donor serum with recipient lymphocytes and complement
b. Donor lymphocytes with recipient serum and complement
c. Donor lymphocytes with recipient lymphocytes
d. Recipient serum with a known panel of multiple donor lymphocytes
e. Recipient serum with donor red blood cells and complement

188. In order to activate helper/inducer T (CD41) lymphocytes, macrophages release

a. Interleukin 1
b. Interleukin 2
c. Interleukin 3
d. Interleukin 4
e. Interferon

189. Which of the following cells cause immunologically restricted tumor cell lysis?

a. Macrophages
b. Cytotoxic T lymphocytes
c. Natural killer cells
d. Polymorphonuclear leukocytes
e. Helper T lymphocytes

190. The primary mechanism of action of cyclosporine A is inhibition of

a. Macrophage function
b. Antibody production
c. Interleukin 1 production
d. Interleukin 2 production
e. Cytotoxic T-cell effectiveness

Items 191–192

A 24-year-old woman presents with lethargy, anorexia, tachypnea, and weakness. Laboratory studies reveal a BUN of 150 mg/dL, serum creatinine of 16 mg/dL, and potassium of 6.2 meq/L. Chest x-ray shows increased pulmonary vascularity and a dilated heart.

191. Management of this patient would include

a. Emergency kidney transplantation
b. Creation and immediate use of a forearm arteriovenous fistula
c. Sodium polystyrene sulfonate (Kayexalate) enemas
d. A 100-g protein diet
e. Cardiac biopsy via femoral vein catheterization

192. In the course of 3 mo of treatment, the patient's congestive heart failure resolves, the lethargy and weakness diminish markedly, and she is able to return to work part-time. Family immune profile studies reveal that her mother and her father both are haplotype identical with regard to HLA antigens and that her sister is a six-antigen match. The patient at this time should be urged to

a. Continue hemodialysis three times a week
b. Undergo cadaveric renal transplantation
c. Accept a kidney transplant from her sister
d. Accept a kidney transplant from her father
e. Accept a kidney transplant from her mother

193. After the first postoperative year of cardiac transplantation, the most common cause of death is

a. Infection
b. Arrhythmia
c. Accelerated graft arteriosclerosis
d. Acute rejection episode
e. Cancer

194. Which of the following precludes cadaveric renal transplantation?
a. Positive cross-match
b. Donor blood type O
c. Two-antigen HLA match with donor
d. Blood pressure of 180/100 mm Hg
e. Hemoglobin level of 8.2 g/dL

195. Which of the following statements regarding hyperacute rejection of a transplanted kidney is true?

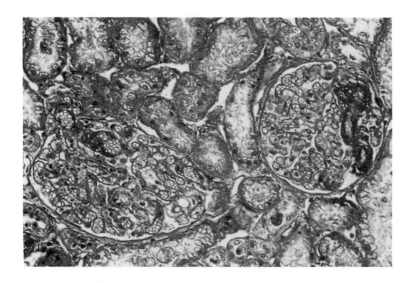

a. It is mediated by preformed donor antibodies against recipient HLA antigens
b. It can be prevented by performing lymphocytotoxicity cross-match testing
c. It is manifest grossly by a swollen, pale kidney at the time of transplant surgery
d. This form of rejection is associated with disseminated intravascular coagulation (DIC)
e. The rejection process can be treated with a steroid bolus and OKT3

196. Which of the following statements regarding heart transplantation is true?

a. Heart transplants are matched by size and ABO blood type rather than tissue typing
b. Cadaveric graft survival is significantly lower with heart transplants as compared with renal transplants
c. Cold ischemia time for donor hearts should not be more than 48 h
d. The upper age limit for heart transplant eligibility is 55 years
e. The leading cause of death after the first year of cardiac transplantation is chronic rejection

197. A 47-year-old man with hypertensive nephropathy develops fever, graft tenderness, and oliguria 4 wk following cadaveric renal transplantation. Serum creatinine is 3.1 mg/dL. A renal ultrasound reveals mild edema of the renal papillae but normal flow in both the renal artery and renal vein. Nuclear scan demonstrates sluggish uptake and excretion. The next most appropriate step is

a. Performing an angiogram
b. Decreasing steroid and cyclosporine dose
c. Beginning intravenous antibiotics
d. Performing renal biopsy, steroid boost, and immunoglobulin therapy
e. Beginning FK 506

198. Posttransplant cytomegalovirus infection may cause

a. Plyelonephritis
b. GI ulceration and hemorrhage
c. Cholecystitis
d. Intraabdominal abscess
e. Parotitis

199. In centers with experienced personnel, 1-year liver transplant survival is now approximately

a. 95%
b. 80%
c. 65%
d. 50%
e. 35%

200. Graft-versus-host disease has occurred with the transplantation of which of the following?

a. Kidney
b. Lung
c. Heart
d. Bone marrow
e. Pancreas

201. Which of the following diseases is appropriately treated with combined heart-lung transplantation?

a. Primary pulmonary hypertension
b. Cystic fibrosis
c. End-stage emphysema
d. Idiopathic dilated cardiomyopathy with long-standing secondary pulmonary hypertension
e. End-stage pulmonary fibrosis secondary to sarcoidosis

202. Which of the following is true regarding successful whole-organ pancreas transplantation in type I diabetes?

a. It results in maintenance of normal serum glucose levels
b. Recurrence of diabetic nephropathy in simultaneously transplanted kidneys is not prevented
c. Oral glucose tolerance tests remain abnormal
d. The pathologic changes of diabetic retinopathy are reversed
e. The rate of diabetic ulcers and amputations in the lower extremities is reduced

203. Which of the following is true regarding bone marrow transplantation?

a. Marrow is highly immunogenic and easily rejected by the nonimmunosuppressed host
b. Marrow transplantation has not been successful in the treatment of aplastic anemias
c. Marrow transplantation has not been successful in the treatment of congenital immunodeficiency diseases
d. Marrow transplantation can be used as a successful therapy for stage IV breast cancer following high-dose chemotherapy
e. Marrow transplantation must be performed with low-level immunosuppression to enhance the degree of chimerism

204. Which of the following statements is true of the major histocompatibility complex (MHC) proteins?

a. Only nonnucleated cells express MHC class I proteins
b. B lymphocytes, antigen-presenting cells, and vascular endothelium express only MHC class II proteins
c. MHC class I proteins are encoded by the HLA-D locus (DR, DP, and DQ)
d. MHC class I proteins act as the major targets for antibody-mediated rejection of organ allografts and are detected by cross-matching techniques
e. B cells recognize antigens bound to MHC class II proteins

205. The most useful serum marker for detecting recurrent disease after treatment of nonseminomatous testicular cancer is

a. Carcinoembryonic antigen (CEA)
b. α-fetoprotein (AFP)
c. Prostate-specific antigen (PSA)
d. CA125
e. p53 oncogene

206. An edentulous 72-year-old man with a 50-year history of cigarette smoking presents with a nontender, hard mass in the lateral neck. The simplest way to establish an accurate histological diagnosis of a neck mass suspected to be cancerous is

a. Fine needle aspiration cytology
b. Bone marrow biopsy
c. Nasopharyngoscopy
d. CT scan of the head and neck
e. Sinus x-ray

207. Which of the following is true regarding intravenous administration of chemotherapy?

a. Subcutaneous extravasation of carmustine (BCNU) or 5-fluorouracil (5-FU) usually causes ulceration
b. Extravasation of doxorubicin rarely causes serious ulceration because the agent binds quickly to tissue nucleic acid
c. Serious and progressive ulceration can be expected following extravasation of vincristine or vinblastine
d. Problems of wound healing should be anticipated if systemic 5-FU therapy is begun less than 2 wk postoperatively
e. Administration of folinic acid prevents most of the toxicity of methotrexate, but does not help to normalize wound healing

208. For which of the following malignancies does histologic grade best correlate with prognosis?

a. Lung cancer
b. Melanoma
c. Colonic adenocarcinoma
d. Hepatocellular carcinoma
e. Soft tissue sarcoma

209. A mother notices an abdominal mass in her 3-year-old son while giving him a bath. There is no history of any symptoms, but the boy's blood pressure is elevated at 105/85 mm Hg. Metastatic workup is negative and the patient is explored. The mass below is found within the left kidney. Which of the following statements concerning this disease is correct?

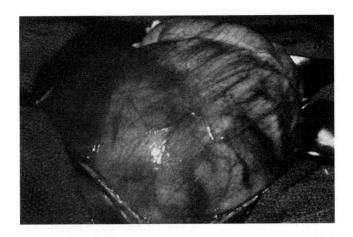

a. This tumor is associated with aniridia, hemihypertrophy, and cryptochidism
b. The majority of patients present with an asymptomatic abdominal mass and hematuria
c. Treatment with surgical excision, radiation, and chemotherapy results in survival of less than 60% even in histologically low-grade tumors
d. Surgical excision is curative and no further treatment is ordinarily advised
e. This tumor is the most common malignancy in childhood

210. An 11-year-old girl presents to your office because of a family history of medullary carcinoma of the thyroid. Physical examination is normal. Which of the following tests would you perform?

a. Urine vanillylmandelic acid (VMA) level
b. Serum insulin level
c. Serum gastrin level
d. Serum glucagon level
e. Serum somatostatin level

211. A 37-year-old woman has developed a 6-cm mass on her anterior thigh over the past 10 mo. The mass appears to be fixed to the underlying muscle, but the overlying skin is movable. The next most appropriate step in management is

a. Above-knee amputation
b. Excisional biopsy
c. Incisional biopsy
d. Bone scan
e. Abdominal CT scan

212. A 50-year-old man is incidentally discovered to have non-Hodgkin's lymphoma confined to the submucosa of the stomach during esophagogastroduodenoscopy for dyspepsia. Which of the following statements is true regarding his condition?

a. Surgery alone cannot be considered adequate treatment
b. Combined chemotherapy and radiation therapy, without prior resecton, are not effective
c. Combined chemotherapy and radiation therapy, without prior resection, result in a high risk of severe hemorrhage and perforation
d. Outcome (freedom from progression and overall survival) is related to the histological grade of the tumor
e. The stomach is the most common site for non-Hodgkin's lymphoma of the gastrointestinal tract

213. Interferons are correctly characterized by which of the following statements?

a. They are a group of complex phospholipids
b. They are produced by virus-infected cells
c. They enhance viral replication
d. They cause Burkitt's lymphoma cell lines to divide
e. They have not been effective in the treatment of hairy cell leukemias

214. Which of the following statements regarding malignant parotid tumors is correct?

a. Acinar carcinoma is a highly aggressive malignant tumor of the parotid gland
b. Squamous carcinoma of the parotid gland exhibits only moderately malignant behavior
c. Regional node dissection for occult metastases is not indicated for malignant parotid tumors because of their low incidence and the morbidity of lymphadenectomy
d. Facial nerve preservation should be attempted when the surgical margins of resection are free of tumor
e. Total parotidectomy (superficial and deep portions of the gland) is indicated for malignant tumors

215. Which of the following potentially operable complications is a common occurrence among patients receiving systemic chemotherapy?

a. Acute cholecystitis
b. Perirectal abscess
c. Appendicitis
d. Incarcerated femoral hernia
e. Diverticulitis

216. Which of the following statements regarding testicular cancer is true?

a. Lymph node dissection after radical orchiectomy is useful for staging but does not increase survival
b. Seminomas and choriocarcinomas are best treated with orchiectomy and retroperitoneal lymph node dissection
c. Seminomas are extremely resistant to radiotherapy
d. Orchiectomy for a testicular mass is approached via the scrotum
e. Cryptorchidism is associated with an increased risk of testicular cancer

217. Advantages of dialysis over renal transplantation include

a. Less expense if the treatment continues for less than 2 years
b. Increased number of pregnancies in female dialysis patients
c. Return of normal menses in female dialysis patients
d. Less anemia in dialysis patients
e. Increased 1-year survival of dialysis patients

Items 218–219

A 30-year-old primigravida complains of headaches, restlessness, sweating, and tachycardia. She is 18 wk pregnant and her blood pressure is 200/120 mm Hg.

218. Appropriate workup might include

a. Exploratory laparotomy
b. Mesenteric angiography
c. Head CT scan
d. Abdominal CT scan
e. Abdominal ultrasonogram

219. Appropriate treatment might consist of

a. Therapeutic abortion
b. Urgent excision of the tumor and a therapeutic abortion
c. Phenoxybenzamine and propranolol followed by a combined cesarean section and excision of the tumor
d. Metyrosine (Demser) blockade followed by a combined cesarean section and excision of the tumor
e. Phenoxybenzamine and propranolol followed by a combined vaginal delivery at term and excision of the tumor

220. Which of the following statements regarding radiation therapy is true?

a. Damage to DNA occurs primarily by the direct effect of ionizing radiation
b. Cellular hypoxia decreases sensitivity to radiation
c. Cells in the S phase of the cell cycle are most radiosensitive
d. Radiation therapy following lumpectomy of a breast cancer provides rates of local control equal to those of mastectomy
e. Skin, gastrointestinal mucosa, and bone marrow are relatively insensitive to radiotherapy

221. Which of the following statements regarding cancer therapy with interleukin 2 (IL-2) is true?

a. It is a B-cell growth factor
b. It induces a major response in patients with metastatic breast cancer
c. It induces a major response in patients with metastatic colon cancer
d. It induces a major response in patients with metastatic melanoma
e. It induces a major response in patients with lymphoma

222. Which statement concerning cancer and nutrition is correct?

a. Levels of nitrates in food and drinking water are positively correlated with the incidence of bladder cancer
b. Regular ingestion of vitamin D from childhood probably inhibits formation of carcinogens
c. Consumption of excessive amounts of animal dietary fats is associated with increased incidences of colon cancer
d. Nutritional support of cancer patients improves response of the tumor to chemotherapy
e. Alcohol ingestion is associated with pancreatic cancer

223. How do cardiac allografts differ from renal allografts?

a. Cardiac allografts are matched by HLA tissue typing and renal allografts are not
b. Cardiac allografts can tolerate a longer period of cold ischemia than renal allografts
c. One-year graft survival for cardiac allografts is substantially lower than that for renal allografts
d. Cardiac allografts are matched only by size and ABO blood type
e. Cyclosporine is a critical component of the immunosuppressive regimen for cardiac allografts but not renal allografts

224. Five-year survival rates in excess of 20% may be expected following resection of pulmonary metastases if

a. Other organ metastases are present
b. Lung lesions are solitary
c. Local tumor recurrence is found
d. The tumor doubling time is less than 20 days
e. The patient has received prior chemotherapy

225. Which statement about transmission of HIV in the health care setting is true?

a. A freshly prepared solution of dilute chlorine bleach will not adequately decontaminate clothing
b. All needles should be capped immediately after use
c. Cuts and other open skin wounds are believed to act as portals of entry for HIV
d. Double gloving reduces the risk of intraoperative needle sticks
e. The risk of seroconversion following a needle stick with a contaminated needle is greater for HIV than for hepatitis B

226. Regarding the risk of breast cancer, which of the following statements is true?

a. Breast cancer occurs more commonly among women of the lower social classes
b. A history of breast cancer in a first-degree family relative is associated with a fourfold increase in risk
c. Women with a first birth after age 30 years have approximately twice the risk of those with a first birth before age 18
d. Cigarette smoking increases the risk of breast cancer
e. Hair dyes have been shown to increase the risk of breast cancer

227. Human immunodeficiency virus (HIV) has been isolated from many body fluids. Which of the following is a major source of transmission?

a. Tears
b. Sweat
c. Semen
d. Urine
e. Breast milk

228. What is the primary toxicity of doxorubicin (Adriamycin)?

a. Cardiomyopathy
b. Pulmonary fibrosis
c. Peripheral neuropathy
d. Uric acid nephropathy
e. Hepatic dysfunction

229. What is the most common cause of cancer death among women?

a. Breast cancer
b. Ovarian cancer
c. Colon cancer
d. Endometrial cancer
e. Lung cancer

230. Which of the following agents causes hemorrhagic cystitis?

a. Bleomycin
b. 5-fluorouracil
c. Cisplatin
d. Vincristine
e. Cyclophosphamide

231. What is the major barrier to successful transplantation across animal species (xenotransplantation)?

a. Acute rejection
b. Chronic rejection
c. Hyperacute rejection
d. Infection
e. ABO incompatibility

232. Which of the following are efficient antigen-presenting cells found in the epidermis?

a. Macrophages
b. T cells
c. Langerhans cells
d. Dendritic cells
e. B cells

233. Which of the following statements is true regarding carcinoembryonic antigen (CEA)?

a. CEA is an accurate screening test for primary colorectal cancer
b. CEA levels have not been helpful in the diagnosis of recurrent colorectal cancer
c. CEA levels, when elevated, are highly specific for colon cancer
d. CEA is present in normal colonic mucosa
e. Postoperative CEA assay is 70% accurate in predicting the appearance of liver metastases within 1 year

DIRECTIONS: Each group of questions below consists of lettered options followed by numbered items. For each numbered item, select the appropriate lettered option(s). Each lettered option may be used once, more than once, or not at all. **Choose exactly the number of options indicated following each item.**

Items 234–236

For each stage in the treatment of the patient below, select the appropriate next step.

a. Left hemicolectomy
b. Right hemicolectomy
c. Subtotal colectomy
d. Total colectomy
e. Hepatic wedge resection
f. External beam irradiation
g. 5-fluorouracil and leucovorin
h. External beam irradiation and chemotherapy
i. Abdominal MRI
j. No further treatment

234. A 65-year-old man is admitted to the hospital with complaints of intermittent constipation and microcytic anemia. Barium enema reveals a nonobstructing "apple-core" lesion of the proximal sigmoid colon. Colonoscopy confirms the location of the mass and reveals no other synchronous lesions. **(SELECT 1 STEP)**

235. The patient undergoes surgery and recovers uneventfully. Pathology of the resected specimen is reported as Dukes C with negative surgical margins. **(SELECT 1 STEP)**

236. In 6-mo follow-up an abdominal CT scan shows a 2-cm isolated lesion in the right lobe of the liver. Repeat colonoscopy shows no evidence of recurrent or metachronous lesions. Chest x-ray and bone scan are normal. **(SELECT 1 STEP)**

Items 237–240

A 32-year-old man with diabetic nephropathy undergoes an uneventful renal transplant from his sister (two-haplotype match). His immunosuppressive regimen includes azathioprine, steroids, and cyclosporine. For each development in the postoperative period, select the most appropriate next step.

a. Begin gancyclovir
b. Administer steroid boost
c. Withhold steroids
d. Decrease cyclosporine
e. Increase cyclosporine
f. Decrease azathioprine
g. Obtain renal ultrasound
h. Begin broad-spectrum antibiotics
i. Administer filgrastim (Neupogen)
j. Administer FK50

237. On postoperative day 3 the patient is doing well, but you notice on his routine laboratory tests that his white blood cell count is 2.0. (**SELECT 1 STEP**)

238. The patient's WBC count gradually returns to normal, but on postoperative day 7 he develops a fever of 39.44°C (103°F) and a nonproductive cough. A chest x-ray reveals diffuse interstitial infiltrates, and a "buffy coat" is positive for viral inclusions. (**SELECT 1 STEP**)

239. The patient recovers from the above illness and is discharged home on postoperative day 18. At 3-mo follow-up he is doing well, but you notice that his creatinine is 2.8 mg/dL. He has no fever, his graft is not tender, and his renal ultrasound is normal. (**SELECT 1 STEP**)

240. Six months following his transplant, the patient begins to develop fever, malaise, and pain of the right lower quadrant. Upon palpation, the graft is tender. Chest x-ray and urine and blood cultures are normal. Renal ultrasound shows an edematous graft. (**SELECT 1 STEP**)

TRANSPLANTS, IMMUNOLOGY, AND ONCOLOGY

Answers

186. The answer is c. (*Greenfield, 2/e, pp 113–114.*) Tumor necrosis factor (TNF) is a peptide hormone produced by endotoxin-activated monocytes/macrophages and has been postulated to be the principal cytokine mediator in gram-negative shock and sepsis-related organ damage. Biologic actions of TNF include polymorphonuclear neutrophil (PMN) activation and degranulation; increased nonspecific host resistance; increased vascular permeability; lymphopenia; promotion of interleukins 1, 2, and 6; capillary leak syndrome; microvascular thrombosis; anorexia and cachexia; and numerous other protective and adverse effects in sepsis. Its role in sepsis is providing a fertile field for research in critical care.

187. The answer is b. (*Greenfield, 2/e, pp 553–554.*) The purpose of a cross-match is to determine whether the recipient has circulating antibodies against donor HLA antigens. Such antibodies do not occur naturally, but rather are the result of prior sensitization during pregnancy, blood transfusions, or previous transplantation. A complement-dependent lymphocytotoxicity cross-match is performed by adding recipient serum and complement to donor cells (T cells, B cells, or monocytes). If specific anti-donor antibodies are present, antibody binding results in complement fixation and cell lysis. This is detected by addition of a vital dye, which is taken up by the damaged cell membrane, resulting in a positive cross-match. If a positive cross-match is detected to donor T cells (HLA class I), transplantation will result in hyperacute rejection.

188. The answer is a. (*Greenfield, 2/e, pp 114–115.*) Interleukin 1 (IL-1) is a thymocyte mitogen produced by activated macrophages as well as many other types of cells (e.g., monocytes, dendritic cells, Langerhans cells, neutrophils, microglial cells). It induces interleukin 2 production by the helper T cell, which initiates a cascade of immunoregulatory and inflammatory functions.

189. The answer is b. *(Greenfield, 2/e, pp 529–546.)* Unlike the granulocyte line, T lymphocytes express the T-cell receptor. This receptor imports antigen specificity to T cells. The helper T cell, when stimulated by interleukin 1 and antigens, produces various lymphokines that ultimately produce effector cells. One of these effector cells is the cytotoxic T cell, which kills cells that express specific antigens, including viral, tumor, and nonbiologic antigens. Macrophages and natural killer cells have some tumoricidal activity; however, this is not specific for tumors.

190. The answer is d. *(Greenfield, 2/e, pp 548–549.)* Cyclosporine is a highly effective immunosuppressive agent produced by fungi. It is more specific than the anti-inflammatory agents such as steroids or the antiproliferative agents such as azathioprine. The effectiveness of cyclosporine in preventing allograft rejection is related to its ability to inhibit interleukin 2 production. Without interleukin 2 from helper T cells, there is no clonal expansion of alloantigen-directed cytotoxic T cells and no stimulation of antibody production by B cells.

191–192. The answers are 191-c, 192-c. *(Greenfield, 2/e, pp 571–581.)* Hemodialysis, rather than management by dietary manipulation alone, should be instituted in patients with end-stage renal failure whose serum creatinine is over 15 mg/dL or whose creatinine clearance is less than 3 mL/min. It is important that hemodialysis be initiated prior to the onset of uremic complications. These complications include hyperkalemia, congestive heart failure, peripheral neuropathy, severe hypertension, pericarditis, bleeding, and severe anemia. The uremic hyperkalemic patient in congestive heart failure may require emergency dialysis in addition to the standard conservative measures, which include (1) limitation of protein intake to less than 60 g/day and restriction of fluid intake and (2) reduction of elevated serum potassium levels by insulin-glucose or sodium polystyrene sulfonate (Kayexalate) enema treatment. Arteriovenous fistulas require about 2 wk to develop adequate size and flow. While awaiting maturation, temporary dialysis can be satisfactorily performed using either an external arteriovenous shunt or the peritoneal cavity. Renal biopsy would be performed in an attempt to obtain a diagnosis of the underlying renal disease.

Patients who are acceptable candidates for kidney transplantation usually should undergo this form of treatment, after they are stabilized, rather than chronic hemodialysis, the mortality for which is now higher than for transplantation. Despite adequate dialysis, problems of neuropathy, bone disease, anemia, and hypertension remain difficult to manage. Compared with chronic dialysis, transplantation restores more patients to happier and more productive lives. It had been conjectured that, all other issues being equal, sex matching was important in the graft survival and that a mother-daughter graft was preferred to a father-daughter graft. Review of the current data does not support such a conclusion. The best graft survival rates for living related transplants—over 90% at 5 years—are obtained when all six histocompatibility loci are identical. All family members of potential transplant recipients should be tissue typed and the donor should be selected on the basis of closest match, if psychological and medical evaluation makes this feasible. With the development of cyclosporine-based immunosuppression, cadaveric kidney graft survival has approached that of living-related transplantation. There are some transplanters who believe that the slight improvement with living-related kidneys does not justify the risk to the donor and that these transplantations should no longer be performed.

193. The answer is c. *(Greenfield, 2/e, pp 602–606.)* Chronic graft rejection is manifested in cardiac allografts as chronic vascular rejection of main and intramuscular coronary arteries. Myointimal proliferation and medial scarring result in diffuse and eccentric arterial narrowing referred to as accelerated graft atherosclerosis. Infection remains the primary cause of death within the first year of cardiac transplant, but accelerated graft arteriosclerosis is the most common cause of mortality thereafter. Percutaneous transluminal coronary angioplasty, coronary artery bypass grafting, and retransplantation are the current options for combating this problem.

194. The answer is a. *(Greenfield, 2/e, pp 553–554.)* A positive crossmatch means that the recipient has circulating antibodies that are cytotoxic to donor-strain lymphocytes. This incompatibility, which almost always leads to an acute humoral rejection of the graft, precludes transplantation. Blood type matching prior to organ allograft is similar to cross-matching prior to transfusion; O is the universal donor and AB the universal recipient. Minor blood group factors do not appear to act as histocompatibility antigens. Matching of HLA antigens in cadaveric renal transplants may improve graft survival, but the impact is relatively minor. While attempts are made to pair recipient and donor by tissue typing, a two-antigen match is perfectly acceptable and even zero-antigen matches can be transplanted with good results. Neither hypertension nor anemia is a contraindication to transplantation; indeed, hypertension may be cured or ameliorated following successful transplantation. Patients with end-stage renal failure generally are anemic and can be transfused, if necessary, intra- or postoperatively. Anemia generally also improves following transplantation because of increased erythropoietin production by the graft.

195. The answer is c. (*Greenfield, 2/e, pp 578–581.*) Hyperacute rejection is mediated by cytotoxic antibodies with subsequent triggering of the complement, coagulation, and kinin systems. It can occur during surgery after the clamps are released from the vascular anastomosis and the recipient's antibodies are exposed to the donor's passenger lymphocytes and kidney tissue. Typically, the kidney will become swollen and pale. Hyperacute rejection is the cause of immediate and early oliguria and biopsies should be performed intraoperatively or early postoperatively. Hyperacute rejection is characterized pathologically by fibrin and platelet thrombosis and necrosis of the glomerular tufts, renal arterioles, and small arteries. Massive polymorphonuclear infiltrate with tubular necrosis occurs 24–36 h after transplantation. The intravascular coagulation rarely results in a systemic coagulopathy. Careful cross-matching can test for cytotoxic antibodies. Although plasmapheresis and cyclophosphamide can transiently decrease the preformed antibody load, to date there exists no adequate prevention or treatment for hyperacute rejection.

196. The answer is a. (*Greenfield, 2/e, pp 599–606.*) Cardiac transplantation has become an acceptable clinical treatment modality for selected patients with end-stage cardiac failure. Allograft survivals are now comparable to those of cadaveric renal transplants—approximately 70% at 1 year and 50% at 5 years as reported by the Stanford group. Although kidneys can be safely preserved by either hypothermic storage or hypothermic perfusion for periods up to 48 h, donor hearts protected by simple hypothermia should be transplanted within 4 h. For this reason the usual tissue-typing procedures used in kidney transplantation are impractical in cardiac transplantation, and indeed there is no correlation between match and outcome. In pairing donor and recipient for heart transplants there must be at least ABO blood group compatibility. Cyclosporine has improved results in both cardiac and renal transplantation despite its major drawback of dose-related nephrotoxicity. Eligibility for cardiac transplantation has evolved from strict age criteria to more flexible guidelines based on a patient's likelihood of surviving and resuming a normally functional life after transplantation. Many centers, however, observe age 65 as the upper limit for transplantation. The leading cause of death in patients surviving more than 1 year after transplantation is infection, followed by graft atherosclerosis.

197. The answer is d. *(Greenfield, 2/e, pp 578–581.)* The patient is experiencing an acute rejection episode. Seventy-four percent of all acute rejection episodes occur between 1 and 6 mo after transplantation. For cadaveric renal transplant recipients, 63% of patients will never have an acute rejection episode, 17% will have only one rejection episode, and 19% will have two or more rejections. In order to grade the rejection as well as to follow the response to treatment, a percutaneous renal biopsy should be performed. The three treatment modalities used for acute rejection are high-dose steroids alone, high-dose steroids plus antilymphocyte globulin (equine serum hyperimmunized to human lymphocytes), or high-dose steroids plus OKT3 (murine monoclonal antibody to the human CD3 complex).

198. The answer is b. *(Greenfield, 2/e, pp 552–553, 560.)* Overall, 30% of all infections contracted in the posttransplant period are viral. The most common viral infections are DNA viruses of the herpesvirus family and include cytomegalovirus (CMV), Epstein-Barr virus, herpes simplex virus, and varicella zoster virus. CMV infections may occur as either primary or reactive infections and have a peak incidence at about 6 wk post transplant. The classic signs include fever, malaise, myalgia, arthralgia, and leukopenia. CMV infection can affect several organ systems and result in pneumonitis; ulceration and hemorrhage in the stomach, duodenum, or colon; hepatitis; esophagitis; retinitis; encephalitis; or pancreatitis. The risk of developing posttransplant CMV depends on donor-recipient serology, with the greatest risk in seronegative patients who receive organs from seropositive donors. Pyelonephritis, cholecystitis, intraabdominal abscesses, and parotitis are caused by bacterial infections or GI perforation and not primarily by CMV infection.

199. The answer is b. (*Greenfield, 2/e, pp 548–553.*) With the introduction of cyclosporine in the early 1980s and the rapidly accumulated experience with liver transplantation, graft and patient survivals have improved markedly. In the azathioprine and steroid era, 1-year graft survival was in the range of 25%. More recently, most centers are experiencing 1-year graft survival rates of approximately 80%.

200. The answer is d. (*Greenfield, 2/e, p 553.*) Donor-type lymphoid cells transplanted within a graft may recognize the host's tissue as foreign and mount an immune response against the host. This response, termed graft-versus-host disease (GVHD), is common in bone marrow transplantation and is an important source of morbidity and mortality. Treatment requires more aggressive immunosuppression. Current clinical practice includes depletion of lymphocytes from the marrow graft in order to prevent the development of GVHD. GVHD has been documented following liver transplantation, presumably because of the large amount of lymphoid tissue in the donor liver. GVHD has not been described following heart, lung, pancreas, or kidney transplantation.

201. The answer is d. (*Greenfield, 2/e, pp 606–615.*) Many causes of end-stage lung disease have been appropriately treated with lung transplantation. Whether one lung or both lungs are replaced at the time of transplantation depends on recipient factors. Patients with restrictive processes like primary pulmonary fibrosis do well with a single lung transplant. For patients with primary pulmonary hypertension, unloading of the right ventricle with single lung transplantation has been adequate and replacement of both lungs has not been necessary in most cases. Cystic fibrosis patients do well after lung transplantation but double lung transplant is frequently necessary because of chronic infections. Secondary pulmonary hypertension is due to left ventricular failure with concomitant increases in pulmonary pressures secondary to increases in left ventricular end-diastolic pressures. Reactive secondary pulmonary hypertension is best treated with heart transplantation. Long-standing secondary pulmonary hypertension that is chiefly fixed is best treated with combined heart-lung transplantation.

202. The answer is d. (*Greenfield, 2/e, pp 615–627.*) Whole-organ pancreas transplantation is the only therapy for type I insulin-dependent diabetes that maintains normal serum glucose levels and normal glucose tolerance tests. When the pancreas is transplanted along with a kidney, the tight glucose control generally prevents the recurrence of diabetic nephropathy. No series has shown the reversal of diabetic retinopathy or reduction in the rate of diabetic ulcers or of amputations, although some parameters of diabetic retinopathy may improve after pancreas transplantation.

203. The answer is a. *(Sabiston, 15/e, pp 501–502.)* Bone marrow cells are highly immunogenic. Successful engraftment requires the use of powerful immunosuppressants that permit the transplanted cells not only to survive the host's immune response, but also to mount a graft-versus-host response against recipient tissues. The graft-versus-host response is the major impediment to more widespread clinical use of this technique. Despite these barriers, human bone marrow transplantation has had important clinical application in the treatment of aplastic anemias and congenital immunodeficiency diseases and several hematologic malignancies. Stem cell transplantation involves harvesting of a patient's own pleuripotent bone marrow cells and subsequent reestablishment of the marrow following high-dose, toxic chemotherapy for advanced cancer. This modality has been used in the treatment of recurrent breast cancer, but recent meta-analyses of the results have failed to show any significant survival benefit. In experimental models, work with bone marrow transplantation for the induction of tolerance to organ allografts has proved highly promising. This may provide a key for the development of treatment protocols in organ transplant recipients that would avoid or reduce the need for toxic systemic immunosuppressants.

204. The answer is d. *(Schwartz, 7/e, pp 366–368.)* Major histocompatibility complex (MHC) proteins are polymorphic cell surface molecules that are important in lymphocyte-lymphocyte and lymphocyte-target interactions. All nucleated cells express MHC class I proteins. B lymphocytes, macrophages, antigen-presenting cells, vascular endothelium, and activated T lymphocytes express both MHC class I and class II. MHC class I proteins are encoded by the HLA-A, B, and C loci, and MHC class II proteins are encoded by the HLA-D locus. Classically, MHC class I molecules with a bound antigen are recognized by the T-cell receptor on CD81 cells, and MHC class II molecules with a bound antigen are recognized by the T-cell receptor on CD41 cells.

205. The answer is b. *(Schwartz, 7/e, pp 323–324.)* In following patients with nonseminomatous testicular tumors, elevated serum levels of the β subunit of human chorionic gonadotropin (hCG), α-fetoprotein, and lactic dehydrogenase have been found to be useful indicators of tumor activity or recurrence. The discovery of prostate-specific antigen has recently been touted as a major breakthrough in screening for prostate cancer, though some clinicians feel that early diagnosis may have no impact on survival in this disease. CA125 has been used to follow ovarian cancers; it is fairly nonspecific but can alert the physician to the need for a more aggressive search for persistent disease when relative increases are noted in a patient after therapy. The p53 oncogenes have been found in soft tissue sarcomas, osteogenic sarcomas, and colon cancers. Their significance is unknown.

206. The answer is a. *(Schwartz, 7/e, pp 329–331.)* Isolated enlarged cervical lymph nodes in the adult are malignant nearly 80% of the time (excluding benign tumors of the thyroid gland). They are usually metastatic squamous cell carcinomas arising from primary sources above the clavicles in the aerodigestive tract. Fine-needle aspiration cytology is commonly used to obtain histological confirmation of suspected cancer. Aspiration cytology can usually diagnose carcinoma accurately, but lymphoma may be difficult to identify by this method, and open biopsy is often necessary. Bone marrow biopsy is not indicated prior to lymph node biopsy. It is done as part of the staging process after a diagnosis of lymphoma has been made. Endoscopy and scanning of the oro- and nasopharynx are part of the diagnostic workup of a suspected malignant cervical lymph node, but do not provide histological proof of cancer.

207. The answer is d. *(Schwartz, 7/e, pp 277–278, 348.)* Since chemotherapy is generally most effective in killing rapidly dividing cells, the rapidly dividing cells of a fresh surgical wound should be in jeopardy when chemotherapy is given in the early postoperative period. Each of the phases of normal wound healing is theoretically at risk from one or another class of chemotherapeutic agents. Immediately following wounding, inflammation and vascular permeability lead to fibrin deposition and polymorphonuclear neutrophil (PMN), monocyte, and platelet influx. Macrophages are attracted by the activated complement system. By the fourth day the proliferative phase begins, and for the next 20 days fibroblasts produce mucopolysaccharides and collagen. Cross-linking of the collagen fibers then continues for several months in the maturation phase. It seems logical to delay antineoplastic agents for 10–14 days unless there are compelling clinical indications (e.g., superior vena cava syndrome) for more urgent treatment. Administration of folinic acid simultaneously with methotrexate normalizes wound healing. Extravasation of chemotherapeutic agents during intravenous administration may result in severe ulceration and sloughing. The nature of the injury is largely related to the nucleic-acid-binding characteristics of the agent. Those agents that do not bind to tissue nucleic acid (vincristine, vinblastine, nitrogen mustard, BCNU, 5-FU) generally cause only local damage from the immediate injury. These substances are quickly metabolized or inactivated, and usual patterns of wound healing can be expected. On the other hand, agents that bind the nucleic acid (doxorubicin, dactinomycin, mitomycin C, mithramycin, and daunorubicin) cause not only immediate toxic reaction in the tissues but, unless excised, continuing and progressive tissue damage. Though some authors have reported success with elevation and ice packs, most recommend surgical excision if there is severe pain, any sign of early necrosis, or significant blistering.

208. The answer is e. (*Schwartz, 7/e, pp 320–324.*) The management of malignant tumors may be guided by knowledge obtained by grading and staging the tumors. Histologic grading reflects the degree of anaplasia of tumor cells. Tumors in which histologic grading seems to have prognostic value include soft tissue sarcoma, transitional cell cancers of the bladder, astrocytoma, and chondrosarcoma. Grading has been of little predictive value in melanoma, hepatocellular carcinoma, or osteosarcoma. Staging is based on the extent of spread rather than histologic appearance and is more relevant in predicting the course of lung and colorectal cancers.

209. The answer is a. (*Schwartz, 7/e, pp 1747–1748.*) This is a nephroblastoma (Wilms tumor) adherent to the left kidney. These tumors are associated with aniridia (rarely) and with hemihypertrophy, cryptorchidism, or hypospadias in about 10% of cases. Most patients present with an asymptomatic mass found by a parent. Less than one-third of patients experience hematuria. As would be expected in over half such cases, this child is hypertensive, probably due to compression of the renal artery by the mass. Treatment with excision, radiation, vincristine, and actinomycin D results in survival rates of over 90% in stage I and II tumors. While computed tomography (CT) or magnetic resonance imaging (MRI) evaluates metasta-tic disease, intravenous pyelography (IVP) is better at differentiating this tumor from polycystic kidney or neuroblastoma. Wilms tumor is the most common abdominal malignancy of childhood, but represents only about 10% of childhood malignant tumors.

210. The answer is c. *(Schwartz, 7/e, pp 1686–1688.)* Medullary carcino-mas occur in families as part of syndromes called multiple endocrine neo-plasia (MEN) type 2A and type 2B. MEN 2A consists of multicentric medullary thyroid cancer, pheochromocytomas or adrenal medullary hyperplasia, and hyperparathyroidism. MEN 2B consists of medullary can-cer, pheochromocytoma and mucosal neuromas, gangliomas, and a Marfan-like habitus. These patients may develop medullary carcinoma at a very young age, and any patient with MEN 2B should be assumed to have medullary cancer until proved otherwise. Patients are followed carefully for pheochromocytoma with urine VMA, for hyperparathyroidism with serum calcium, and for medullary carcinoma with serum calcitonin. However, as some patients have a normal basal calcitonin, a pentagastrin or provocative calcium infusion test should be performed in these high-risk patients. Patients thought to have MEN 1 syndrome (pituitary, parathyroid, and pancreatic tumors) or Zollinger-Ellison syndrome should be assayed for serum gastrin, insulin, glucagon, and somatostatin. These assays may prove to be inappropriately high in MEN 1 syndrome due to pancreatic islet cell tumors.

211. The answer is c. *(Schwartz, 7/e, pp 334–335.)* Benign soft tissue tumors far outnumber their malignant counterparts. Because of this, pro-longed delays are common before definitive treatment of soft tissue sarco-mas is instituted. Risk for malignancy is increased for tumors greater than 5 cm in largest diameter, as well as for those lesions that are symptomatic or have enlarged rapidly over a short period of time. Properly performed biopsy is critical in the initial treatment of any soft tissue mass. Improperly performed biopsies can complicate the care of the sarcoma patient, and in rare circumstances even eliminate certain surgical options. Excisional biop-sies should be reserved for small masses for which complete excision would not jeopardize subsequent treatment should a sarcoma be found. For all other masses incisional biopsy should be performed. The incision should be placed directly over the mass and should be oriented along the long axis of the extremity.

212. The answer is e. *[Tondini, Ann Oncol 4(10):831–837, 1993. Gobbi, Cancer 65(11):2528–2536, 1990.]* The stomach is the most common site in the gastrointestinal tract for non-Hodgkin's lymphoma, followed by the small intestine and the colon. Lymphomas constitute 3% of all malignant gastric tumors. Ninety percent of these lymphomas are of the non-Hodgkin's type. Surgery alone can be considered adequate treatment for patients with non-Hodgkin's lymphoma that does not infiltrate beyond the submucosa. However, gastric resection is not considered mandatory, and there are no substantial differences in response to therapy and survival when resection is compared with combined chemotherapy and radiation therapy, including in advanced cases. Moreover, chemotherapy and radiation therapy have been shown to be effective even in unresected bulky cases, and provide minimal risk of hemorrhage and perforation even in this setting.

213. The answer is b. *(Schwartz, 7/e, pp 349–350.)* The interferons are a group of glycoproteins first found as products of virus-infected cells that inhibited viral replication. Subsequently, they have been shown to have a variety of effects both on cells of the immune system and on malignant cells. Interferons cause Burkitt's lymphoma cell lines to differentiate and lose the capacity to divide. Hematologic malignancies are very responsive to interferons; up to 100% of hairy cell leukemias show some degree of remission. Interferon α has been used in the treatment of chronic active hepatitis B and C with promising results in recent clinical trials.

214. The answer is d. *(Schwartz, 7/e, pp 656–662.)* Acinar, adenoid cystic, and low grades of mucoepidermoid carcinomas exhibit moderately malignant behavior. Undifferentiated, squamous, and high grades of mucoepidermoid carcinomas are considered highly malignant tumors. Regional node dissection is indicated for malignant tumors because of the high (up to 50%) incidence of occult regional metastases. Facial nerve preservation should be attempted when the margins are adequate and the tumor is well localized. The minimal appropriate procedure for parotid carcinoma is a superficial parotidectomy with nerve preservation. The nerve must be partially or totally sacrificed if the tumor directly involves the nerve trunk or its branches.

215. The answer is b. *(Schwartz, 7/e, pp 347–348.)* A surgeon is frequently asked to evaluate patients who are receiving systemic chemotherapy. Most complications of chemotherapy do not require surgical therapy. Perirectal abscesses are more common in these immunosuppressed patients. Gastrointestinal bleeding occurs secondary to mucosal irritation and thrombocytopenia. Pancreatitis is uncommon, but is associated with L-asparaginase use. Up to 20% of patients treated with floxuridine by continuous hepatic artery infusion develop some degree of inflammation and obstruction of the bile duct. Systemic chemotherapy does not increase the likelihood of acute cholecystitis, appendicitis, incarcerated femoral hernia, or diverticulitis.

216. The answer is e. *(Schwartz, 7/e, pp 1794–1795.)* After radical orchiectomy, lymph node dissection is indicated in embryonal carcinoma, teratocarcinoma, and adult teratoma if there is no supradiaphragmatic spread. This dissection increases the 5-year survival and helps in staging. Seminoma is extremely radiosensitive and lymph node dissection is unnecessary. Choriocarcinoma is associated with pulmonary metastases in 81% of cases and is treated with chemotherapy. Orchiectomy for a testicular mass is approached via an inguinal incision in order to perform a high ligation of the cord and to eliminate spread of the tumor. Cryptorchidism (undescended testicle) is associated with decreased spermatogenesis and carries a lifelong risk of malignant degeneration even after being surgically corrected.

217. The answer is a. *(Greenfield, 2/e, pp 237–238, 571–572.)* Dialysis is less expensive than renal transplantation if the graft functions for less than 2 years. Recipients with functioning grafts are less anemic because of erythropoietin production by the graft. As more dialysis patients are treated with recombinant erythropoietin, this advantage may disappear. Transplanted females have more normal menses and an increased number of successful pregnancies. The patient survival in the two groups is comparable at 1 year.

218–219. The answers are 218-e, 219-e. *(Schwartz, 7/e, pp 1646–1649.)* This young pregnant woman presents with the symptoms of a pheochromocytoma. These tumors can initially become symptomatic during pregnancy. A noninvasive workup should be performed. Ultrasonography of the abdomen is frequently sufficient to localize the tumor to the right or left adrenal; an abdominal CT scan with its large dose of radiation should be avoided in pregnancy. The treatment can be early excision of the pheochromocytoma, and in three cases in pregnant women this was done with survival of two of the three infants. A therapeutic abortion, especially at 18 wk, is not indicated, and cesarian section would not produce a viable fetus. The current approach is α- and β-adrenergic blockade followed by vaginal delivery or cesarean section with excision of the tumor at the same time as delivery or electively after delivery. Metyrosine (Demser) inhibits tyrosine hydroxylase and results in a decrease in endogenous levels of catecholamines. This form of treatment, coupled with term delivery, is also acceptable.

220. The answer is b. *(Greenfield, 2/e, pp 491–495.)* Only about 30% of the biologic damage from x-rays is due to the direct effects on the target molecule. The remainder is due to an indirect action mediated by free radicals and can be modified by free radical scavengers such as sulfhydryl. The percentage of cells killed by a given dose of x-rays or gamma rays is greatly increased by molecular oxygen; cells deficient in oxygen are resistant to radiation. Among the basic principles of radiation biology is the observation that the sensitivity of mammalian cells to radiation varies with their position in the cell division cycle. M phase (mitotic phase) cells are the most radiosensitive. Radiation is frequently employed for local control of disease. Survival rates for breast lumpectomy and radiation are equal to those of mastectomy, but local control rates (10–15% recurrence at 10 years for stage I and II cancers treated with lumpectomy and radiation versus approximately 5% treated with mastectomy) are nevertheless inferior. Rapidly dividing cells of the gastrointestinal mucosa and bone marrow are particularly sensitive to the effects of radiation.

221. The answer is d. *(Schwartz, 7/e, pp 349–351.)* With the availability of recombinant interleukin-2, multiple trials of cancer therapy with this lymphokine have been undertaken. The most successful trials have documented complete or partial responses in patients with metastatic renal cell carcinoma and melanoma. However, IL-2 therapy has been ineffective in the treatment of breast cancer, colon cancer, and lymphoma. The therapy is not innocuous. All patients exhibit a marked lymphocytosis, eosinophilia, fluid retention, fever, and decrease in peripheral vascular resistance, effects similar to those of septic shock.

222. The answer is c. *(Heys, Br J Surg 79:614–623, 1992.)* Malignant tumors require energy substrates to grow and ordinarily claim these substrates from the host. In animal studies, withholding dietary proteins diminishes the rate of tumor growth. There is no evidence in the human to suggest acceleration of tumor growth when nutritional support is provided. There is also no evidence that nutritional therapy improves the response of the tumor to therapy. For nearly a century, the association of stomach cancer and diet has been recognized. Among the wide variety of substances incriminated are nitrates and nitrosamides in food and drinking water. There is evidence that regular ingestion of vitamin C from childhood may reduce the formation of carcinogens, though reduction in the incidence of cancer has not been demonstrated. Excess amounts of dietary fat and deficiency of fiber have been clearly associated with colon cancer. Animal fats have also been associated with cancer of the exocrine pancreas, the prostate, and the endometrium. Alcohol consumption, especially when combined with cigarette smoking, increases the incidence of esophageal cancer. Consumption of alcohol also increases the incidence of pancreatitis, but not pancreatic cancer.

223. The answer is d. *(Greenfield, 2/e, pp 599–606.)* Cardiac allograft has become an accepted treatment for end-stage heart disease. One-year cardiac allograft survival approaches 90% and is equivalent to 1-year renal allograft survival. Cardiac allografts have a cold ischemia preservation time of 4–5 h and therefore tissue typing is not practical. Cardiac donors are matched to recipients only by size and ABO blood type. Tissue typing remains an important component of cadaveric kidney allograft matching. The mainstay of immunosuppression for both cardiac and renal allografts continues to include cyclosporine, azathioprine (Imuran), and steroids.

224. The answer is b. *(Schwartz, 7/e, pp 340–341, 352–353.)* Resection of metastases of lung, liver, and brain can result in occasional 5-year cures. In general, surgery should be undertaken only when the primary tumor is controlled, diffuse metastatic disease has been ruled out, and the affected patient's condition and the location of the metastasis permit safe resection. Five-year survival rates as high as 18% have been reported for selected patients with liver metastases from colorectal primary tumors. However, the best results have come from resection of pulmonary metastases, in which 5-year survival rates exceed those of resection for primary bronchogenic carcinoma. Autopsy reviews have demonstrated that many patients with pulmonary metastases have no other evidence of tumor, which suggests that resectional treatment may be justified even when the lung foci are not solitary. Selection of patients for pulmonary resections may be aided by measurement of tumor doubling times; patients with doubling times greater than 40 days appear to benefit most, while those with doubling times less than 20 days are not significantly helped.

225. The answer is c. *(Rhame, Postgrad Med 91:141–152, 1992. Wilson, Postgrad Med 88:193–201, 1990.)* The risk of contracting HIV is much less than the risk of contracting hepatitis B from a patient. Although the risk of transmission of HIV in the health care setting is very low, there are reported cases of seroconversion after parenteral exposure. Particular precautions should be taken in operating upon patients who are known to be seropositive for HIV or who have known risk factors. Recommendations include elimination of inexperienced personnel or personnel with open lesions on body surfaces from the operating room. Disposable gowns, drapes, masks, and eye shields should be used. Contaminated clothing should be soaked in a dilute solution (1:10) of chlorine bleach prior to washing. Double gloving does not reduce the major intraoperative risk of needle puncture, which is the primary source of risk to the operating team. Needles should never be capped; an uncapped needle is less dangerous than are the maneuvers to recap needles.

226. The answer is c. *(Harris et al, pp 159–167.)* Risk factors for breast cancer include family history, nulliparity, previous breast cancer, early menarche, and late menopause. A late age at first birth (after age 30) doubles the risk of breast cancer compared with early parity (age 18 or earlier). Having one first-degree relative (mother, sister, or daughter) with breast cancer also doubles the risk. Women of the upper social classes, as measured by either education or income, have been found to have the highest incidence of breast cancer. Neither cigarette smoking nor the use of hair dye has been correlated with breast cancer.

227. The answer is c. *(Recommendations for prevention of HIV transmission in health care settings. NY State J Med 88:25–31, 1988. Rhame, Postgrad*

Med 91:141–144, 1992.) HIV has been isolated from blood, semen, vaginal secretions, saliva, tears, breast milk, CSF, amniotic fluid, and urine. It is an extremely fastidious virus that ordinarily is transmitted only after repeated admixture of body fluids. Blood and semen are by far the major transmission fluids.

228. The answer is a. (*Greenfield, 2/e, p 502.*) Doxorubicin, an antibiotic derived from *Streptomyces* species, has activity against sarcomas and carcinomas of the breast, liver, bladder, prostate, head and neck, esophagus, and lung. Its major side effect is production of a dilated cardiomyopathy. Patients receiving this agent should have echocardiography before and after treatment in order to monitor potential cardiac toxicity.

229. The answer is e. (*Greenfield, 2/e, pp 455–459.*) Cancer remains the second most common cause of mortality in the United States after heart disease, accounting for 22% of all deaths. Both sexes have demonstrated dramatic increases in the death rate observed from lung cancer from 1930 to 1990 owing to increases in cigarette smoking. Lung cancer is the leading cause of cancer death in both men and women.

230. The answer is e. (*Greenfield, 2/e, p 501.*) Cyclophosphamide is an alkylating agent used in the treatment of a variety of solid tumors. Its major side effect is hemorrhagic cystitis. Bleomycin can cause pulmonary fibrosis. Vincristine is an alkaloid that can cause peripheral and central neuropathies. Cisplatin is an alkylating agent that can lead to ototoxity, neurotoxicity, and nephrotoxicity. 5-fluorouracil is an antimetabolite that can cause mucositis, dermatitis, and cerebellar dysfunction.

231. The answer is c. (*Greenfield, 2/e, p 555.*) The major barrier to successful xenotransplantation has been hyperacute rejection, which refers to the binding of preformed human antibodies to donor endothelial cells. This results in the activation of complement, cell lysis, and eventually vascular thrombosis.

232. The answer is c. (*Greenfield, 2/e, p 537.*) Processing and presentation of antigen in association with class II molecules is critical for activation of T cells. Langerhans cells are potent antigen-presenting cells (APCs) found in skin. Macrophages are the major APCs in the body. Dendritic cells are APCs found in lymphoid tissue.

233. The answer is e. (*Greenfield, 2/e, pp 1138, 1144.*) CEA is a glycoprotein that is present in early embryonic and fetal cells (an oncofetal antigen) and in colon cancer. It is not found in normal colon mucosa. It is not tumor specific and may be elevated in a variety of benign and malignant conditions, including cirrhosis, ulcerative colitis, renal failure, pancreatitis, pancreatic cancer, stomach cancer, breast cancer, and lung cancer. The CEA assay is, however, a sensitive serologic tool for identifying recurrent disease. In about two-thirds of patients with recurrent disease, an increased CEA level is the first indicator of tumor reappearance. A rising CEA following colon cancer surgery, in the absence of other conditions associated with an elevated CEA, predicts the appearance of liver metastases within 1 year with an accuracy approaching 70%.

234–236. The answers are 234-a, 235-g, 236-e. (*Greenfield, 2/e, pp 1137–1144.*) The patient has a left colon cancer. In order to resect the tumor with a margin of 3–5 cm on its proximal and distal ends as well as to remove the draining lymph node basin, a left hemicolectomy should be performed. A Dukes C tumor is one that extends through the bowel wall and involves adjacent lymph nodes. In a study of 1166 patients with stage B and C colon cancer, the National Surgical Adjuvant Breast and Bowel Project (NSABP) reported an improved survival in patients randomized to receive adjuvant chemotherapy compared with no further treatment after resection. Adjuvant radiation therapy has only been useful in preventing local recurrence in rectal cancers with positive surgical margins.

The liver is the most common site of bloodborne metastases from primary colorectal cancers. In a subgroup of patients, the liver may be the only site of disease. Overall, surgical resection is associated with a 25–30% 5-year survival rate.

237–240. The answers are 237-f, 238-a, 239-d, 240-b. (*Greenfield, 2/e, pp 577–581.*) Routine postoperative immunosuppression for a renal transplant recipient includes cyclosporine, azathioprine, and steroids. Cyclosporine is nephrotoxic and is frequently withheld in the postoperative period until the creatinine returns to normal following transplantation.

Azathioprine has bone marrow toxicity as its major side effect and both WBC and platelet counts need to be monitored in the immediate post-transplant period. The patient's decrease in WBCs is secondary to azathioprine toxicity, and the most appropriate step is to decrease the dose of azathioprine.

Viral infections are a serious cause of morbidity following transplantation. A "buffy coat" is the supernatant of a centrifuged blood sample that contains the WBCs. Viral cultures from this supernatant as well as localization of inclusion bodies can identify transplant patients infected with cytomegalovirus (CMV). This patient has CMV pneumonitis and needs to be treated with high-dose gancyclovir.

An elevation in creatinine at 3-mo follow-up can be secondary to rejection, anastomotic problems, urologic complications, infection, or nephrotoxicity of various medications. With a normal ultrasound, no fever, and no graft tenderness, the most likely cause is cyclosporine-induced nephrotoxicity and the most appropriate step is a reduction in the cyclosporine dose.

Finally, at 6 mo with graft tenderness, fever, and an edematous kidney on ultrasound, rejection must be suspected. Negative cultures make infection unlikely, and a steroid boost is appropriate. Addition of monoclonal antibodies to CD3 (OKT3) or pooled antibodies against lymphocytes (ALG) is also appropriate in the treatment of a first rejection.

ENDOCRINE PROBLEMS AND BREAST

Questions

DIRECTIONS: Each item below contains a question or incomplete statement followed by suggested responses. Select the **one best** response to each question.

241. Which of the following statements regarding adrenal cortical insufficiency is true?

a. Treatment with exogenous steroids is usually ineffective

b. It is commonly seen as a consequence of metastasis of distant cancers, such as lung or breast, to the adrenal glands

c. Chronic adrenal insufficiency (Addison's disease) in the preoperative patient should be recognizable by a constellation of findings, including hyperglycemia, hypernatremia, and hypokalemia

d. Death from untreated chronic adrenal insufficiency may occur within hours of surgery

e. The most common underlying cause today is infection with resistant tuberculosis

242. The thyroid scan shown below exhibits a pattern that is most consistent with which of the following disorders?

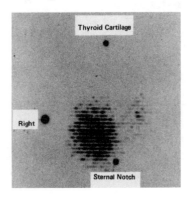

a. Hypersecreting adenoma
b. Graves' disease
c. Lateral aberrant thyroid
d. Papillary carcinoma of thyroid
e. Medullary carcinoma of thyroid

243. A 17-year-old girl presents with an anterior neck mass. Her thyroid scan, shown below, is most consistent with which of the following disorders?

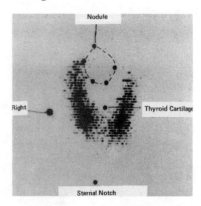

a. Hypersecreting adenoma
b. Parathyroid adenoma
c. Thyroglossal duct cyst
d. Graves' disease
e. Carcinoma

244. A 35-year-old woman undergoes her first screening mammogram. Which of the following mammographic findings would require a breast biopsy?

a. Breast calcifications larger than 2 mm in diameter
b. Five or more clustered breast microcalcifications per square centimeter
c. A density that effaces with compression
d. Saucer-shaped microcalcifications
e. Multiple round well-circumscribed breast densities

245. Estrogen receptor activity is clinically useful in predicting

a. The presence of ovarian cancer
b. The presence of metastatic disease
c. Response to chemotherapy
d. Response to hormonal manipulation
e. The likelihood of development of osteoporosis

246. When galactorrhea occurs in a high school student, a diagnostic associated finding would be

a. Gonadal atrophy
b. Bitemporal hemianopia
c. Exophthalmos and lid lag
d. Episodic hypertension
e. "Buffalo hump"

247. The diagnosis of primary hyperparathyroidism is most strongly suggested by

a. Serum acid phosphatase above 120 IU/L
b. Serum alkaline phosphatase above 120 IU/L
c. Serum calcium above 11 mg/dL
d. Urinary calcium below 100 mg/day
e. Parathyroid hormone levels below 5 pmol/L

248. Somatostatin contributes to which of the following processes?

a. Inhibition of adrenocortical cells
b. Inhibition of pancreatic α cells
c. Stimulation of antral gastrin cells
d. Stimulation of secretin-producing cells in the duodenum
e. Stimulation of GI motility

249. Which of the following statements concerning Cushing syndrome secondary to adrenal adenoma is true?

a. Adrenal adenomas cause 40–60% of all cases of Cushing syndrome
b. Biochemical and x-ray procedures are generally unsuccessful in lateralizing the tumors preoperatively
c. Exploration of both adrenal glands is indicated
d. For uncomplicated tumors, an open transperitoneal surgical approach is usually employed
e. Postoperative corticoid therapy is required to prevent hypoadrenalism

250. A 40-year-old woman is found to have a 1- to 2-cm, slightly tender cystic mass in her breast; she has no perceptible axillary adenopathy. What course would you follow?

a. Reassurance and reexamination in the immediate postmenstrual period
b. Immediate excisional biopsy
c. Aspiration of the mass with cytologic analysis
d. Fluoroscopically guided needle localization biopsy
e. Mammography and reevaluation of options with new information

251. Which statement concerning radiation-induced thyroid cancer is true?

a. It usually follows high-dose radiation to the head and neck
b. A patient with a history of radiation is safe if no cancer has been found 20 years after exposure
c. Approximately 25% of patients with a history of head and neck irradiation develop thyroid cancer
d. Most radiation-induced thyroid cancers are follicular
e. The treatment of choice is a near-total (or total) thyroidectomy

252. The course of papillary carcinoma of the thyroid is best described by which of the following statements?

a. Metastases are rare; local growth is rapid; erosion into the trachea and large blood vessels is frequent
b. Local invasion and metastases almost never occur, which makes the term *carcinoma* misleading
c. Bony metastases are frequent and produce an osteolytic pattern particularly in vertebrae
d. Metastases frequently occur to cervical lymph nodes; distant metastases and local invasion are rare
e. Rapid, widespread metastatic involvement of the liver, lungs, and bone marrow results in a 5-year survival rate of approximately 10%

253. Fibrocystic disease of the breast has been associated with elevated blood levels of

a. Testosterone
b. Progesterone
c. Estrogen
d. Luteinizing hormone
e. Aldosterone

254. A 14-year-old black girl had her right breast removed because of a large mass. The tumor weighed 1400 g and was found to have a bulging, very firm, lobulated surface with a whorl-like pattern, as illustrated below. This neoplasm is most likely

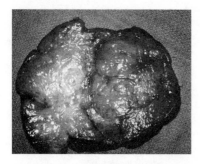

a. Cystosarcoma phylloides
b. Intraductal carcinoma
c. Malignant lymphoma
d. Fibroadenoma
e. Juvenile hypertrophy

255. As an incidental finding during an upper abdominal CT scan, a 3-cm mass in the adrenal gland is noted. The appropriate next step in analysis and management of this finding would be

a. Observation
b. CT-guided needle biopsy
c. Excision of the mass
d. Measurement of urine catecholamine excretion
e. Cortisol provocation test

Items 256–257

A 53-year-old woman presents with complaints of weakness, anorexia, malaise, constipation, and back pain. While being evaluated, she becomes somewhat lethargic. Laboratory studies include a normal chest x-ray; serum albumin 3.2 mg/dL; serum calcium 14 mg/dL; serum phosphorus 2.6 mg/dL; serum chloride 108 mg/dL; BUN 32 mg/dL; and creatinine 2.0 mg/dL.

256. Appropriate initial management would include

a. Intravenous normal saline infusion
b. Administration of thiazide diuretics
c. Administration of intravenous phosphorus
d. Use of mithramycin
e. Neck exploration and parathyroidectomy

257. After appropriate immediate management, the patient's symptoms resolve. Diagnostic tests to perform at this point would include which of the following?

a. Abdominal angiogram
b. Measurement of serum gastrin hormone levels
c. Kveim test
d. Serum and urine protein electrophoresis
e. Neck exploration

258. A woman sustains an injury to her chest after striking the steering wheel of her automobile during a collision. Which of the following statements concerning fat necrosis of the breast is true?

a. Most patients report a history of trauma
b. The lesion is usually nontender and diffuse
c. It predisposes patients to the development of breast cancer
d. It is difficult to distinguish from breast cancer
e. Excision exacerbates the process

Items 259–260

259. The most likely diagnosis in a patient with hypertension, hypokalemia, and a 7-cm suprarenal mass is

a. Hypernephroma
b. Cushing's disease
c. Adrenocortical carcinoma
d. Pheochromocytoma
e. Carcinoid

260. Appropriate treatment of this condition would include which of the following?

a. Embolization of the arterial blood supply, including the suprarenal artery
b. Metronidazole
c. Mitotane
d. Phentolamine
e. Phenoxybenzamine

261. For pregnant women who are found to have breast cancer

a. Termination of a first-trimester pregnancy is mandatory
b. Carcinoma of the breast behaves more aggressively in pregnant women owing to hormonal stimulation
c. Breast conservation is inappropriate for third-trimester pregnancies
d. Most have hormonally sensitive tumors
e. Administration of adjuvant chemotherapy is safe for the fetus during the second and third trimesters

262. True statements regarding Paget's disease of the breast include that it

a. Usually precedes development of Paget's disease of bone
b. Presents with nipple-areolar eczematous changes
c. Does not involve axillary lymph nodes because it is a manifestation of intraductal carcinoma only
d. Accounts for 10–15% of all newly diagnosed breast cancers
e. Is adequately treated with wide excision when it presents as a mass

263. A 40-year-old man who has a long history of peptic ulcer disease that has not responded to medical therapy is admitted to the hospital. His serum gastrin levels are markedly elevated; at celiotomy, a small, firm mass is palpated in the tail of the pancreas. Correct statements concerning this patient's condition include which of the following?

a. Histamine or a protein meal will markedly increase basal acid secretion
b. Secretin administration will suppress acid secretion
c. The pancreatic mass will probably be benign
d. Distal pancreatectomy is the treatment of choice
e. H_2 receptor antagonists have not been beneficial in the treatment of this condition

264. Of the common complications of thyroidectomy, the one that may be avoided through prophylaxis is

a. Injury to the recurrent laryngeal nerve
b. Injury to the superior laryngeal nerve
c. Symptomatic hypocalcemia
d. Thyroid storm
e. Postoperative hemorrhage and wound hematoma

Items 265–266

265. Following correction of the patient's hypercalcemia with hydration and gentle diuresis with furosemide, the most likely therapeutic approach would be

a. Administration of maintenance doses of steroids
b. Radiation treatment for bony metastases
c. Neck exploration and resection of three out of four parathyroid glands
d. Neck exploration and resection of a parathyroid adenoma
e. Avoidance of sunlight, vitamin D, and calcium-containing dairy products

266. This 30-year-old woman presented with weakness, bone pain, an elevated parathormone level, and a serum calcium level of 15.2 mg/dL. Skeletal survey films were taken, including the hand films and chest x-ray shown. The most likely cause of these findings is

a. Sarcoidosis
b. Vitamin D intoxication
c. Paget's disease
d. Metastatic carcinoma
e. Primary hyperparathyroidism

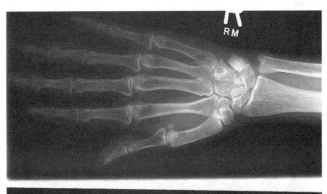

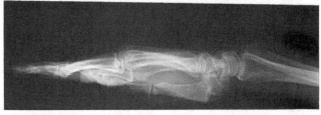

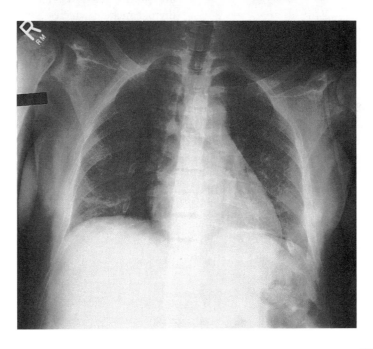

267. A 25-year-old woman is found to have an anterior neck mass. Her thyroid scan, shown below, exhibits findings that are consistent with which of the following disorders?

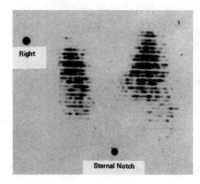

a. Carcinoma
b. Toxic adenoma
c. Toxic multinodular goiter
d. Graves' disease
e. de Quervain's (subacute) thyroiditis

268. Incisional biopsy of a breast mass in a 35-year-old woman demonstrates a hypercellular fibroadenoma (cystosarcoma phylloides) at the time of frozen section. Appropriate management of this lesion could include

a. Wide local excision with a rim of normal tissue
b. Lumpectomy and axillary lymphadenectomy
c. Modified radical mastectomy
d. Excision and postoperative radiotherapy
e. Excision, postoperative radiotherapy, and systemic chemotherapy

269. A 36-year-old woman, 20 wk pregnant, presents with a 1.5-cm right thyroid mass. Fine-needle aspiration is consistent with a papillary neoplasm. The mass is "cold" by scan and solid by ultrasound. Which method of treatment would be contraindicated?

a. Right thyroid lobectomy
b. Subtotal thyroidectomy
c. Total thyroidectomy
d. Total thyroidectomy with lymph node dissection
e. ^{131}I radioactive ablation of the thyroid gland

270. Correct statements concerning Hürthle-cell carcinoma of the thyroid include which of the following?

a. It is a form of anaplastic thyroid cancer
b. It metastasizes via the lymphatics to regional lymph node basins
c. Treatment consists of a near-total (or total) thyroidectomy
d. Microscopically, it consists of clusters of cells separated by areas of collagen and amyloid
e. Once treated appropriately, it has a low rate of recurrence

271. A 28-year-old man presents with a 2.5-cm mass in the anterior triangle of the left neck. The mass moves with swallowing and has slowly enlarged over the past 1–2 years. The patient's past medical history is notable for high-dose irradiation to the chest and abdomen for Hodgkin's lymphoma 8 years prior to presentation. Thyroid scan shows a "cold" lesion. Fine-needle aspiration cytology is "suspicious." Core-needle biopsy shows features suggestive of a follicular neoplasm. True statements regarding this patient's condition include

a. Thyroid nodules in men are rarely malignant

b. Prior radiation to the chest, if anything, would diminish the risk of subsequent thyroid cancer

c. In the setting of abnormal cytology, an initial course of TSH suppression by thyroid hormone is recommended

d. In the setting of a possible follicular neoplasm, radioactive iodine (^{131}I) ablation is recommended

e. Total thyroidectomy is an acceptable treatment for this patient

272. True statements about discharge from the nipple include

a. Intermittent thin or milky discharge can be physiologic

b. Expressible nipple discharge is an indication for open biopsy

c. Bloody discharge is indicative of an underlying malignancy

d. Galactorrhea is indicative of an underlying malignancy

e. Pathologic discharge is usually bilateral

273. True statements regarding Cushing's disease and Cushing syndrome include which of the following?

a. Adrenocortical hyperplasia is the most common cause of Cushing's disease

b. Overproduction of ACTH is pathognomonic of Cushing syndrome

c. Clinical manifestations of Cushing's disease and Cushing syndrome are identical

d. Cushing syndrome is caused only by neoplasms of either the pituitary or adrenal glands

e. Cushing's disease is incurable

274. A 34-year-old woman has recurrent fainting spells induced by fasting. Her serum insulin levels during these episodes are markedly elevated. Correct statements regarding this patient's condition include which of the following?

a. The underlying lesion is probably an α-cell tumor of the pancreas
b. The underlying lesion is usually multifocal
c. These lesions are usually malignant
d. Serum calcium levels may be elevated
e. She should be screened for a coexistent pheochromocytoma

275. The incidence of breast cancer

a. Increases with increasing age
b. Has declined since the 1940s
c. Is related to dietary fat intake
d. Is related to coffee intake
e. Is related to vitamin C intake

DIRECTIONS: Each group of questions below consists of lettered options followed by numbered items. For each numbered item, select the appropriate lettered option(s). Each lettered option may be used once, more than once, or not at all. **Choose exactly the number of options indicated following each item.**

Items 276–280

For each clinical description select the appropriate stage of breast cancer.

a. Stage I
b. Stage II
c. Stage III
d. Stage IV
e. Inflammatory carcinoma

276. Tumor not palpable, clinically positive lymph nodes fixed to one another, no evidence of metastases **(SELECT 1 STAGE)**

277. Tumor 5.0 cm; clinically positive, movable ipsilateral lymph nodes; no evidence of metastases **(SELECT 1 STAGE)**

278. Tumor 2.1 cm, clinically negative lymph nodes, no evidence of metastases **(SELECT 1 STAGE)**

279. Tumor not palpable but breast diffusely enlarged and erythematous, clinically positive supraclavicular nodes, and evidence of metastases **(SELECT 1 STAGE)**

280. Tumor 0.5 cm, clinically negative lymph nodes, pathological rib fracture **(SELECT 1 STAGE)**

Items 281–285

A 43-year-old man presents with signs and symptoms of peritonitis in the right lower quadrant. The clinical impression and supportive data suggest acute appendicitis. At exploration, however, a tumor is found; frozen section suggests carcinoid features. For each tumor described, choose the most appropriate surgical procedure.

a. Appendectomy
b. Segmental ileal resection
c. Cecectomy
d. Right hemicolectomy
e. Hepatic wedge resection and appropriate bowel resection

281. A 2.5-cm tumor at the base of the appendix **(SELECT 1 PROCEDURE)**

282. A 1.0-cm tumor at the tip of the appendix **(SELECT 1 PROCEDURE)**

283. A 0.5-cm tumor with serosal umbilication in the ileum (SE-LECT 1 PROCEDURE)

284. A 1.0-cm tumor of the midappendix; 1-cm firm, pale lesion at the periphery of the right lobe of the liver (SELECT 1 PRO-CEDURE)

285. A 3.5-cm tumor encroaching onto the cecum and extensive liver metastases (SELECT 1 PROCE-DURE)

Items 286–290

For each clinical problem out-lined, select acceptable treatment options.

a. No further surgical intervention
b. Wide local excision
c. Wide local excision with adjuvant radiation therapy
d. Wide local excision with axillary lymph node dissection and radia-tion therapy
e. Simple mastectomy (without axil-lary lymph node dissection)
f. Modified radical mastectomy (sim-ple mastectomy with in-continuity axillary lymph node dissection)
g. Radical mastectomy
h. Bilateral prophylactic simple mas-tectomies

286. A 49-year-old woman under-goes biopsy of a 1.0-cm breast mass. Pathology shows extensive comedo ductal carcinoma in situ. (SELECT 2 CHOICES)

287. A 42-year-old woman with a familial breast cancer (mother, four sisters, and additional relatives) undergoes her fifth breast biopsy for a palpable mass. Pathology shows ductal hyperplasia with severe atypia. (SELECT 2 CHOICES)

288. A 51-year-old (pre-menopausal) woman undergoes needle localization biopsy for microcalcifications. Pathology reveals sclerosing adenosis with microcalcifications and extensive lobular carcinoma in situ. (SELECT 1 CHOICE)

289. A 35-year-old woman pre-sents with a palpable 1.5-cm tumor in the upper outer quadrant of her left breast. Biopsy reveals invasive ductal carcinoma with 10% intra-ductal carcinoma. (SELECT 2 CHOICES)

290. A neglected 82-year-old woman presents with a locally advanced breast cancer that is invading the pectoralis major mus-cle over a broad base. She is other-wise in good health. (SELECT 1 CHOICE)

ENDOCRINE PROBLEMS AND BREAST

Answers

241. The answer is d. (*Greenfield, 2/e, pp 204–205.*) Failure to recognize adrenal cortical insufficiency, particularly in the postoperative patient, may be a fatal error. This error is especially regrettable because therapy (exogenous steroids) is effective and easy to administer. Adrenal insufficiency may occur in a host of settings including tuberculosis (formerly the most common cause), autoimmune states, severe infections (classically, meningococcal septicemia), pituitary insufficiency, after burns, during anticoagulant therapy, and—most commonly today—after interruption of chronically administered exogenous steroids. Although the adrenal gland is an occasional site for distant metastases, such as from lung or breast, it is rare for there to be enough destruction of the glands to produce clinical adrenal insufficiency. Chronic adrenal insufficiency (classic Addison's disease) should be recognizable preoperatively by the constellation of skin pigmentation, weakness, weight loss, hypotension, nausea, vomiting, abdominal pain, hypoglycemia, hyponatremia, and hyperkalemia. Death may occur within hours of surgery if a patient with Addison's disease is operated on without cognizance of adrenal insufficiency and pretreatment with exogenous steroids. Patients who have adrenal insufficiency as a result of interruption of chronically administered exogenous steroids may not develop the classic electrolyte abnormalities until the preterminal period. Adrenal insufficiency may also develop insidiously in the postoperative period, progressing over a course of several days. This insidious course is seen when adrenal injury occurs in the perioperative period, as would be the case with adrenal damage from hemorrhage into the gland in a patient receiving postoperative anticoagulant therapy. Measurement of blood corticosteroid levels, urinary corticosteroid secretion, urinary sodium levels, and the response to exogenous steroids is helpful in establishing the diagnosis of adrenal insufficiency.

242. The answer is a. (*Schwartz, 7/e, pp 1672, 1680.*) The thyroid scan illustrated in the question shows a single focus of increased isotope uptake, often referred to as a "hot" nodule; the remainder of the thyroid gland has not taken up radioactive iodine. Hyperfunctioning adenomas become independent of thyroid stimulating hormone (TSH) control and secrete thyroid hormone autonomously, which results in clinical hyperthyroidism. The elevated thyroid hormone levels ultimately diminish TSH levels severely and thus depress function of the remaining normal thyroid gland. An isolated focus of increased uptake on a thyroid scan is virtually diagnostic of a hyperfunctioning adenoma. Carcinomas usually display diminished uptake and are called "cold" nodules. Graves' disease would probably manifest as a diffusely hyperactive gland without nodularity. Multinodular goiter would display many nodules with varying activity.

243. The answer is c. (Schwartz, 7/e, pp 601–602, 1717.) The thyroid gland originates embryologically from the foramen cecum at the base of the tongue. Normally, the thyroglossal duct becomes obliterated and resorbed, but portions may remain patent and become filled with serous fluid, which produces a midline cervical mass. Observe that in the scan of the patient described in the question, the mass is central and appears not to be part of the gland itself.

244. The answer is b. (Schwartz, 7/e, pp 543–546.) Breast biopsies have traditionally been performed to obtain histology for clinically suspicious palpable masses. In more recent years the advent of screening mammography has led to the discovery of nonpalpable but radiographically suspicious breast lesions that have a strong correlation with breast cancer. These nonpalpable, mammographically detected lesions are (1) breast calcifications that are (a) smaller than 2 mm, (b) punctate, microlinear, or branching, and (c) clustered along ducts or concentrated in clusters greater than five calcifications per square centimeter; (2) stellate-shaped lesions; (3) masses with ill-defined borders or nodular contours; (4) solitary dominant masses that are significantly larger than any other mass in either breast; and (5) areas of increased noneffacing tissue density or distorted breast architecture. A parenchymal density that effaces with compression represents normal glandular tissue. Saucer-shaped microcalcifications are seen in patients with microscopic cystic disease, a benign condition. Multiple round well-circumscribed densities are usually cysts, whose nature may be confirmed with breast sonography.

245. The answer is d. *(Schwartz, 7/e, pp 586–588.)* The likelihood of response of a breast cancer to hormonal therapy is dependent on the presence of hormone receptors in the cytoplasm of the breast cancer cells. Receptors for corticosteroids, progesterone, prolactin, and estrogen have been identified. Eighty percent of patients with tumors that exhibit receptors to both estrogen and progesterone respond favorably to hormonal manipulation. Estrogen receptor activity has no predictive value in diagnosing ovarian cancer or metastatic disease, forecasting the development of osteoporosis, or determining the likelihood of a beneficial response to chemotherapy.

246. The answer is b. *(Schwartz, 7/e, pp 1620–1628.)* Prolactin-secreting tumors in the pituitary gland (previously called *chromophobe adenomas*) may grow to large size and cause bitemporal hemianopia because of proximity to the optic chiasm. They are typically associated with amenorrhea and galactorrhea (the "A/G syndrome") in women. In both sexes lack of libido and impotence or infertility may be noted. Sexual vigor is usually restored after removal of the adenomas. These tumors are not life threatening; if their physical size is not an issue or the relative sexual dysfunction is not a problem, benign neglect is sometimes recommended.

247. The answer is c. *(Norton, Ann Surg 215:297–299, 1992. Potts, Ann Intern Med 114:593–597, 1991.)* Primary hyperparathyroidism is a common disease, with over 100,000 new cases diagnosed each year in the United States, usually in women. Essential to the diagnosis of hyperparathyroidism is the finding of hypercalcemia. Though there are many causes of hypercalcemia, hyperparathyroidism is by far the most prevalent. With rare exceptions, operations for primary hyperparathyroidism should not be performed unless the patient is hypercalcemic. Parathyroid hormone (PTH) is not invariably elevated, but it should be elevated relative to the serum calcium level. Ordinarily, high serum calcium levels suppress parathyroid secretion. Therefore, in the presence of hypercalcemia, normal levels of PTH are "abnormal." Patients with primary hyperparathyroidism have either normal or elevated urinary calcium. As the name suggests, patients with familial hypocalciuric hypercalcemia (FHH) have hypercalcemia. They also usually have elevated PTH, but surgery is not indicated in this relatively rare setting of hypercalcemia.

248. The answer is b. (*Greenfield, 2/e, pp 751–752, 869–870.*) Somatostatin is produced by D cells in the pancreatic islets and in a variety of other tissue sites in the central nervous system, gut, and elsewhere. It is a potent inhibitory regulator of intestinal hormones and motility. Because it was originally found in the hypothalamus, somatostatin earned its name because it was believed to be a major inhibitor of secretion of growth hormone. It has now been shown to inhibit the secretion of most GI hormones, particularly insulin and glucagon, as well as gastrin, secretin, VIP, PP, gastric acid, pepsin, pancreatic enzymes, thyroid-stimulating hormone, renin, and calcitonin. It also inhibits intestinal, biliary, and gastric motility, and is occasionally of value in controlling bowel fistulas by sharply reducing the amount of drainage. It has no known effect on adrenocortical cells.

249. The answer is e. (*Greenfield, 2/e, pp 1344–1345.*) Primary adrenal pathology causes 10–20% of all cases of Cushing syndrome. A hyperfunctioning adrenal adenoma can usually be lateralized by preoperative radiologic studies, eliminating the need to explore both adrenal glands. In 10–15% of cases, adenomas are bilateral. The favored surgical approach today is via transabdominal laparoscopy or by a posterior unilateral flank route. The anterior transperitoneal approach should be reserved for complicated cases such as large or obviously malignant lesions. After tumor excision, corticosteroid therapy to correct postoperative hypoadrenalism is necessary.

250. The answer is c. (*Greenfield, 2/e, p 1373.*) Most clinicians would recommend aspiration and cytologic examination of the cyst fluid in this situation. Cysts are common lesions in the breasts of women in their thirties and forties; malignancies are relatively rare. All such lesions justify attention, however, and physicians must not underestimate the fear associated with the discovery of a mass in the breast, even in low-risk situations. If the lesion does not completely disappear after aspiration, excision is advised. In young women the breast parenchyma is dense, which limits the diagnostic value of mammography. The American Cancer Society (ACS) does not suggest a baseline mammographic examination until age 35 unless a suspicious lesion exists.

251. The answer is e. (*Greenfield, 2/e, pp 1301–1303.*) Radiation-induced thyroid cancer was first recognized in 1950 by Duffy and Fitzgerald. It usually follows low-dose external radiation. Most cancers occur after exposure to 1500 rads or less to the neck, but an increase in thyroid cancer has been noted after as little as 6 rads. Salivary gland tumors and possibly parathyroid adenomas are also associated with radiation. The latent period for these tumors is 30 years or longer. Of all patients who have low-dose radiation, about 9% have been found to have thyroid cancer, usually of the papillary type. Treatment consists of a near-total thyroidectomy because there is a high incidence of bilaterality and because there is a greater incidence of complications if a second operation is necessary.

252. The answer is d. *(Greenfield, 2/e, pp 1301–1303.)* Papillary carcinoma of the thyroid frequently metastasizes to cervical lymph nodes, but distant metastasis is uncommon. The nonaggressive nature of this tumor locally and the infrequency of distant metastases combine to produce an 80–95% 5-year survival rate. A contributing factor to the success of thyroid surgery for papillary carcinoma is the easy accessibility of cervical nodes for examination and dissection. Slow growth and a predilection for local extension are characteristics of this tumor that contribute to a high survival rate in affected persons. This is true even of patients who have limited surgery, which has led to considerable controversy regarding the extent of the indicated surgical procedure.

253. The answer is c. *(Greenfield, 2/e, pp 1372–1374.)* Fibrocystic disease (chronic cystic mastitis) is a common disorder of the adult female breast. It is rare after cessation of ovarian function, either natural or induced. Its association with estrogens is inferential. In postmenopausal women it only occurs when replacement estrogen therapy is in use. Its main clinical significance relates to the need to differentiate irregular breast tissue from cancer. Patients afflicted with this disorder are often frustrated by the repeated biopsies that may be recommended.

254. The answer is d. *(Schwartz, 7/e, pp 552–553.)* Fibroadenomas occur infrequently before puberty but are the most common breast tumors between puberty and the early thirties. They usually are well demarcated and firm. Although most fibroadenomas are no larger than 3 cm in diameter, giant or juvenile fibroadenomas frequently are very large. The bigger fibroadenomas (greater than 5 cm) occur predominantly in adolescent black girls. The average age at onset of juvenile mammary hypertrophy is

16 years. This disorder involves a diffuse change in the entire breast and does not usually manifest clinically as a discrete mass; it may be unilateral or bilateral and can cause an enormous and incapacitating increase in breast size. Regression may be spontaneous and sometimes coincides with puberty or pregnancy. Cystosarcoma phylloides may also cause a large lesion. Together with intraductal carcinoma, it characteristically occurs in older women. Lymphomas are less firm than fibroadenomas and do not have a whorl-like pattern. They display a characteristic fish-flesh texture.

255. The answer is a. *(Gajraj, Br J Surg 80:422–426, 1993.)* With the increasing use of CT and MRI scans for other purposes, small "incidentalomas" of the adrenal gland are becoming a frequent finding. In the absence of any clinical signs or symptoms of endocrine dysfunction, most experts now recommend observation and a search for evidence of endocrine dysfunction for lesions less than 5 cm in diameter. Lesions below that size are common and are usually asymptomatic, nonfunctional adenomas or adrenal cysts. Functional neoplasms secrete an excess of hormones, which produces clinical signs and symptoms. All functional tumors and solid tumors greater than 5.0 cm in diameter should be removed. Cystic masses greater than 5 cm may be aspirated with a fine needle. Clear fluid suggests a benign lesion; if the fluid is bloody or aspiration produces solid tissue, then the lesion should be resected.

Cystic tumors ranging from 3.5 to 5.0 cm may also be aspirated. If bloody fluid is obtained or if the lesion is solid, then resection should be considered in a patient who is otherwise a healthy surgical candidate. Both solid and cystic masses less than 3.5 cm may be followed and can be considered benign if they do not increase in size or become functional.

256. The answer is a. *(Schwartz, 7/e, pp 1679–1707.)* The patient described is exhibiting classic signs and symptoms of hyperparathyroidism. In addition, if a history is obtainable, frequently the patient will relate a history of renal calculi and bone pain—the syndrome characterized as "groans, stones, and bones." The acute management of the hypercalcemic state includes vigorous hydration to restore intravascular volume, which is invariably diminished. This will establish renal perfusion and thus promote urinary calcium excretion. Thiazide diuretics are contraindicated because they frequently cause patients to become hypercalcemic. Instead, diuresis should be promoted with the use of "loop" diuretics such as furosemide (Lasix). The use of intravenous phosphorus infusion is no longer recommended because precipitation in the lungs, heart, or kidney can lead to serious morbidity. Mithramycin is an antineoplastic agent that in low doses inhibits bone resorption and thus diminishes serum calcium levels; it is used only when other maneuvers fail to decrease the calcium level. Calcitonin is useful at times. Bisphosphonates are newer agents particularly useful for lowering calcium levels in resistant cases, such as those associated with humoral malignancy. Finally, "emergency" neck exploration is seldom warranted. In unprepared patients, the morbidity is unacceptably high.

257. The answer is d. *(Schwartz, 7/e, pp 64, 1698.)* The mechanism of hypercalcemia of malignancy is thought to be due to either elaboration of a "PTH-like" humoral factor or, many times, direct bone destruction by metastatic disease. Breast, prostatic, pulmonary, and hematologic malignancy all may give rise to hypercalcemia. Serum and urine electrophoresis may identify a malignancy that causes bone destruction, such as multiple myeloma. Sarcoidosis may produce hypercalcemia, but the presence of the normal chest x-ray essentially rules out this possibility. Thus, a Kveim test is not indicated. An abdominal angiogram would not be expected to identify a likely cause of hypercalcemia. Serum gastrin is not implicated in the differential diagnosis of hypercalcemia. A neck exploration would not be indicated unless a parathyroid adenoma or carcinoma was suspected.

258. The answer is d. *(Schwartz, 7/e, p 552.)* Injury to breast tissue may cause necrosis of mammary adipose tissue and lead to the formation of a tender, localized, firm mass. A history of trauma is often elicited from affected patients, but less apparent factors, such as prolonged pressure, may also produce fat necrosis. Half the patients in whom the diagnosis is made do not recall a history of trauma. The pathophysiology of this lesion seems to involve early development of liquefaction of mammary fat with the formation of a cystic mass. Through a process of fibrosis, this lesion evolves into a firm, sometimes calcified lump that may be difficult to distinguish from carcinoma. There is, however, no relation between fat necrosis and the subsequent development of breast cancer. Excisional biopsy is usually required for definitive diagnosis; if the diagnosis of fat necrosis is confirmed, simple excision removes and terminates the process.

259–260. The answers are 259-c, 260-c. *(Schwartz, 7/e, pp 1642–1645.)* The constellation of symptoms in this patient is typical of a functional adrenocortical tumor. Masculinization in females is also a common finding. Elevated urine 17-ketosteroids will be found in this patient. Any adrenocortical tumor larger than 6 cm should be considered a carcinoma rather than an adenoma. Treatment should include resection, not embolization, of as much tumor as possible. This would include invaded adjacent organs such as the kidney or the tail of the pancreas. Symptoms related to hormone production can be minimized by complete resection despite the inability to cure advanced disease. The most effective adjuvant therapy is mitotane, which is toxic for functional adrenocortical cells. When mitotane is used, therefore, glucocorticoids must be administered. Ketoconazole (not metronidazole) has been found to inhibit the production of various steroid hormones and may be useful in the treatment of hormone-related symptoms. The overall 5-year survival of patients with adrenocortical carcinoma treated with resection and mitotane is 20%. Phentolamine and phenoxybenzamine are α-adrenergic blockers that are sometimes useful in the preoperative management of pheochromocytomas.

261. The answer is e. *(Barnavon, Surg Gynecol Obstet 171:347–352, 1990.)* Approximately 2% of American women who develop carcinoma of the breast are pregnant at the time of diagnosis. The therapeutic approach to these patients has changed considerably in recent years. Though changes in the breast that occur during pregnancy often lead to a delay in diagnosis of breast carcinoma, there is no convincing evidence that breast carcinoma in pregnant women behaves differently or is histologically different from that in nonpregnant women. Furthermore, when patients are matched for age and stage of disease, no significant differences in survival rates are found. The majority of breast cancers in these patients, as with most premenopausal patients, are estrogen-receptor negative and not hormonally sensitive. Therefore, elective termination of pregnancy is generally no longer indicated to decrease estrogen stimulation of the tumor. Since radiation exposure endangers the fetus and there is no evidence that general anesthesia and nonabdominal surgery increase premature labor, modified radical mastectomy is recommended for stage I or II carcinoma (tumor less than 4 cm in diameter). Patients in later stages of pregnancy, however, can start radiation therapy shortly after delivery, and some may be candidates for breast-conserving surgery and adjuvant radiotherapy. Chemotherapy does not appear to increase the risk of congenital malformation when given in the second or third trimester of pregnancy. Patients who require adjuvant chemotherapy during the first trimester may opt for a therapeutic abortion, however, since there is a slightly increased risk of fetal malformation in that circumstance.

262. The answer is b. (*Harris, pp 870–876.*) Paget's disease of the breast is unrelated to Paget's bone disease. It represents a small percentage (1–3%) of all breast cancers and is thought to originate in the retroareolar lactiferous ducts. It progresses toward the nipple-areola complex in most patients, where it causes the typical clinical finding of nipple eczema and erosion. Up to 20% of patients with Paget's disease have an associated breast mass, and these patients are more likely to have involvement of axillary nodes. Nipple-areolar disease alone usually represents in situ cancer; these patients have a 10-year survival rate of over 80%. In contrast, if Paget's disease presents with a mass, the mass is likely to be an infiltrating ductal carcinoma. The generally recommended surgical procedure for Paget's disease is currently a modified radical mastectomy. The validity of breast-saving surgery and adjuvant radiation therapy for patients without an associated mass is under investigation.

263. The answer is d. (*Schwartz, 7/e, pp 1190–1196.*) The syndrome of a gastrin-secreting non-β-cell pancreatic tumor is a rare entity first described by Zollinger and Ellison. They originally described a triad of (1) fulminant, complicated peptic ulceration; (2) extreme gastric hypersecretion; and (3) a non-β-cell tumor of pancreatic islets. Over 50% of the tumors are malignant, and 40% have metastases at the time of surgery. Until recently, total gastrectomy was the primary operation for this tumor; however, it is now believed that operative exploration of the patient with resection of the tumor should be done if possible. H_2 receptor antagonists have also proved very promising in the management of these patients. Patients with Zollinger-Ellison tumors have very high basal gastric acid (greater than 35 meq/h) and serum gastrin levels (usually greater than 200 pg/mL). A protein meal or histamine usually does not increase acid and gastrin levels as it would in conventional duodenal ulcer patients. A paradoxical rise in serum gastrin after intravenous secretin is diagnostic of Zollinger-Ellison syndrome.

264. The answer is d. (*Schwartz, 7/e, pp 1692–1693.*) The incidence of complications with thyroidectomy or parathyroidectomy is relatively low in most series. Thyroid storm, a manifestation of severe thyrotoxicosis, is avoided by prophylactic treatment with propylthiouracil or methimazole prior to surgery. The remaining complications listed are complications of technique. The likelihood of serious complications increases with the extent of resection ("total thyroidectomy" versus "subtotal thyroidectomy") and with the number of neck explorations (initial exploration versus reexploration). Injury to the recurrent laryngeal nerve can compromise the airway, as can hemorrhage into the wound. Superior laryngeal nerve injury causes annoying voice "fatigue," but is rarely of significant consequence. Hypocalcemia is usually transient, but can at times necessitate permanent calcium supplementation. Perforation of hollow neck structures very seldom occurs, and, unless it is massive or not appreciated, usually causes no morbidity.

265–266. The answers are 265-d, 266-e. (*Schwartz, 7/e, pp 1697–1707.*) This patient's presentation and films are consistent with primary hyperparathyroidism. The elevated parathormone level (PTH) confirms the diagnosis. Her chest film demonstrates marked osteopenia and the hand films are classic for this disease with severe demineralization and periosteal bone resorption most prominent in the middle phalanges. The films show no evidence of malignant lesions or mediastinal adenopathy consistent with sarcoidosis, and an elevated PTH level is not found in Paget's disease or vitamin D intoxication.

Treatment for primary hyperparathyroidism in this setting is resection of the diseased parathyroid glands after initial correction of the severe hypercalcemia. A neck exploration would yield a single parathyroid adenoma in about 85% of cases. Two adenomata are found less often (approximately 5%) and hyperplasia of all four glands occurs in about 10–15% of patients. If hyperplasia is found, treatment includes resection of three and one-half glands. The remnant of the fourth gland can be identified with a metal clip in case reexploration becomes necessary. Alternatively, all four glands can be removed with autotransplantation of a small piece of parathyroid tissue into the forearm or sternocleidomastoid muscle. Subsequent hyperfunction, should it develop, can then be treated by removal of this tissue. A patient with osteopenia this severe will need calcium supplementation postoperatively. Vitamin D supplementation may also be necessary if hypocalcemia develops and persists despite treatment with oral calcium.

267. The answer is a. (*Schwartz, 7/e, pp 1678–1689.*) The thyroid scan of the patient discussed in the question shows a discrete area of decreased radioactive iodine uptake with the remainder of the gland accepting iodine normally. This means the tissue that composes the nodule is not endocrinologically active for thyroid hormone. The two major mass lesions of the thyroid that can produce this pattern are a nonfunctioning follicular adenoma and a carcinoma. Carcinomas seldom produce thyroid hormone. Adenomas may be very active (toxic) and suppress the remaining gland. Most thyroid adenomas, however, are not hormone producing and appear as "cold" nodules on a thyroid scan. Graves' disease produces a diffusely hyperactive gland without nodularity. de Quervain's thyroiditis presents as a painful, swollen thyroid gland rather than as a discrete nodule. A large parathyroid adenoma could conceivably displace the thyroid gland and produce a pattern similar to the one shown, but it would be unusual. A localized infectious process also could produce such a pattern. The essential point is that a "cold" thyroid nodule may represent a carcinoma, and needle biopsy or surgical excision is indicated to rule out this possibility.

268. The answer is a. *(Schwartz, 7/e, pp 552–553.)* Cystosarcoma phylloides is a tumor most often seen in younger women. It can grow to enormous size and at times ulcerate through the skin. Still, it is a lesion with low propensity toward metastasis. Local recurrence is common, especially if the initial resection was inadequate. Simple reexcision with adequate margins is curative. Very large lesions may necessitate simple mastectomy to achieve clear margins. Axillary lymphadenectomy, however, is seldom indicated without biopsy-positive demonstration of tumor in the nodes. The low incidence of metastatic disease suggests that adjunctive therapy is indicated only for known metastatic disease, even when the tumors are quite large and ulcerated.

269. The answer is e. *(Schwartz, 7/e, pp 1681–1684.)* This patient has cytologic evidence of a papillary lesion, possibly papillary carcinoma. Papillary carcinoma is a relatively nonaggressive lesion with long-term survival (>20 years) of more than 90%. The lesion is frequently multicentric, which argues for more complete resection. Metastases, when they occur, are usually responsive to surgical resection or radioablation therapy. Removal of the involved lobe, and possibly the entire thyroid gland, is appropriate. Central and lateral lymph node dissection is performed for clinically suspect lymph nodes. Papillary carcinoma is frequently multifocal. Bilateral disease mandates total thyroidectomy. The use of radioactive ^{131}I, however, is contraindicated in pregnancy and should be used with caution in women of childbearing age.

270. The answer is c. *(Schwartz, 7/e, pp 1685–1686.)* Hürthle-cell cancer is a type of follicular cancer, but it tends to recur more often than other types. Follicular cancer spreads hematogenously to distant sites. This is unlike papillary cancer, which metastasizes via the lymphatics. Amyloid deposits in the stroma of a thyroid tumor are diagnostic of medullary carcinoma. The treatment of choice is a near-total thyroidectomy to facilitate later body scanning for metastases and treatment with ^{131}I.

271. The answer is e. *(Schwartz, 7/e, pp 1681–1689.)* Thyroid nodules are somewhat less common in men and should always suggest malignancy. The history of irradiation to the chest and the findings on biopsy mandate resection of the lesion in this patient, since prior exposure to radiation, even at low dosage, is a strong risk factor for the subsequent development of thyroid cancer. The optimum management of thyroid carcinoma remains controversial. Thyroid lobectomy, subtotal thyroidectomy, and total thyroidectomy are all acceptable techniques for treatment. Removal of the gland permits more accurate histologic diagnosis, particularly with regard to the relatively radioresistant Hürthle-cell follicular variant. Removal of the gland also makes subsequent treatment of metastases with radioactive iodine more effective. Suppression with thyroid hormone (Synthroid) in the setting of abnormal cytology is not recommended.

272. The answer is a. *(Harris, pp 106–110.)* Nipple discharge from the breast may be classified as pathologic, physiologic, or galactorrhea. Galactorrhea may be due to hormonal imbalance (hyperprolactinemia, hypothyroidism), drugs (oral contraceptives, phenothiazines, antihypertensives, tranquilizers), or trauma to the chest. Physiologic nipple discharge is intermittent, nonlactational (usually serous), and due to stimulation of the nipple or to drugs (estrogens, tranquilizers). Both galactorrhea and physiologic discharge are frequently bilateral and arise from multiple ducts. Pathologic nipple discharge may be caused by benign lesions of the breast (duct ectasia, papilloma, fibrocystic disease) or by cancer. It may be bloody, serous, or gray-green. It is spontaneous and unilateral and can often be localized to a single nipple duct. When pathologic discharge is diagnosed, an effort should be made to identify the source. If an associated mass is present, it should be biopsied. If no mass is found, a terminal duct excision of the involved duct(s) should be performed. Only 10 percent of patients with pathologic nipple discharge are found to have breast cancer.

273. The answer is c. (*Schwartz, 7/e, pp 1622–1623, 1635–1639.*) Cushing's disease is caused by hypersecretion of ACTH by the pituitary gland. This hypersecretion, in turn, is caused by either a pituitary adenoma (90% of cases) or diffuse pituitary corticotrope hyperplasia (10% of cases) due to hypersecretion of CRH (corticotropin-releasing hormone) by the hypothalamus. A high cure rate is achieved with surgery, occasionally followed by adjuvant radiotherapy for large pituitary adenomas. Cushing syndrome refers to the clinical manifestations of glucocorticoid excess due to any cause (Cushing's disease, administration of exogenous glucocorticoids, adrenocortical hyperplasia, adrenal adenoma, adrenal carcinoma, ectopic ACTH-secreting tumors) and includes truncal obesity, hypertension, hirsutism, moon facies, proximal muscle wasting, ecchymoses, skin striae, osteoporosis, diabetes mellitus, amenorrhea, growth retardation, and immunosuppression. The most common cause of Cushing syndrome is iatrogenic, via administration of synthetic corticosteroids.

274. The answer is d. (*Schwartz, 7/e, pp 1493–1494, 1686–1688.*) Insulin-secreting β-cell tumors of the pancreas produce paroxysmal nervous system manifestations that may be a consequence of hypoglycemia, although the blood glucose level may bear little relation to the severity of the symptoms, even in the same patient from episode to episode. Most insulinomas are single discrete tumors. Patients with insulinoma in the setting of the MEN 1 syndrome (synchronous islet cell tumors of the pancreas, pituitary hyperplasia or adenomas, and parathyroid chief cell hyperplasia), however, are more likely to have multiple tumors throughout the pancreas. If a careful examination of the pancreas reveals one or more specific adenomas, these can be locally excised. Excision of these tumors may be difficult in MEN 1, when the tumors are small and multiple (10–15% of cases). The finding of an elevated serum calcium level would raise the suspicion of MEN 1 and parathyroid hyperplasia. Insulinomas are not associated with MEN 2, which comprises coexistent medullary thyroid cancer, parathyroid hyperplasia, and pheochromocytoma. About one in seven of these tumors is malignant. Streptozotocin, a potent antibiotic that selectively destroys islet cells, can be useful in controlling symptoms from unresectable malignant tumors of the islet cells but probably has little to offer in the definitive management of the typical benign islet cell insulinoma.

275. The answer is a. (*Harris, pp 159–167.*) Breast cancer is rarely seen before the age of 20, but thereafter its incidence increases inexorably. While the prevalence of breast cancer (the raw number of patients alive with disease) is greatest among perimenopausal women, the incidence of breast cancer (the number of new cases per 100,000 population) rises so sharply that it is twice as common among women between 80 and 85 years of age as among those 60 to 65. In addition, the age-adjusted incidence has increased steadily since the mid-1940s. No data is presently available consistently linking the incidence of breast cancer to dietary factors. A possible linkage between breast cancer and alcohol consumption at an early age is being studied.

276–280. The answers are 276-c, 277-b, 278-b, 279-e, 280-d.
(*Schwartz, 7/e, p 321.*) The American Joint Committee on Cancer has defined a four-tiered staging system for breast cancer based on the clinical criteria of tumor size, involvement of lymph nodes, and metastatic disease. In one version of this system, a separate category is reserved for inflammatory breast cancer. While the grouping of breast cancers into stages provides a useful shorthand for expressing a patient's survival probability, it is noteworthy that considerable heterogeneity exists both with respect to tumor size and nodal characteristics among tumors that are classified within a given stage.

The TNM stage of breast cancer is assigned by measuring the greatest diameter of the tumor ("T"), assessing the axillary and clavicular lymph nodes for enlargement and fixation ("N"), and judging whether metastatic disease is present ("M"). In general, the worst of the three TNM parameters will determine the stage assignment.

Tumors that are not palpable are classified T0; tumors 2 cm or less, T1; tumors greater than 2 but not more than 5 cm, T2; tumors greater than 5 cm, T3; and tumors with extension into the chest wall or skin, T4.

Clinically negative lymph nodes are classified N0; positive, movable ipsilateral axillary nodes, N1; fixed ipsilateral axillary nodes, N2; and clavicular nodes, N3.

Absence of evidence of metastatic disease is classified M0; distant metastatic disease, M1.

The patient in question 276 has a T0, N2, M0 lesion. This is stage III (fixed or matted nodes are a poor prognostic sign).

The patient in question 277 has a T2, N1, M0 lesion. This is stage II.

The patient in question 278 has a T2, N0, M0 lesion. Though smaller than the tumor in question 277 and without clinically involved nodes, this tumor is also stage II.

The patient in question 279 has findings compatible with inflammatory breast cancer. A biopsy of the involved skin and a mammogram would confirm the diagnosis. The patient in question 280 has a T1, N0, M1 lesion. This is stage IV (stage IV is any T, any N, M1).

281–285. The answers are 281-d, 282-a, 283-b, 284-e, 285-c. *(Schwartz, 7/e, pp 1244–1246.)* Carcinoid tumors are most commonly found in the appendix and small bowel, where they may be multiple. They have a tendency to metastasize, which varies with the size of the tumor. Tumors < 1 cm uncommonly metastasize. Tumors > 2.0 cm are more often found to be metastatic. Metastasis to the liver and beyond may give rise to the carcinoid syndrome. The tumors cause an intense desmoplastic reaction. Spread into the serosal lymphatics does not imply metastatic disease; local resection is potentially curative. When metastatic lesions are found in the liver, they should be resected when technically feasible to limit the symptoms of the carcinoid syndrome. When extensive hepatic metastases are found, the disease is not curable. Resection of the appendix and cecum may be performed to prevent an early intestinal obstruction by locally encroaching tumor.

286–290. The answers are 286-c, f; 287-a, h; 288-a; 289-d, e; 290-g. *(Schwartz, 7/e, pp 572–586.)* Generally accepted treatment for stage I breast cancer in premenopausal women includes lumpectomy (wide excision, partial mastectomy, quadrantectomy) combined with axillary lymph node dissection and adjuvant radiation therapy, and modified radical mastectomy. Both approaches offer equivalent chances of cure; there is a higher incidence of local recurrence with lumpectomy, axillary dissection, and radiation, but this observation has not been found to affect the overall cure rate in comparison with mastectomy.

Patients with familial breast cancer (multiple first-degree relatives and penetrance of breast cancer through several familial generations) have extremely high risks of developing breast cancer in the course of their lifetimes. A subset of patients with familial breast cancer has been identified by a specific gene mutation (*BRCA1*); however, the genetic basis of most cases of familial breast cancer has yet to be elucidated. A patient with a history of familial breast cancer and multiple biopsies showing atypia may reasonably request bilateral prophylactic simple mastectomies. Alternatively, she may continue with routine surveillance.

Lobular carcinoma in situ is a histologic marker that identifies patients who are at increased risk for the development of breast cancer. It is not a precancerous lesion in itself, and there is no benefit to widely excising it because the risk of subsequent cancer is equal for both breasts. As the risk for the future development of breast cancer is now estimated to be approximately 1% per year, prophylactic mastectomy is no longer recommended. Proper management would consist of close surveillance for cancer by twice yearly examinations and yearly mammography. Sclerosing adenosis is a benign lesion.

Ductal carcinoma in situ is the precursor of invasive ductal carcinoma. It is described in four histologic variants (papillary, cribriform, solid, and comedo type), of which the comedo subtype shows the greatest tendency to recur after wide excision alone. For years, ductal carcinoma in situ was treated by simple mastectomy. In recent years, studies have shown equally good results with wide excision alone (for small noncomedo lesions) or wide excision plus radiation therapy. For a 1.0-cm comedocarcinoma (which may extend microscopically wider still), most experts would favor simple mastectomy or wide excision with radiation therapy.

There are few indications for radical mastectomy as it is both more traumatic and disfiguring than any other method of local control of breast cancer and offers no greater survival benefit. One indication for radical mastectomy, however, is locally advanced breast cancer with wide invasion of the pectoralis major in a patient who is physiologically able to tolerate general anesthesia.

GASTROINTESTINAL TRACT, LIVER, AND PANCREAS

Questions

DIRECTIONS: Each item below contains a question or incomplete statement followed by suggested responses. Select the **one best** response to each question.

291. Omeprazole has been added to the H$_2$ antagonists as a therapeutic approach to the management of acute gastric and duodenal ulcers. It acts by

a. Blocking breakdown of mucosal-damaging metabolites of NSAIDs
b. Providing a direct cytoprotective effect
c. Buffering gastric acids
d. Inhibiting parietal cell hydrogen-potassium-ATPase
e. Inhibiting gastrin release and parietal cell acid production

292. Evidence that a splenectomy might benefit a patient with immune (idiopathic) thrombocytopenic purpura (ITP) includes

a. A significant enlargement of the spleen
b. A high reticulocyte count
c. Megakaryocytic elements in the bone marrow
d. An increase in the platelet count on cortisone therapy
e. Patient age of less than 5 years

293. An 18-year-old woman presents with abdominal pain, fever, and leukocytosis. With the presumptive diagnosis of appendicitis, a right lower quadrant (McBurney) incision is made and the lesion pictured below is delivered. The process is 50 cm proximal to the ileocecal valve. This lesion

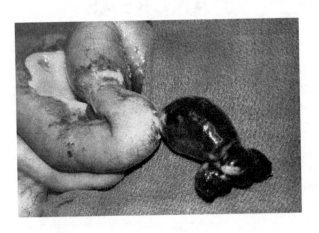

a. Can best be diagnosed by preoperative angiogram, which should be done whenever the diagnosis is suspected
b. Should routinely be removed when incidentally discovered during celiotomy
c. Is embryologically derived from a persistent vitelline duct (omphalomesenteric duct)
d. Often contains ectopic adrenal tissue
e. Is frequently associated with cutaneous flushing and episodic tachycardia

294. A 41-year-old man complains of regurgitation of saliva and of ingested but undigested food. An esophagram reveals a "bird's beak" deformity. Which of the following statements is true about this condition?

a. Chest pain is common in the advanced stages of this disease
b. More patients are improved by forceful dilation than by surgical intervention
c. Manometry can be expected to show high resting pressures of the lower esophageal sphincter
d. Surgical treatment primarily consists of resection of the distal esophagus with reanastomosis to the stomach above the diaphragm
e. Patients with this disease are at no increased risk for the development of carcinoma

295. Which of the following statements concerning imperforate anus is true?

a. Imperforate anus affects males more frequently than females
b. In 90% of males, but only 50% of females, the rectum ends below the level of the levator ani complex
c. The rectum usually ends in a blind pouch
d. The chance for eventual continence is greater when the rectum has descended to below the levator ani muscles
e. Immediate definitive repair of the anatomic defect is required to maximize the chance of eventual continence

Items 296–297

A previously healthy 80-year-old woman presents with early satiety and abdominal fullness. The CT scan shown below is obtained.

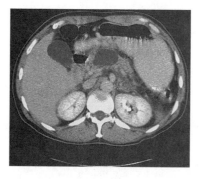

296. The lesion is most likely a

a. Pancreatic pseudocyst
b. Pancreatic adenocarcinoma
c. Pancreatic cystadenocarcinoma
d. Retroperitoneal lymphoma
e. Pancreatic serous cystadenoma

297. Which of the following statements about this lesion is true?

a. Clinical and laboratory findings together establish a preoperative diagnosis
b. Significant weight loss and back pain are the typical presentation
c. The lesion may be multilocular or calcified
d. It is unlikely to be cured by resection if large
e. It is associated with a history of pancreatitis

298. A patient with a history of familial polyposis undergoes a diagnostic polypectomy. Which of the following types of polyps is most likely to be found?

a. Villous adenoma
b. Hyperplastic polyp
c. Adenomatous polyp
d. Retention polyp
e. Pseudopolyp

299. What is the most common serious complication of an end colostomy?

a. Bleeding
b. Skin breakdown
c. Parastomal hernia
d. Colonic perforation during irrigation
e. Stomal prolapse

300. Which of the following statements regarding pancreatic carcinoma is true?

a. The majority of cases present with jaundice alone
b. CT scan, angiography, and laparoscopy have been unsuccessful in predicting resectability
c. If a patient is jaundiced, the resectability rate is less than 5%
d. 99% of patients with pancreatic cancer have metastatic disease at the time of diagnosis
e. The 5-year survival rate after a Whipple procedure (pancreaticoduodenectomy) performed for cure is 30–40%

Items 301–302

A 45-year-old woman is explored for a perforated duodenal ulcer 6 h after onset of symptoms. She has a history of chronic peptic ulcer disease treated medically with minimal symptoms.

301. The procedure of choice is

a. Simple closure with omental patch
b. Truncal vagotomy and pyloroplasty
c. Antrectomy and truncal vagotomy
d. Highly selective vagotomy
e. Hemigastrectomy

302. Six weeks after surgery, the patient returns complaining of postprandial weakness, sweating, light-headedness, crampy abdominal pain, and diarrhea. The best management would be

a. Antispasmodic medications (e.g., Lomotil)
b. Dietary advice and counseling that symptoms will probably abate within 3 mo of surgery
c. Dietary advice and counseling that symptoms will probably not abate but are not dangerous
d. Workup for neuroendocrine tumor (e.g., carcinoid)
e. Preparation for revision to Roux-en-Y gastrojejunostomy

Items 303–304

A 60-year-old male alcoholic is admitted to the hospital with hematemesis. His blood pressure is 100/60 mm Hg, the physical examination reveals splenomegaly and ascites, and the initial hematocrit is 25%. Nasogastric suction yields 300 mL of fresh blood.

303. A 55-year-old man complains of chronic intermittent epigastric pain, and gastroscopy demonstrates a 2-cm ulcer of the distal lesser curvature. Endoscopic biopsy yields no malignant tissue. After a 6-wk trial of H_2 blockade and antacid therapy, the ulcer is unchanged. Proper therapy at this point is

a. Repeat trial of medical therapy
b. Local excision of the ulcer
c. Billroth I partial gastrectomy
d. Billroth I partial gastrectomy with vagotomy
e. Vagotomy and pyloroplasty

304. After initial resuscitation, this man should undergo

a. Esophageal balloon tamponade
b. Barium swallow
c. Selective angiography
d. Esophagogastroscopy
e. Exploratory celiotomy

305. A diagnosis of bleeding esophageal varices is made in this patient. Appropriate initial therapy would be

a. Intravenous vasopressin
b. Endoscopic sclerotherapy
c. Emergency portacaval shunt
d. Emergency esophageal transection
e. Esophageal balloon tamponade

306. During an operation for carcinoma of the hepatic flexure of the colon, an unexpected discontinuous 3-cm metastasis is discovered in the edge of the right lobe of the liver. The surgeon should

a. Terminate the operation, screen the patient for evidence of other metastases, and plan further therapy after the reevaluation
b. Perform a right hemicolectomy and a right hepatic lobectomy
c. Perform a right hemicolectomy and a wedge resection of the metastasis
d. Perform a cecostomy and schedule reoperation after a course of systemic chemotherapy
e. Perform local resection of the primary colon cancer and plan radiation therapy for the lesion on the liver

307. A 42-year-old man with no history of use of nonsteroidal anti-inflammatory drugs (NSAIDs) presents with recurrent gastritis. Infection with *Helicobacter pylori* is suspected. Which of the following statements is true?

a. Morphologically, the bacteria is a gram-positive, tennis-racket-shaped organism
b. Diagnosis can be made by serologic testing or urea breath tests
c. Diagnosis is most routinely achieved via culturing endoscopic scrapings
d. The most effective way to treat and prevent recurrence of this patient's gastritis is through the use of single-drug therapy aimed at eradicating *H. pylori*
e. The organism is easily eradicated

308. Which of the following hernias follows the path of the spermatic cord within the cremaster muscle?

a. Femoral
b. Direct inguinal
c. Indirect inguinal
d. Spigelian
e. Interparietal

309. A spry octogenarian who has never before been hospitalized is admitted with signs and symptoms typical of a small bowel obstruction. Which of the following clinical findings would give the most help in ascertaining the diagnosis?

a. Coffee-grounds aspirate from the stomach
b. Aerobilia
c. A leukocyte count of $40,000/\mu L$
d. A pH of 7.5, P_{CO_2} of 50 kPa, and paradoxically acid urine
e. A palpable mass in the pelvis

310. Which of the following colonic pathologies is thought to have no malignant potential?

a. Ulcerative colitis
b. Villous adenomas
c. Familial polyposis
d. Peutz-Jeghers syndrome
e. Crohn's colitis

311. A 70-year-old woman has nausea, vomiting, abdominal distention, and episodic, crampy midabdominal pain. She has no history of previous surgery but has a long history of cholelithiasis for which she has refused surgery. Her abdominal radiograph reveals a spherical density in the right lower quadrant. Correct treatment should consist of

a. Ileocolectomy
b. Cholecystectomy
c. Ileotomy and extraction
d. Nasogastric tube decompression
e. Intravenous antibiotics

312. Which of the following statements concerning Hirschsprung's disease is true?

a. It is initially treated by colostomy
b. It is best diagnosed in the newborn period by barium enema
c. It is characterized by the absence of ganglion cells in the transverse colon
d. It is associated with a high incidence of genitourinary tract anomalies
e. It is the congenital disease that most commonly leads to subsequent fecal incontinence

313. Spontaneous closure of which of the following congenital abnormalities of the abdominal wall generally occurs by the age of 4?

a. Umbilical hernia
b. Patent urachus
c. Patent omphalomesenteric duct
d. Omphalocele
e. Gastroschisis

314. Laparoscopic cholecystectomy is indicated for symptomatic gallstones in which of the following conditions?

a. Cirrhosis
b. Prior upper abdominal surgery
c. Suspected carcinoma of the gallbladder
d. Morbid obesity
e. Coagulopathy

315. Infants with anorectal anomalies tend to have other congenital anomalies. Associated abnormalities include which of the following?

a. Abnormalities of the cervical spine
b. Hydrocephalus
c. Duodenal atresia
d. Heart disease
e. Corneal opacities

316. A 48-year-old woman develops pain of the right lower quadrant while playing tennis. The pain progresses and the patient presents to the emergency room later that day with a low-grade fever, a white blood count of 13,000, and complaints of anorexia and nausea as well as persistent, sharp pain of the right lower quadrant. On examination she is tender in the right lower quadrant with muscular spasm and there is a suggestion of a mass effect. An ultrasound is ordered and shows an apparent mass in the abdominal wall. Which of the following is the most likely diagnosis?

a. Acute appendicitis
b. Cecal carcinoma
c. Hematoma of the rectus sheath
d. Torsion of an ovarian cyst
e. Cholecystitis

317. A 36-h-old infant presents with bilious vomiting and an increasingly distended abdomen. At exploration the segment below is found as the point of obstruction. Which of the following statements regarding this finding is true?

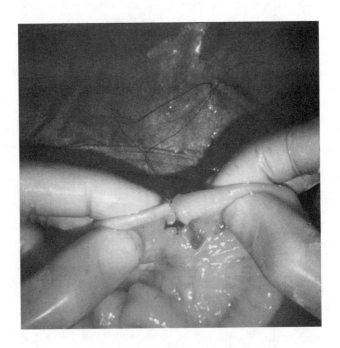

a. Resection with primary anastomosis should not be performed
b. Gentle, persistent traction on the specimen usually corrects the defect and removes the need for a resection
c. The lesion is much more common in the jejunum than in the ileum in this age group
d. This problem is probably related to mesenteric vascular insufficiency
e. A properly monitored barium enema might have corrected this defect and removed the need for an operation

318. In determining the proper treatment for a sliding hiatal hernia, the most useful step would be

a. Barium swallow with cinefluoroscopy during Valsalva maneuver
b. Flexible endoscopy
c. 24-h monitoring of esophageal pH
d. Measuring the size of the hernia
e. Assessing the patient's smoking and drinking history

319. Which of the following statements regarding the etiology of obstructive jaundice is true?

a. A markedly elevated SGOT and SGPT are usually associated with obstructive jaundice
b. When extrahepatic biliary obstruction is suspected, the first test should be endoscopic ultrasonography (EUS)
c. A Klatskin tumor will result in extrahepatic ductal dilation only
d. A liver-spleen scan will add significantly to the diagnostic workup for obstructive jaundice
e. Carcinoma of the head of the pancreas can cause deep epigastric or back pain in as many as 80% of patients

320. A previously healthy 9-year-old child comes to the emergency room because of fulminant upper gastrointestinal bleeding. The hemorrhage is most likely to be the result of

a. Esophageal varices
b. Mallory-Weiss syndrome
c. Gastritis
d. A gastric ulcer
e. A duodenal ulcer

321. Intragastric pressure remains steady near 2–5 mm Hg during slow gastric filling, but rises rapidly to high levels after reaching a volume of

a. 400–600 mL
b. 700–900 mL
c. 1000–1200 mL
d. 1300–1500 mL
e. 1600–1800 mL

322. Which of the following statements is true regarding the effects of colon resection?

a. Net absorption of water by the rectum has been demonstrated in humans
b. Patients who undergo major colon resections suffer little change in their bowel habits following operation
c. The left colon is better adapted for water absorption than the right colon
d. The right colon is better adapted for electrolyte absorption than the left colon
e. The role of the ileocecal valve in normal fluid homeostasis is well established

323. Operative planning and preoperative counseling for a patient with a rectal carcinoma can be best provided if the patient is staged before surgery by

a. Rigid proctoscopy
b. Barium enema
c. MRI of the pelvis
d. CT scanning of the pelvis
e. Rectal endosonography

324. Which statement regarding absorption by the small intestine is true?

a. All but the fat in milk is digested and absorbed in humans by the end of the duodenum
b. Complete absorption of carbohydrates in a normal meal occurs in the ileum
c. In short gut syndrome, much of the dietary carbohydrate appears in the stool
d. Aldosterone markedly decreases sodium transport across the gut mucosa
e. Enzymes of the brush border of the small intestine can digest and absorb less than 5% of an average protein meal in the absence of the pancreas

325. Local stimuli that inhibit the release of gastrin from the gastric mucosa include which of the following?

a. Small proteins
b. 20-proof alcohol
c. Caffeine
d. Acidic antral contents
e. Antral distention

326. Which statement regarding fat absorption is true?

a. Half of neutral fat can be absorbed in the complete absence of bile and pancreatic lipase
b. Fifty percent of the total bile salt pool is lost in the stool and replaced daily by synthesis in the liver
c. Glycerol, short-chain fatty acids, and medium-chain triglycerides exit the mucosal cell in chylomicrons
d. Conjugated bile salts are actively resorbed in the colon and returned to the liver via the portal vein
e. Water-insoluble dietary lipid is rendered into soluble micelles through mixing with pancreatic amylase

327. For a symptomatic partial duodenal obstruction secondary to an annular pancreas, the operative treatment of choice is

a. A Whipple procedure
b. Gastrojejunostomy
c. Vagotomy and gastrojejunostomy
d. Partial resection of the annular pancreas
e. Duodenojejunostomy

328. A previously healthy 15-year-old boy is brought to the emergency room with complaints of about 12 h of progressive anorexia, nausea, and pain of the right lower quadrant. On physical examination, he is found to have a rectal temperature of 38.18°C (100.58°F) and has direct and rebound abdominal tenderness localizing to McBurney's point as well as involuntary guarding in the right lower quadrant. At operation through a McBurney-type incision, the appendix and cecum are found to be normal, but the surgeon is impressed with the marked edema of the terminal ileum, which also has an overlying fibrinopurulent exudate. The correct procedure is to

a. Close the abdomen after culturing the exudate
b. Perform a standard appendectomy
c. Resect the involved terminal ileum
d. Perform the ileocolic resection
e. Perform an ileocolostomy to bypass the involved terminal ileum

329. A 32-year-old woman undergoes a cholecystectomy for acute cholecystitis and is discharged home on the sixth postoperative day. She returns to the clinic 8 mo after the operation for a routine visit and is noted by the surgeon to be jaundiced. Laboratory values on readmission show total bilirubin 5.6 mg/dL; direct bilirubin 4.8 mg/dL; alkaline phosphatase 250 IU (normal 21–91 IU); SGOT 52 KU (normal 10–40 KU); SGPT 51 KU (normal 10–40 KU). An ultrasonogram shows dilated intrahepatic ducts. The patient undergoes the transhepatic cholangiogram seen below. Appropriate management is

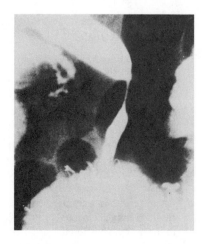

a. Choledochoplasty with insertion of a T tube
b. End-to-end choledochocholedochal anastomosis
c. Roux-en-Y choledochojejunostomy
d. Percutaneous transhepatic dilatation
e. Choledochoduodenostomy

330. After complete removal of a sessile polyp of 2.0 × 1.5 cm found one fingerlength above the anal mucocutaneous margin, the pathologist reports it to have been a villous adenoma that contained carcinoma in situ. You would recommend that this patient undergo

a. Reexcision of the biopsy site with wider margins
b. Abdominoperineal rectosigmoid resection
c. Anterior resection of the rectum
d. External radiation therapy to the rectum
e. No further therapy

331. A 55-year-old woman with cancer of the cervix undergoes hysterectomy and is found to have pelvic lymph nodes involved with cancer. She then receives a course of external beam radiation (4500 rads). When the physician counsels her prior to her radiation treatment, she should be told of all the possible complications of radiation enteritis. Which of the following is generally not associated with radiation injury?

a. Malabsorption
b. Intussusception
c. Ulceration
d. Fistulization
e. Perforation

332. Which of the following would be expected to stimulate intestinal motility?

a. Fear
b. Gastrin
c. Secretin
d. Acetylcholine
e. Cholecystokinin

333. Which of the following statements concerning carcinoma of the esophagus is true?

a. Alcohol has been implicated as a precipitating factor
b. Squamous carcinoma is the most common type at the cardioesophageal junction
c. It has a higher incidence in males
d. It occurs more commonly in patients with corrosive esophagitis
e. Surgical excision is the only effective treatment

Items 334–335

334. A 30-year-old man with a duodenal ulcer is being considered for surgery because of intractable pain and a previous bleeding episode. Serum gastrin levels are found to be over 1000 pg/mL (normal 40–150) on three separate determinations. The patient should be told that the operation of choice is

a. Vagotomy and pyloroplasty
b. Highly selective vagotomy and tumor resection
c. Subtotal gastrectomy
d. Total gastrectomy
e. Partial pancreatectomy

335. Another 30-year-old man with the identical clinical situation presented in the previous question is being considered for surgery. His serum gastrin level, however, is 150 ± 10 pg/mL on three determinations. The surgeon should perform

a. An arteriogram
b. A secretin stimulation test
c. A total gastrectomy
d. A subtotal gastrectomy
e. A highly selective vagotomy

336. The most common clinical presentation of idiopathic retroperitoneal fibrosis is

a. Ureteral obstruction
b. Leg edema
c. Calf claudication
d. Jaundice
e. Intestinal obstruction

337. A 55-year-old man who is extremely obese reports weakness, sweating, tachycardia, confusion, and headache whenever he fasts for more than a few hours. He has prompt relief of symptoms when he eats. These symptoms are most suggestive of which of the following disorders?

a. Diabetes mellitus
b. Insulinoma
c. Zollinger-Ellison syndrome
d. Carcinoid syndrome
e. Multiple endocrine neoplasia, type II

338. In planning the management of a 2.8-cm epidermoid carcinoma of the anus, the first therapeutic approach should be

a. Abdominoperineal resection
b. Wide local resection with bilateral inguinal node dissection
c. Local radiation therapy
d. Systemic chemotherapy
e. Combined radiation therapy and chemotherapy

339. An 80-year-old man is admitted to the hospital complaining of nausea, abdominal pain, distention, and diarrhea. A cautiously performed transanal contrast study reveals an "apple core" configuration in the rectosigmoid. Appropriate management at this time would include

a. Colonoscopic decompression and rectal tube placement
b. Saline enemas and digital disimpaction of fecal matter from the rectum
c. Colon resection and proximal colostomy
d. Oral administration of metronidazole and checking a *Clostridium difficile* titer
e. Evaluation of an electrocardiogram and obtaining an angiogram to evaluate for colonic mesenteric ischemia

340. Indications for operation in Crohn's disease include which of the following?

a. Intestinal obstruction
b. Enterovesical fistula
c. Ileum–ascending colon fistula
d. Enterovaginal fistula
e. Free perforation

341. A 50-year-old man presents to the emergency room with a 6-h history of excruciating abdominal pain and distention. The abdominal film shown below is obtained. The next diagnostic maneuver should be

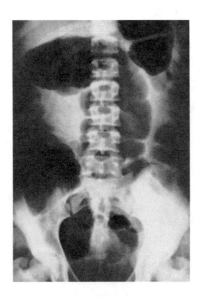

a. Emergency celiotomy
b. Upper gastrointestinal series with small-bowel follow-through
c. CT scan of the abdomen
d. Barium enema
e. Sigmoidoscopy

342. Which of the following organisms is most closely associated with gastric and duodenal ulcer disease?

a. *Campylobacter*
b. *Cytomegalovirus*
c. *Helicobacter*
d. *Mycobacterium avium-intracellulare*
e. *Yersinia enterocolitica*

343. On Monday morning, a septuagenarian man has a moderate-sized abdominal aneurysm resected. On Friday, he is noted to be markedly distended with an abdominal radiograph on which the cecum is measured as 12 cm across. Proper management at this time would be

a. Decompression of the large bowel via colonoscopy
b. Replacement of the nasogastric tube and administration of low-dose cholinergic drugs
c. Continued nothing-by-mouth orders, administration of a gentle saline enema, and encouragement of ambulation
d. Immediate return to the operating room for operative decompression by transverse colostomy
e. Right hemicolectomy

344. In the management of echinococcal liver cysts

a. A large cyst should be treated by percutaneous aspiration of its contents
b. Medical treatment with albendazole usually preempts the need for surgical drainage
c. Negative serologic tests suggest that the cyst is chronic and inactive and that no treatment is indicated
d. Leakage of cyst fluid puts the patient at risk for anaphylactic reaction
e. Coexistent extrahepatic cysts are uncommon

345. Which of the following statements regarding appendicitis during pregnancy is correct?

a. Appendicitis is the most prevalent extrauterine indication for celiotomy during pregnancy
b. Appendicitis occurs more commonly in pregnant women than in nonpregnant women of comparable age
c. Suspected appendicitis in a pregnant woman should be managed with a period of observation of due to the risks of laparotomy to the fetus
d. Noncomplicated appendicitis results in a 20% fetal mortality and premature labor rate
e. The severity of appendicitis correlates with increased gestational age of the fetus

346. Which of the following is most likely to require surgical correction?
a. Large sliding esophageal hiatal hernia
b. Paraesophageal hiatal hernia
c. Traction diverticulum of esophagus
d. Schatzki's ring of distal esophagus
e. Esophageal web

347. A 65-year-old man who is hospitalized with pancreatic carcinoma develops abdominal distention and obstipation. The following abdominal radiograph is obtained. Appropriate management would best be achieved by

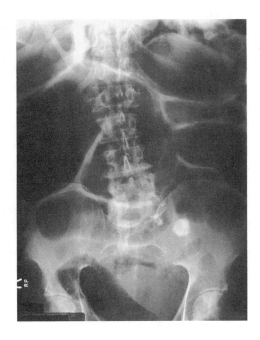

a. Urgent colostomy or cecostomy
b. Discontinuation of anticholinergic medications and narcotics and correction of metabolic disorders
c. Digital disimpaction of a fecal mass in the rectum
d. Diagnostic and therapeutic colonoscopy
e. Detorsion of the volvulus and colopexy or resection

348. True statements regarding Zenker's diverticulum include

a. Aspiration pneumonitis is unlikely
b. It is a congenital abnormality
c. The most common symptom is a sensation of high obstruction on swallowing
d. It is a traction-type diverticulum
e. Treatment is restriction of certain foods

349. True statements regarding hemobilia include which of the following?

a. The classic presentation includes biliary colic, jaundice, and gastrointestinal bleeding
b. Spontaneous bleeding secondary to hematologic disorders is the major cause of this disorder
c. Percutaneous transhepatic catheter placement of an absorbable gelatin sponge (Gelfoam) is the preferred treatment in cases of significant intrahepatic bleeding
d. Angiography and endoscopy have no role in the treatment of intrahepatic bleeding
e. Arterial embolization is advocated for hemobilia from the extrahepatic bile ducts

Items 350–351

350. A 30-year-old female patient who presents with bleeding per rectum is found at colonoscopy to have colitis confined to the transverse and descending colon. A biopsy is performed. Which of the following statements is true about this patient?

a. The inflammatory process is likely to be confined to the mucosa and submucosa
b. The inflammatory reaction is likely to be continuous
c. Superficial as opposed to linear ulcerations can be expected
d. Noncaseating granulomata can be expected in up to 50% of patients with similar disease
e. Microabcesses within crypts are common

351. Regarding potential complications in this patient, which of the following statements is true?

a. The occurrence of toxic megacolon is common
b. Perforation occurs in about 25% of patients with similar disease
c. Fistulas between the colon and segments of intestine, bladder, vagina, urethra, and skin may develop
d. Extraintestinal manifestations including uveitis and erythema nodosum would be exceedingly rare in this patient
e. This patient would be at no increased risk for the development of cancer of the colon as compared with an age-matched population

352. An upper GI series is performed on a 71-year-old woman who presented with several months of chest pain that occurred when she was eating. The film below is obtained. Investigation reveals a microcytic anemia and erosive gastritis on upper endoscopy. Which of the following statements about the patient's condition is true?

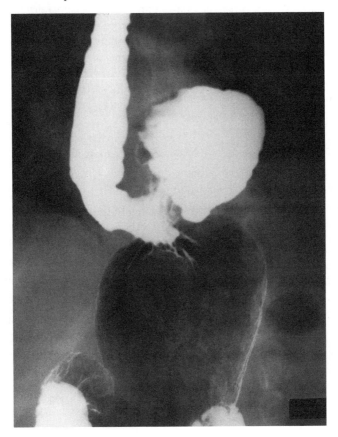

a. It is congenital
b. The gastroesophageal junction is above the diaphragm
c. Ulceration, gastritis, and anemia are common
d. It usually is controlled by medical therapy
e. Surgical treatment, if indicated, should be delayed up to 3 mo to allow inflammation around the gastroesophageal junction to subside

353. Which statement regarding adenocarcinoma of the pancreas is true?

a. It occurs most frequently in the body of the gland
b. It carries a 1–2% 5-year survival rate
c. It is nonresectable if it presents as painless jaundice
d. It can usually be resected if it presents in the body or tail of the pancreas and does not involve the common bile duct
e. It is associated with diabetes insipidus

354. Correct statements concerning intussusception in infants include which of the following?

a. Recurrence rates following treatment are high
b. It is frequently preceded by a gastrointestinal viral illness
c. A 1- to 2-wk period of parenteral alimentation should precede surgical reduction when surgery is required
d. Hydrostatic reduction without surgery rarely provides successful treatment
e. The most common type occurs at the junction of the descending colon and sigmoid colon

355. A 32-year-old woman presents to the hospital with a 24-h history of abdominal pain of the right lower quadrant. She undergoes an uncomplicated appendectomy for acute appendicitis and is discharged home on the fourth postoperative day. The pathologist notes the presence of a carcinoid tumor (1.2 cm) in the tip of the appendix. Which of the following statements is true?

a. The patient should be advised to undergo ileocolectomy
b. The most common location of carcinoids is in the appendix
c. The carcinoid syndrome occurs in more than half the patients with carcinoid tumors
d. The tumor is an apudoma
e. Carcinoid syndrome is seen only when the tumor is drained by the portal venous system

356. Which of the following statements regarding direct inguinal hernias is true?

a. They are the most common inguinal hernias in women
b. They protrude medially to the inferior epigastric vessels
c. They should be opened and ligated at the internal ring
d. They commonly protrude into the scrotal sac in men
e. They incarcerate more commonly than indirect hernias

357. A 35-year-old woman presents with pancreatitis. Subsequent endoscopic retrograde cholangiopancreatography (ERCP) reveals the congenital cystic anomaly of her biliary system illustrated in the film below. Which of the following statements regarding this problem is true?

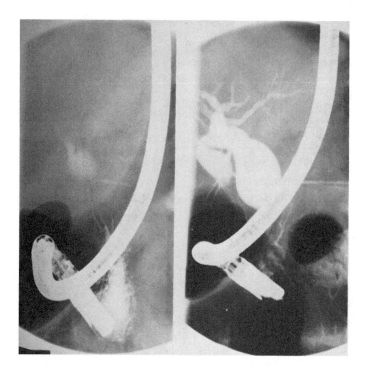

a. Treatment consists of internal drainage via choledochoduodenostomy
b. Malignant changes may occur within this structure
c. Most patients present with the classic triad of epigastric pain, an abdominal mass, and jaundice
d. Cystic dilation of the intrahepatic biliary tree may coexist and is managed in a similar fashion
e. Surgery should be reserved for symptomatic patients

358. Which of the following statements regarding stress ulceration is true?

a. It is true ulceration, extending into and through the muscularis mucosa
b. It classically involves the antrum
c. Increased secretion of gastric acid has been shown to play a causative role
d. It frequently involves multiple sites
e. It is seen following shock or sepsis, but for some unknown reason does not occur following major surgery, trauma, or burns

359. Which statement concerning cholangitis is correct?

a. The most common infecting organism is *Staphylococcus aureus*
b. The diagnosis is suggested by the Charcot triad
c. The disease occurs primarily in young, immunocompromised patients
d. Cholecystostomy is the procedure of choice in affected patients
e. Surgery is indicated once the diagnosis of cholangitis is made

360. An 88-year-old man with a history of end-stage renal failure, severe coronary artery disease, and brain metastases from lung cancer presents with acute cholecystitis. His family wants "everything done." The best management option in this patient would be

a. Tube cholecystostomy
b. Open cholecystectomy
c. Laparoscopic cholecystectomy
d. Intravenous antibiotics followed by elective cholecystectomy
e. Lithotripsy followed by long-term bile acid therapy

361. After a weekend drinking binge, a 45-year-old alcoholic man presents to the hospital with abdominal pain, nausea, and vomiting. On physical examination the patient is afebrile and is noted to have a palpable tender mass in the epigastrium. Laboratory tests reveal an amylase of 250 U/dL (normal < 180). A CT scan done on the second hospital day is pictured below. Which of the following statements concerning this patient's condition is true?

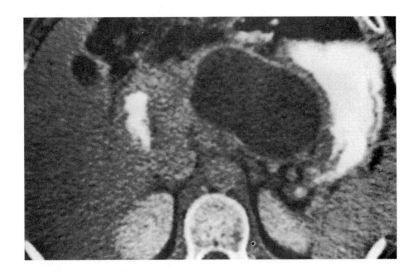

   a. The mass may cause gastric outlet or extrahepatic biliary obstruction
   b. Spontaneous resolution almost never occurs
   c. The mass is seen only with acute pancreatitis
   d. The mass has an epithelial lining
   e. Malignant degeneration occurs in about 25% of cases if left untreated

362. Dieulafoy's lesion of the stomach is characterized by

   a. A large mucosal defect with underlying, friable vascular plexus
   b. Frequent rebleeding after endoscopic treatment
   c. Massive bleeding that requires subtotal gastrectomy
   d. Location in the proximal stomach
   e. Acid-peptic changes of the gastric mucosa

363. During an appendectomy for acute appendicitis, a 4-cm mass is found in the midportion of the appendix. Frozen section reveals this lesion to be a carcinoid tumor. Which of the following statements is true?

a. No further surgery is indicated
b. A right hemicolectomy should be performed
c. There is about a 50% chance that this patient will develop the carcinoid syndrome
d. Carcinoid tumors arise from islet cells
e. Carcinoid syndrome can occur only in the presence of liver metastases

364. Correct statements regarding rectal carcinoid tumors include

a. Endoscopic resection is sufficient for tumors smaller than 2 cm
b. Patients frequently present with the carcinoid syndrome
c. They are rapidly growing tumors
d. Local recurrence is rare with complete resection of the primary lesion
e. They can develop the carcinoid syndrome even in the absence of liver metastases

365. Indications for surgical removal of polypoid lesions of the gallbladder include

a. Size greater than 0.5 cm
b. Presence of clinical symptoms
c. Patient age of over 25 years
d. Presence of multiple small lesions
e. Absence of shadowing on ultrasound

366. A patient who has a total pancreatectomy might be expected to develop which of the following complications?

a. Diabetes mellitus
b. Hypercalcemia
c. Hyperphosphatemia
d. Constipation
e. Weight gain

367. A 28-year-old previously healthy woman arrives in the emergency room complaining of 24 h of anorexia and nausea and lower abdominal pain that is more intense in the right lower quadrant than elsewhere. On examination she has peritoneal signs of the right lower quadrant and a rectal temperature of 38.38°C (101.8°F). At exploration through incision of the right lower quadrant, she is found to have a small, contained perforation of a cecal diverticulum. Which of the following statements regarding this situation is true?

a. Cecal diverticula are acquired disorders
b. Cecal diverticula are usually multiple
c. Cecal diverticula are mucosal herniations through the muscularis propria
d. Diverticulectomy, closure of the cecal defect, and appendectomy may be indicated
e. An ileocolectomy is indicated even with well-localized inflammation

368. True statements regarding cavernous hemangiomata of the liver in adults include

a. The majority become symptomatic
b. They may undergo malignant transformation
c. They enlarge under hormonal stimulation
d. They should be resected to avoid spontaneous rupture and life-threatening hemorrhage
e. A liver/spleen radionucleotide scan is the most sensitive and specific way to make the diagnosis

369. Correct statements regarding carcinoembryonic antigen (CEA) and colorectal tumors include which of the following?

a. Elevated CEA is indicative of a tumor of gastrointestinal origin
b. A low CEA level after resection of a colon tumor is a poor marker of disease control
c. Ninety percent of colorectal tumors produce CEA
d. There is a high likelihood of liver involvement if the CEA level is high (greater than 100 ng/mL)
e. CEA levels are unusually low in cigarette smokers

DIRECTIONS: Each group of questions below consists of lettered options followed by numbered items. For each numbered item, select the appropriate lettered option(s). Each lettered option may be used once, more than once, or not at all. **Choose exactly the number of options indicated following each item.**

Items 370–373

Select the appropriate surgical procedure for each patient.

a. Vagotomy and antrectomy
b. Antrectomy alone
c. Vagotomy and pyloroplasty
d. Vagotomy and gastrojejunostomy
e. Proximal gastric vagotomy

370. A 72-year-old patient with an intractable type I ulcer along the incisura with a significant amount of scarring along the entire length of the lesser curvature (**SELECT 1 PROCEDURE**)

371. A 46-year-old patient with gastric outlet obstruction secondary to ulcer disease and severe inflammation around the pylorus and first and second portions of the duodenum (**SELECT 1 PROCEDURE**)

372. A 90-year-old patient with a bleeding duodenal ulcer (**SELECT 1 PROCEDURE**)

373. A 36-year-old patient with a type III (pyloric) ulcer that is refractory to medical treatment (**SELECT 1 PROCEDURE**)

Items 374–376

Match each description with the correct abnormality.

a. Rupture of the diaphragm
b. Paraesophageal hiatal hernia
c. Sliding hiatal hernia
d. Foramen of Bochdalek hernia
e. Foramen of Morgagni hernia

374. The most common congenital diaphragmatic hernia in infants (**SELECT 1 ABNORMALITY**)

375. The hernia most likely to cause acute respiratory distress in infants (**SELECT 1 ABNORMALITY**)

376. A congenital hernia that is most frequently discovered as an incidental finding in adults (**SELECT 1 ABNORMALITY**)

Items 377–378

For each patient listed below, select the likely diagnosis.

a. Spontaneous bacterial peritonitis
b. Perforated diverticulum
c. Perforated gastric ulcer
d. Ruptured spleen
e. Ruptured echinococcal liver cyst
f. Sigmoid volvulus
g. Cecal volvulus
h. Perforated transverse colon carcinoma
i. Strangulated hernia with necrotic bowel

377. A 65-year-old previously healthy man presents with severe abdominal pain that came on suddenly. He has abdominal tenderness and guarding in all four quadrants on physical examination. A radiograph is obtained and demonstrates a radiolucency under the right hemidiaphragm. **(SELECT 4 DIAGNOSES)**

378. An 82-year-old nursing home patient presents to the emergency room with vomiting, abdominal pain, and distention. A radiograph is obtained and demonstrates a grossly dilated loop of intestine overlying the sacrum in the shape of an upside down U. **(SELECT 1 DIAGNOSIS)**

Items 379–380

For each patient, select the best course of action.

a. Administration of intravenous vasopressin
b. Administration of intraarterial vasopressin
c. Left thoracotomy, full-thickness suture ligation, and drainage of the pleural cavity
d. Balloon tamponade
e. Endoscopic control of bleeding
f. Gastrotomy and suture ligation
g. Insertion of a chest tube
h. Pulmonary arteriogram and streptokinase infusion
i. Cardiac catheterization and intraarterial infusion of tissue plasminogen activator

379. A 72-year-old man with severe coronary artery disease presents with painless hematemesis following a prolonged bout of vomiting. Upper endoscopy reveals a tear just below the gastroesophageal junction, which is actively bleeding. **(SELECT 3 ACTIONS)**

380. A 56-year-old man complains of the onset of severe substernal pain after a night of heavy drinking followed by uncontrolled retching. He states that there was a small amount of blood in his vomit. A chest x-ray shows a moderate-sized left pleural effusion. **(SELECT 1 ACTION)**

GASTROINTESTINAL TRACT, LIVER, AND PANCREAS

Answers

291. The answer is d. (*McQuaid, Surg Clin North Am 72:285–316, 1992.*) Omeprazole (Prilosec) irreversibly inhibits the hydrogen-potassium-ATPase (proton pump) in the secretory canaliculus of the gastric parietal cell. This blocks the last step in the acid-secretory process. Omeprazole's duration of action exceeds 24 h and doses of 20–30 mg per day inhibit more than 90% of 24-h acid secretion. Omeprazole provides excellent suppression of meal-stimulated and nocturnal acid secretion. It seems very safe for short-term therapy. However, its safety for long-term use is uncertain since it produces significant hypergastrinemia, hyperplasia of enterochromaffin-like cells, and carcinoid tumors in laboratory animals with prolonged administration.

292. The answer is d. (*Schwartz, 7/e, pp 1507–1508.*) Patients with ITP who have mild symptoms need no therapy, but they are usually advised to avoid contact sports and elective surgery. When symptoms (e.g., easy bruising, menorrhagia, bleeding gums) are troublesome, the bleeding time will be prolonged, capillary fragility greatly increased, and clot retraction poor. Corticosteroid therapy will increase the platelet count in over 75% of cases and provides the best indication that splenectomy will be of lasting benefit. The platelet count can be expected to rise shortly after splenectomy and prolonged remissions are anticipated in 80% of cases. The size of the spleen and the state of function in the bone marrow have no predictive value in assessing the likelihood of response to splenectomy. In children, complete spontaneous remissions are common (80% of cases) and surgical intervention should be avoided.

293. The answer is c. (*Schwartz, 7/e, pp 1249, 1387.*) This is an inflamed Meckel's diverticulum. This common lesion is often clinically indistinguishable from acute appendicitis. It is the remnant of the vitelline duct.

Meckel's diverticula are usually located 50–75 cm proximal to the ileocecal valve, are antimesenteric, and may contain either gastric and pancreatic or pancreatic tissue. Hemorrhage or obstruction is a more common presentation than inflammation. ^{99m}Tc pertechnetate has affinity for gastric mucosa and a scan with this isotope can aid in the diagnosis of this anomaly as a cause of lower gastrointestinal hemorrhage in a child. Angiography is more useful when looking for arteriovenous malformations. Since complications are relatively rare, most authors do not recommend removing asymptomatic diverticula when they are incidentally discovered during abdominal procedures. Those diverticula with a narrow neck, palpable heterotopic tissue, or nodularity are prone to obstruction and should be excised. In addition, patients explored for abdominal pain of unknown etiology should also undergo diverticulectomy, as should those operated on for appendicitis who are to be left with a scar of the right lower quadrant.

294. The answer is c. *(Schwartz, 7/e, pp 1126–1137.)* Patients with achalasia typically present with distal esophageal obstruction, which leads to regurgitation of saliva and undigested food. The characteristic appearance of the esophagram is the tapered "bird's beak" deformity at the level of the esophagogastric junction. Chest pain may be seen in the early stages of the disease. Manometry yields high resting pressures of the lower esophageal sphincter, which fails to relax or only partially relaxes. The absence of peristaltic deglutitory contractions in the body of the esophagus is also noted during manometry. Although both surgical intervention and forceful dilation have been used to treat this disease, surgery results in improvement in over 90% of patients, compared with only 70% of patients treated by forceful dilation. Surgical treatment is an esophagomyotomy. Patients with achalasia have seven times the risk of developing squamous cell carcinoma as compared with the general population. This dreaded complication can occur even after successful treatment for the disease.

295. The answer is d. *(Schwartz, 7/e, pp 1736–1737, 1768.)* Imperforate anus affects males and females with equal frequency, occurring in 1 of each 20,000 live births. It is due to failure of descent of the urorectal septum. Imperforate anus may be broadly classified into "high" or "low," depending on whether the rectum ends above or below the level of the levator ani complex. In 90% of females, but only 50% of males, the lesion is of the low variety. The rectal fistula may end in the prostatic urethra or vagina in the high cases, while the low cases terminate in a perineal fistula. For the low cases, only a perineal operation may be required and these children will be expected to be continent. A pull-through procedure will be required for the high imperforate anus and the likelihood of continence is smaller. If there is doubt about the level or location of the termination of the rectum, it is better to perform a temporary colostomy than to compromise the ultimate chances of continence by an injudicious perineal approach.

296–297. The answers are 296-c, 297-e. (*Greenfield, 2/e, p 916.*) This woman has a cystadenocarcinoma arising from the pancreatic body and tail, which was successfully resected. About 90% of primary malignant neoplasms of the exocrine pancreas are adenocarcinomas of duct cell origin. The remaining neoplasms include adenosquamous carcinoma, mucinous carcinomas, microadenocarcinoma, giant cell carcinoma, and cystadenocarcinoma of uncertain histogenesis. The clinical presentation is usually quite subtle, with symptoms related primarily to the enlarging mass. There are no diagnostic laboratory findings and definitive preoperative diagnosis is rare. An elderly patient with no history of pancreatitis is unlikely to have a pseudocyst and a benign neoplasm is also less likely in this age group. These less common carcinomas are often several times the size of typical ductal cancers and often arise in the body or tail of the pancreas. They may become very large without invading adjacent viscera and do not generally cause significant pain or weight loss. Therefore, even large tumors may be cured by resection, and aggressive surgical management is indicated.

298. The answer is c. (*Greenfield, 2/e, pp 1109–1127.*) Varying types of colonic polyps can be distinguished on pathologic examination. Adenomatous polyps are distributed throughout the entire large bowel, more commonly in the right and left colon than the rectum. They are often pedunculated and show an increased number of glands compared with normal mucosa. Although polyps that appear in familial polyposis are indistinguishable from single adenomatous polyps, they are manifested much earlier in life. Carcinomatous changes in patients who have familial polyposis occur approximately 20 years before carcinomatous changes of the bowel occur among patients in the general population.

299. The answer is c. (*Schwartz, 7/e, pp 472–473.*) According to the United Ostomy Association Data Registry, the most frequent serious complication of end colostomies is parastomal herniation, which commonly occurs when the stoma is placed lateral to, rather than through, the rectus muscle. Symptomatic herniation requires operative relocation of the stoma or mesh herniorrhaphy. Minor problems are frequently encountered with colostomies. They include irregularity of function, irritation of the skin due to leakage of enteric contents, or bleeding from the exposed mucosa following trauma. Prolapse occurs most frequently with transverse loop colostomies and is likely due to the use of the transverse loop to decompress distal colon obstructions. As the intestine decompresses, it retracts from the edge of the surrounding fascia, which allows prolapse or herniation of the mobile transverse colon. Optimal treatment of stomal prolapse is restoration of intestinal continuity or conversion to an end colostomy. Perforation of a stoma is usually due to careless instrumentation with an irrigation catheter. Perforations that cause minimal peritoneal contamination may be treated with observation and antibiotics, while more extensive leaks require operative closure.

300. The answer is d. *(Greenfield, 2/e, pp 901–915.)* The prognosis for a patient with carcinoma of the pancreas is dismal. The plurality of cases (46%) present as pain without jaundice; 34% present as pain with jaundice; and only 13% present with jaundice alone. Tumors over 1–2 cm may be seen by ultrasonography, computed tomography, or magnetic resonance imaging, but none of these methods can visualize smaller tumors. Endoscopic retrograde pancreaticocholangiography is helpful in distinguishing the more favorable tumors of the duodenum, ampulla, and common bile duct and lymphomas from cancer of the head of the pancreas. A combination of techniques including CT, angiography, and laparoscopy will accurately determine resectability in 97% of cases. Overall, the rate of resectability for possible cure is dismal: 5–10% of all patients and 10–25% of patients who present with jaundice alone, the latter due to earlier diagnosis of small tumors obstructing the common bile duct in the head of the pancreas. Ninety-nine percent of patients have metastatic disease at the time of diagnosis, and only 5–20% will be alive at 5 years following a pancreaticoduodenectomy.

301. The answer is c. *(Greenfield, 2/e, pp 759–773.)* Perforation of a duodenal ulcer is an indication for emergency celiotomy and closure of the perforation. In patients with no prior history of peptic ulcer disease, simple closure with an omental patch is recommended. Seventy-two percent of patients who are asymptomatic preoperatively will remain so postoperatively. Patients with long-standing ulcer disease require a definitive acid-reducing procedure, except in high-risk situations. The choice of procedure is made by weighing the risk of recurrence against the incidence of undesirable side effects of the procedure, and considerable controversy persists about this issue. Antrectomy and truncal vagotomy offers a recurrence rate of 1%, but carries a 15–25% incidence of sequelae such as diarrhea, dumping syndrome, bloating, and gastric stasis. Highly selective vagotomy, if technically feasible, offers a 1–5% incidence of side effects but carries a recurrence rate of 10–13% in some series, although results are better when gastric and prepyloric ulcers are excluded. In general, definitive acid-reducing procedures should be postponed if the perforation is more than 12 h old or if there is extensive peritoneal soilage. Pyloroplasty and truncal vagotomy carries intermediate rates of recurrence and side effects, but has the advantage of speed in the setting of very ill patients with acute perforation.

302. The answer is b. (*Sawyers, Am J Surg 159:8–14, 1990.*) Though reminiscent of the carcinoid syndrome, this patient's complaints in the context of recent gastric surgery are highly suggestive of the "dumping syndrome," seen after gastroenteric bypass such as antrectomy and gastrojejunostomy. Dumping syndrome presents as vasomotor symptoms (weakness, sweating, syncope) and intestinal symptoms (bloating, cramping, diarrhea). The etiology of dumping has best been attributed to the rapid influx of fluid with a high osmotic gradient into the small intestine from the gastric remnant. Medical management consists of reassurance and frequent small meals that are low in carbohydrates (to limit the osmotic load). Antispasmodic medications are sometimes used if dietary adjustments are unsuccessful. The majority of cases will resolve within 3 mo of operation on this regimen. Surgery for intractable dumping consists of creation of an antiperistaltic limb of jejunum distal to the gastrojejunostomy.

303. The answer is c. (*Greenfield, 2/e, pp 779–787.*) Benign gastric ulcers have a peak incidence in the fifth decade, with male predominance. About 95% of gastric ulcers are located near the lesser curvature. It should be recognized that up to 16% of patients with gastric carcinoma pass a 12-wk healing trial and that benign ulcers may enlarge during medical therapy.

Therefore, the possibility of malignancy must be assessed by biopsy despite a 5–10% false negative rate. Six weeks of medical therapy will heal many gastric ulcers, but a recurrence rate as high as 63% and the serious consequence of complications in this older group of patients warrant surgery for recurrent or nonhealing ulcers. A distal gastrectomy with gastroduodenostomy is usually feasible in the absence of duodenal disease. Vagotomy, while advocated by some, is generally not included. Local excision with definitive distal resection or vagotomy and pyloroplasty is appropriate for a proximal ulcer that would otherwise require a subtotal gastrectomy.

304–305. The answers are 304-d, 305-b. *(Greenfield, 2/e, pp 986–1005.)* The diagnosis of bleeding esophageal varices is aided in the adult by stigmata of portal hypertension. Upper gastrointestinal hemorrhage in cirrhotics is due to esophageal varices in less than half of patients. Gastritis and peptic ulcer disease account for the majority of cases. Esophagoscopy is the single most reliable means of establishing the source of bleeding, though variations in transvariceal blood flow may result in nonvisualization of the varices. In addition, endoscopic sclerotherapy is reported to control acute variceal hemorrhage in 80–90% of cases and carries an acute mortality lower than that of other procedures. Barium swallow has a high false negative rate and offers no therapeutic advantage. Celiac angiography will rule out arterial hemorrhage and will demonstrate venous collateral circulation, but will not demonstrate variceal bleeding. Parenteral vasopressin controls variceal hemorrhage by constriction of the splanchnic arteriolar bed and a resultant drop in portal pressure. Intraarterial vasopressin offers no advantage over intravenous administration and requires a mesenteric catheter. The reported control rate is 50–70%. Esophageal balloon tamponade controls variceal hemorrhage in two-thirds of patients, but may also control bleeding ulcers and thereby obscure the diagnosis. Although balloon tamponade has reduced the mortality and morbidity from variceal hemorrhage in good-risk patients, an increased awareness of associated complications (aspiration, asphyxiation, and ulceration at the tamponade site), as well as a rebleeding rate of 40%, has reduced its use. It is indicated as a temporary measure when vasopressin and sclerotherapy fail. Emergency portacaval shunt is advised in good-risk cirrhotic patients whose bleeding is not controlled with vasopressin or sclerosis. The mortality for patients with bleeding varices not subjected to shunting is between 66 and 73%, whereas operative mortality of emergency shunts ranges from 20 to 50%. Esophageal transection with the autostapler carries the same mortality as shunt procedures and the rebleeding rate is estimated to be 50% at 1 year.

306. The answer is c. (*Greenfield, 2/e, pp 1019–1021.*) Because approximately 5% of colorectal cancers are associated with resectable hepatic metastases, appropriate preoperative discussion should include obtaining permission for removal of synchronous peripheral hepatic lesions if they are found. If gross tumor is removed, a 25% "cure" rate can be anticipated. Adequate local resection, either by wedge or by limited partial hepatectomy, may be carried out whenever no extrahepatic disease is found and the hepatic lesion is technically removable. Any option that leaves the potentially obstructing primary cancer unremoved would be unacceptable. Radiation therapy has little to offer in colon cancer or its hepatic metastases. Local infusion of floxuridine (FUDR) via an implantable Infusaid pump for 14 days at 0.3 mg/kg/day has been reported to provide some acceptable palliation in selected patients with unresectable hepatic lesions.

307. The answer is b. (*Schwesinger, Am J Surg 172:411–417, 1996.*) Helicobacter pylori infections have become extremely common. Nearly a third of all American adults are now infected. Morphologically, the organism is a gram-negative, corkscrew-shaped, motile bacillus with three–seven flagella. Noninvasive approaches with simple, relatively inexpensive serologic and urea breath tests can establish the diagnosis of H. pylori infection. Culturing endoscopic scrapings or biopsy specimens has proved to be impractical because of the need for special media and elaborate growth conditions. A rapid urease test is used when endoscopy provides a specimen for analysis. Therapy is problematic because the organism is not easily eradicated. Monotherapy is largely ineffective. However, dual- and triple-drug therapy can achieve eradication in 80–90% of patients. Unfortunately, compliance rates with multidrug therapy are low.

308. The answer is c. (*Zinner, 10/e, pp 479–572.*) An indirect inguinal hernia leaves the abdominal cavity by entering the dilated internal inguinal ring and passing along the anteromedial aspect of the spermatic cord. The internal inguinal ring is an opening in the transversalis fascia for the passage of the spermatic cord; an indirect inguinal hernia, therefore, lies within the fibers of the cremaster muscle. Repair consists of removing the hernia sac and tightening the internal inguinal ring. A femoral hernia passes directly beneath the inguinal ligament at a point medial to the femoral vessels, and a direct inguinal hernia passes through a weakness in the floor of the inguinal canal medial to the inferior epigastric artery. Each is dependent on defects in Hesselbach's triangle of transversalis fascia and neither lies within the cremaster muscle fibers. Repair consists of reconstructing the floor of the inguinal canal. Spigelian hernias, which are rare, protrude through an anatomic defect that can occur along the lateral border of the rectus muscle at its junction with the linea semilunaris. An interparietal hernia is one in which the hernia sac, instead of protruding in the usual fashion, makes its way between the fascial layers of the abdominal wall. These unusual hernias may be preperitoneal (between the peritoneum and transversalis fascia), interstitial (between muscle layers), or superficial (between the external oblique aponeurosis and the skin).

309. The answer is b. (*Zinner, 10/e, pp 581–591.*) The finding of air in the biliary tract of a nonseptic patient is diagnostic of a biliary enteric fistula. When the clinical findings also include small bowel obstruction in an elderly patient without a history of prior abdominal surgery (a "virgin" abdomen), the diagnosis of gallstone ileus can be made with a high degree of certainty. In this condition, a large chronic gallstone mechanically erodes through the wall of the gallbladder into adjacent stomach or duodenum. As the stone moves down the small intestine, mild cramping symptoms are common. When the gallstone arrives in the distal ileum, the caliber of the bowel no longer allows passage and obstruction develops. Surgical removal of the gallstone is necessary. The diseases suggested by each of the other response items (bleeding ulcer, peritoneal infection, pyloric outlet obstruction, pelvic neoplasm) are common in elderly patients, but each of them would probably present with symptoms other than those of small bowel obstruction.

310. The answer is d. (*Zinner, 10/e, pp 1286–1300.*) Cancer of the colon in patients with chronic ulcerative colitis is 10 times more frequent than in the general population. Duration of disease is very important; the risk of developing cancer is low in the first 10 years but thereafter rises about 4% per year. The average age of cancer development in patients with chronic ulcerative colitis is 37 years; idiopathic carcinoma of the colon, however, develops at an average age of 65 years. Crohn's colitis is currently felt to be a precancerous condition as well. The chance of development of carcinoma of the colon in patients with familial polyposis is essentially 100%. Treatment of the patient with familial polyposis generally consists of subtotal colectomy with ileoproctostomy and regular proctoscopic examination of the rectal stump. Villous adenomas have been demonstrated to contain malignant portions in about one-third of affected persons and invasive malignancy in another one-third of removed specimens. Anterior resection is performed for large lesions or those containing invasive carcinomas when the lesion is above the peritoneal reflection. Abdominoperineal resection is indicated for low-lying rectal villous adenomas when they have demonstrated invasive carcinomas. Transrectal excision with regular follow-up examinations is sufficient for lesions without invasive carcinomas. Peutz-Jeghers syndrome is characterized by intestinal polyposis and melanin spots of the oral mucosa. Unlike the adenomatous polyps seen in familial polyposis, the lesions in this condition are hamartomas, which have no malignant potential.

311. The answer is c. *(Greenfield, 2/e, pp 825–826.)* Gallstone ileus is due to erosion of a stone from the gallbladder into the gastrointestinal tract (most commonly into the duodenum). The stone becomes lodged in the small bowel (usually in the terminal ileum) and causes small-bowel obstruction. Plain films of the abdomen that demonstrate small-bowel obstruction and air in the biliary tract are diagnostic of the condition. Treatment consists of ileotomy, removal of the stone, and cholecystectomy if it is technically safe. If there is significant inflammation of the right upper quadrant, ileotomy for stone extraction followed by an interval cholecystectomy is often a safer alternative. Operating on the biliary fistula doubles the mortality rate compared with simple removal of the gallstone from the intestine.

312. The answer is a. *(Greenfield, 2/e, pp 2057–2066.)* Hirschsprung's disease, which is the congenital absence of ganglion cells in the rectum or rectosigmoid colon, is definitively diagnosed by rectal biopsy. The typical findings on barium enema, a distal narrow segment of bowel with markedly distended colon proximally, may not be seen early in life. Symptoms may go unrecognized in the newborn period with consequent development of malnutrition or enterocolitis. Initial treatment is colostomy decompression. Definitive repair is best delayed until nutritional status is adequate and the chronically distended bowel has returned to normal size. Unlike the situation with imperforate anus, which is associated with a high incidence of genitourinary tract anomalies and a 50% incidence of long-term fecal incontinence, in Hirschsprung's disease repair leads to satisfactory bowel function in most affected patients.

313. The answer is a. (*Zinner, 10/e, pp 529–531.*) Omphalocele and gastroschisis result in evisceration of bowel and require emergency surgical treatment to effect immediate or staged reduction and abdominal wall closure. Patent urachal or omphalomesenteric ducts result from incomplete closure of embryonic connections from the bladder and ileum, respectively, to the abdominal wall. They are appropriately treated by excision of the tracts and closure of the bladder or ileum. In most children, umbilical hernias close spontaneously by the age of 4 and need not be repaired unless incarceration or marbled enlargement and distortion of the umbilicus occur.

314. The answer is d. (*Zinner, 10/e, pp 1855–1865.*) Laparoscopic cholecystectomy is now viewed as the treatment of choice for most patients with symptomatic gallstones. This procedure has frequently been performed in obese patients with the same efficiency, morbidity and mortality rates, and length of hospitalization as in the average-weight population. The other conditions listed represent currently accepted relative contraindications, but as experience increases and techniques improve, the safe indications for laparoscopic cholecystectomy are likely to expand.

315. The answer is d. (*Zinner, 10/e, pp 2097–2115.*) Congenital anorectal anomalies are frequently associated with other congenital anomalies including heart disease, esophageal atresia, abnormalities of the lumbosacral spine, double urinary collecting systems, hydronephrosis, and communication between the rectum and the urinary tract, vagina, or perineum. They occur in approximately 1 in 2000 live births. Depending on the type of anomaly (whether the rectum ends above or below the level of the levator ani complex), a variety of surgical procedures has been devised to treat the problem. However, even when anatomic integrity is established, the prognosis for effective toilet training is poor. In 50% of cases continence is never achieved. Cervical spine abnormalities, hydrocephalus, duodenal atresia, and corneal opacities have no significant association with congenital anorectal anomalies.

316. The answer is c. *(Greenfield, 2/e, p 1236.)* Hematomas of the rectus sheath are more common in women and present most often in the fifth decade. A history of trauma, sudden muscular exertion, or anticoagulation can usually be elicited. The pain is of sudden onset and is sharp in nature. The hematoma is most common in the right lower quadrant and irritation of the peritoneum leads to fever, leukocytosis, anorexia, and nausea. Preoperatively the diagnosis can be established with an ultrasound or CT scan showing a mass within the rectus sheath. Management is conservative unless symptoms are severe and bleeding persists, in which case surgical evacuation of the hematoma and ligation of bleeding vessels is required.

317. The answer is d. *(Zinner, 10/e, pp 2083–2087.)* This is an example of an ileal atresia. Whether the atresia is jejunal or ileal does not affect treatment and there is no predilection for one site over the other. Resection and primary anastomosis should be performed if possible, but the bowel should be exteriorized if there is a question of viability or there is a large size discrepancy between two segments. Plain films will reveal a small bowel obstruction with no gas beyond the lesion. A carefully administered meglumine diatrizoate (Gastrografin) enema can help in the differential diagnosis. Midgut volvulus and meconium ileus can be apparent on an enema, which is important as meconium ileus should be managed nonoperatively. The basis of jejunoileal atresia is probably a mesenteric vascular accident during intrauterine growth.

318. The answer is b. *(Greenfield, 2/e, pp 680–694.)* Surgical treatment for sliding esophageal hernias should only be considered in symptomatic patients with objectively documented esophagitis or stenosis. The overwhelming majority of sliding hiatal hernias are totally asymptomatic, even many of those with demonstrable reflux. Even in the presence of reflux, esophageal inflammation rarely develops because the esophagus is so efficient at clearing the refluxed acid. Symptomatic hernias should be treated vigorously by the variety of medical measures that have been found helpful. Patients who do have symptoms of episodic reflux and who remain untreated can expect their disease to progress to intolerable esophagitis or fibrosis and stenosis. Neither the presence of the hernia nor its size is important in deciding on surgical therapy. Once esophagitis has been documented to persist under adequate medical therapy, manometric or pH studies may help determine the optimum surgical treatment.

319. The answer is b. (*Zinner, 10/e, pp 1739–1751.*) While elevation of SGOT and SGPT are indicative of hepatocellular disease, elevated alkaline phosphatase is indicative of biliary obstruction. Based on safety and cost, ultrasonography is the initial diagnostic procedure. Once ductal dilation is identified, a percutaneous transhepatic cholangiogram or ERCP may be performed to localize and characterize the obstruction. If a distal common bile duct obstruction is noted, a CT scan is recommended to image the head of the pancreas. In most instances, a liver-spleen scan adds little to the diagnostic workup. This also applies to the upper gastrointestinal series. Cancer of the head of the pancreas is associated with painless jaundice.

320. The answer is a. (*Schwartz, 7/e, pp 1417–1420.*) Massive hematemesis in children is almost always due to variceal bleeding. The varices usually result from extrahepatic portal vein obstruction consequent to bacterial infection transmitted via a patent umbilical vein during infancy. In spite of this common cause, a history of neonatal omphalitis is infrequently obtainable. Bleeding can be massive but is usually self-limited, and esophageal tamponade or vasopressin is usually not necessary. Elective portal-systemic decompression is recommended for recurrent bleeding episodes.

321. The answer is c. (*Schwartz, 7/e, pp 1181, 1187–1188.*) The proximal stomach can distend or accommodate a large volume without any increase in intragastric pressure. This phenomenon permits solid food to settle along the greater curvature while liquids are propelled along the lesser curvature by slow tonic contractions of the upper stomach. In the normal state, once a volume of 1000–1200 mL is reached, intragastric pressure rises to high levels. While the stomach's ability to accommodate large volumes is necessary for normal gastric motor activity, a potentially deleterious effect is seen in patients with gastric atony. These patients may accumulate several liters of gastric juice in the stomach without sensing fullness, and this often leads to massive emesis and aspiration.

322. The answer is b. (*Schwartz, 7/e, pp 1265–1274.*) Because the reserve capacity of the colon for water absorption greatly exceeds the normal requirements for maintaining stable bowel function, patients may undergo resection of a large fraction of the colon and suffer little change in bowel habits. Neither the right nor the left colon appears to be a site of preferential water and electrolyte absorption, nor does the ileocecal valve play a noticeable role in fluid homeostasis. However, in diseases characterized by increased fluid secretion of the small bowel, the colon is more likely to be overwhelmed by the absorptive demand following partial colectomy than in the intact state. The rectum does not appear to play a role in fluid absorption.

323. The answer is e. (*Zinner, 10/e, pp 1455–1500.*) Workup of a patient with a diagnosed rectal cancer should include CT scan of the upper abdomen in search of liver metastases and assessment of the depth of local invasion by transanal ultrasound. Sonographic staging of the rectal wall and pararectal lymph nodes has become crucial in planning the magnitude of the resection and choice of preoperative treatment. The survival advantages of neoadjuvant radiation therapy now seem clear. Administering radiation preoperatively to large or deeply invasive tumors often reduces the tumor mass and permits clean resection of previously bulky disease. In addition, the cytoreductive effect of preoperative radiation therapy now allows many patients to undergo sphincter-saving procedures and avoid the morbidity of proctectomy and colostomy.

324. The answer is a. (*Greenfield, 2/e, pp 812–816.*) Digestion and absorption of dietary carbohydrate by the duodenum and small intestine are so avid that complete absorption has already occurred by the time ingested food has traversed 200 cm of jejunum. Simple fluids that require minimal digestion, such as milk, are entirely absorbed, save for their fat content, within the duodenum. Even in the short gut syndrome, virtually all dietary carbohydrate is absorbed within the residual jejunum. While pancreatic peptidases are important to protein digestion, redundant digestive enzymes are so widely distributed within the duodenal and jejunal brush border that 95% of a protein meal can be absorbed in the absence of the pancreas. Salt and water flux in the small intestine is influenced by a variety of hormones; aldosterone markedly increases sodium uptake, while prostaglandins stimulate fluid and electrolyte secretion.

325. The answer is d. (*Greenfield, 2/e, pp 749–751.*) Gastrin, an aqueous extract of the antral G cell, stimulates acid and pepsin secretion. A variety of local stimuli cause the release of gastrin. The most potent of these are small proteins, 20-proof alcohol, and caffeine. Acidic antral contents inhibit gastrin secretion; alkalinization of the antrum is stimulatory. Mechanical distention of the antrum also stimulates gastrin secretion.

326. The answer is a. *(Greenfield, 2/e, p 816.)* As it does with carbohydrate digestion, the gastrointestinal tract exhibits remarkable redundancy and alternative pathways to facilitate fat uptake. In the normal state, water-insoluble dietary lipid is rendered into soluble micelles through mixing with pancreatic and intestinal lipase and with bile. However, lipases of the stomach and small intestine permit absorption of approximately half of neutral dietary fat in the absence of bile and pancreatic secretion. Small breakdown products of complex fats—such as glycerol, short-chain fatty acids, and medium-chain triglycerides—can be transported directly from the jejunal mucosal cell into the portal venous system, whereas larger triglycerides, resynthesized by the mucosal cells from fatty acids, are deposited in chylomicrons and released into the lymphatic system. Enterohepatic recirculation of bile with active resorption in the ileum and secretion into the portal venous system yields an effective bile salt pool 6–8 times its actual volume. Normal daily losses of bile into the stool represent 10–15% of the total bile salt pool; these losses can usually be replaced by new synthesis in the liver. However, bile salt-wasting states, such as inflammatory bowel disease or ileal resection, may exceed the liver's capacity to maintain an adequate volume of bile.

327. The answer is e. *(Schwartz, 7/e, pp 1728–1729.)* A bypass procedure is the operation of choice for obstruction secondary to an annular pancreas. A Whipple procedure is too radical a therapy for this benign disease, and a partial resection of the annular pancreas often is complicated by fistula. Duodenojejunostomy is much more physiologic than gastrojejunostomy and does not require a vagotomy to prevent marginal ulceration; it is therefore the procedure of choice.

328. The answer is b. *(Schwartz, 7/e, pp 1231–1232, 1387.)* Patients with regional enteritis usually have a chronic and slowly progressive course with intermittent symptom-free periods. The usual symptoms are anorexia, abdominal pain, diarrhea, fever, and weight loss. There are extraintestinal syndromes that may be seen, such as ankylosing spondylitis; polyarthritis; erythema nodosum; pyoderma gangrenosum; gallstones; hepatic fatty infiltration; and fibrosis of the biliary tract, pancreas, and retroperitoneum. However, in about 10% of patients, especially those who are young, the onset of the disease is abrupt and may be mistaken for acute appendicitis. Appendectomy is indicated in such patients as long as the cecum at the base of the appendix is not involved; otherwise the risk of fecal fistula must be considered. Interestingly, about 90% of patients who present with the acute appendicitis-like form of regional enteritis will not progress to development of the full-blown chronic disease. Thus, resection or bypass of the involved areas is not indicated at this time.

329. The answer is c. *(Moosa, Arch Surg 125:1028–1031, 1990. Schwartz, 7/e, p 1446.)* The scenario in the question is a typical course of a patient with iatrogenic injury of the common bile duct. These injuries commonly occur in the proximal portion of the extrahepatic biliary system. The transhepatic cholangiogram documents a biliary stricture, which in this clinical setting is best dealt with surgically. Choledochoduodenostomy generally cannot be performed because of the proximal location of the stricture. The best results are achieved with end-to-side choledochojejunostomy (Roux-en-Y) performed over a stent. Percutaneous transhepatic dilation has been attempted in select cases, but follow-up is too short to make an adequate assessment of this technique. Primary repair of the common bile duct may result in recurrent stricture.

330. The answer is e. *(Schwartz, 7/e, pp 1341–1346.)* Many authorities now recommend abandonment of the phrase *carcinoma in situ* because it gives a misleading impression to the patient and family regarding the true implications of severe dysplasia. Almost all agree that no further treatment is indicated when a polyp has been adequately removed and such changes are found. Only when malignant cells penetrate the muscularis mucosae is there any potential for metastases, and only when that depth of penetration is seen should the term *carcinoma* be used. Even then resection is probably not indicated if the gross and microscopic margins are clear, the tumor is well differentiated, and the stalk is not invaded.

331. The answer is b. *(Schwartz, 7/e, pp 1253–1255.)* The effects of radiation on the intestine depend on a variety of factors, which include the age of the patient, temperature, degree of oxygenation, and metabolic activity. Acute intestinal radiation injury is manifested in the bowel by the cessation of viable cell production and is seen clinically as diarrhea or gastrointestinal bleeding. Progressive vasculitis and fibrosis are seen in the latter stages of radiation injury and may result in malabsorption, ulceration, fistulization, or perforation. Intussusception is generally not associated with radiation injury.

332. The answer is d. (*Greenfield, 2/e, pp 757–758, 807–808.*) Drugs, hormones, or emotional states (e.g., fear) that stimulate or simulate sympathetic activity inhibit intestinal motility. Those factors that arouse parasympathetic activity (acetylcholine) stimulate motility. Gastrin has specific delaying effects on gastric emptying. Secretin and cholecystokinin are potent regulators of intestinal and digestive activities but probably have no effect on motility per se.

333. The answer is d. (*Greenfield, 2/e, pp 698–712.*) Carcinoma of the esophagus occurs primarily in the sixth and seventh decades of life in a male:female ratio of 3:1. Although the cause is unknown; alcohol, tobacco, and dietary factors have been implicated as causative agents. A high incidence is reported in patients with corrosive esophagitis. The malignant tumors arising in the esophagus are usually squamous cell carcinomas except those involving the esophagogastric junction, which are usually adenocarcinomas. Even though squamous cell carcinomas are weakly radiosensitive, surgical extirpation affords reasonable, if short-term, palliation. Some authorities recommend radiotherapy for palliation alone or in combination with surgery to treat this lesion. Adenocarcinomas are not particularly radiosensitive and surgical treatment is generally employed. Following resection for esophageal carcinoma among the highly select group of patients whose tumors are still resectable when the diagnosis is made, survival is only about 14% at 5 years. The overall 5-year survival is under 5%.

334–335. The answers are 334-b, 335-b. (*Greenfield, 2/e, pp 919–925.*) Total gastrectomy was formerly the procedure of choice for patients with Zollinger-Ellison syndrome (ZES). However, with the knowledge that most patients will die of metastatic disease and that the symptoms can often be controlled with H_2 receptor antagonists, the role for surgery has changed. Initial surgical exploration is aimed at curative resection of the tumor. Unfortunately metastatic disease is often present or will develop at a later date despite tumor resection. Therefore, highly selective vagotomy is also added to the procedure to reduce the required dose of H_2 receptor antagonists.

The second patient has a gastrin level suggestive of but not diagnostic of ZES. A secretin stimulation test will cause a significant rise in serum gastrin levels in patients with ZES.

336. The answer is a. (*Greenfield, 2/e, pp 1243–1244.*) Idiopathic retroperitoneal fibrosis is a nonsuppurative inflammatory process of the retroperitoneum that causes problems by extrinsic compression of retroperitoneal structures. The ureters, aorta, and inferior vena cava are most at risk; however, the aorta is quite resistant to compression and the inferior vena cava has multiple collaterals, so that ureteral obstruction is the most common presentation of this disease process. The common bile duct and duodenum may be compressed and obstructed, but this occurs much less frequently. Treatment of ureteral obstruction includes conservative therapy with steroids. Surgical intervention is often required and ureterolysis with intraperitoneal transplantation is the current procedure of choice. Biopsies must also be taken to exclude a malignant process as the cause of the fibrosis.

337. The answer is b. (*Greenfield, 2/e, pp 919–923.*) Tumors arising from the pancreatic β cells give rise to hyperinsulinism. Seventy-five percent of these tumors are benign adenomas and in 15% of affected patients the adenomas are multiple. Symptoms relate to a rapidly falling blood glucose level and are due to epinephrine release triggered by hypoglycemia (sweating, weakness, tachycardia). Cerebral symptoms of headache, confusion, visual disturbances, convulsions, and coma are due to glucose deprivation of the brain. Whipple's triad summarizes the clinical findings in patients with insulinomas: (1) attacks precipitated by fasting or exertion; (2) fasting blood glucose concentrations below 50 mg/dL; (3) symptoms relieved by oral or intravenous glucose administration. These tumors are treated surgically and simple excision of an adenoma is curative in the majority of cases.

338. The answer is e. (*Greenfield, 2/e, pp 1148–1150.*) Epidermoid cancers of the anal canal metastasize to inguinal nodes as well as to the perirectal and mesenteric nodes. The results of local radical surgery have been disappointing. Combined external radiation (dose range 3500–5000 cG) with synchronous chemotherapy (fluorouracil and mitomycin) is now recommended as the means for controlling the disease. Radical surgical approaches are now generally reserved for treatment failures and recurrences.

339. The answer is c. (*Greenfield, 2/e, pp 1137–1141.*) A markedly distended colon could have many causes in this 80-year-old man. The contrast study, however, reveals a classic "apple core" lesion in the distal colon, which is diagnostic of colon cancer. No further diagnostic studies are appropriate prior to relief of this large bowel obstruction. After medical preparation (e.g., hydration, normalization of electrolytes), this patient should undergo prompt surgical management of his mechanical obstruction; conservative management by resection and proximal colostomy would generally be preferred in this elderly patient with an obstructed, unprepared bowel.

340. The answer is e. (*Greenfield, 2/e, pp 831–843.*) Surgical treatment of Crohn's disease is aimed at correcting complications that are causing symptoms. Intestinal obstruction is usually partial and secondary to a fixed stricture that is not responsive to anti-inflammatory agents. When the obstruction causes symptoms that compromise nutritional status, surgery is warranted. Fistula formation in itself is not an indication for surgery. Fistulas between the intestine and the bladder and the intestine and the vagina, however, generally cause significant symptoms and warrant surgical intervention, while an ileum–ascending colon fistula is very common yet rarely symptomatic. Perforation of bowel into the free abdominal cavity is obviously a surgical emergency.

341. The answer is e. (*Greenfield, 2/e, pp 827, 1092–1093.*) The film shows a markedly distended colon. The differential diagnosis includes tumor, foreign body, and colitis, but far more likely is either cecal or sigmoid volvulus. Sigmoid volvulus may be ruled out quickly by proctosigmoidoscopy, which is preferable to barium enema, since sigmoid volvulus may be treated successfully by rectal tube decompression via the sigmoidoscope. If sigmoidoscopy is negative, the working diagnosis, based on this classic film, must be cecal volvulus; barium enema would clinch the diagnosis, but the colon might rupture in the intervening 1–2 h. Emergency celiotomy should be done.

342. The answer is c. (*Graham, Gastroenterology 105:279–282, 1993.*) *Helicobacter pylori* is a spiral-shaped, gram-negative bacterium that is found in the viscous gastric mucus layer and has an affinity for epithelial cells. It was originally classified as a form of *Campylobacter,* but its genomic and phenotypic characteristics were subsequently found to be unique and it was given a new genus name. Urease and other peptides released by H. *pylori* may be toxic and cause direct gastroduodenal injury. Evidence is strong that H. *pylori* plays a role in the etiology of ulcer disease. There is an almost 100% association between gastric H. *pylori* infection and duodenal ulcer disease, and about 70% of patients with gastric ulcers are also infected with H. *pylori*. Furthermore, colonization with H. *pylori* increases the risk of developing a duodenal ulcer by up to 20-fold. Eradication of H. *pylori* from the stomach markedly decreases the rate of ulcer recurrence. This generally requires "triple therapy" with colloidal bismuth (Pepto-Bismol), an antibiotic (amoxicillin or ampicillin), and a nitroimidazole such as metronidazole. Recent studies have also demonstrated a possible association between H. *pylori* infection and gastric carcinoma.

343. The answer is e. *(Schwartz, 7/e, pp 1275–1277.)* The history, x-ray, and clinical findings are typical of a postoperative cecal volvulus, a condition in which the cecum is twisted on its mesentery (often, after aneurysm resection, a neomesentery) and becomes acutely obstructed. At 12 cm, the cecum is in imminent danger of perforation. Particularly in the presence of a prosthetic graft, cecal perforation is a catastrophe. Urgent decompression is needed. To attempt colonoscopic decompression would necessitate insufflation of additional air and increase the stress on the already compromised cecal wall. A transverse colostomy "decompression" would not decompress the cecum nor would it provide detorsion of the cecal mesentery to allow restoration of adequate blood supply to the right colon. While untwisting the cecum and fixing it to the lateral abdominal wall (to inhibit recurrence) by a decompressing cecostomy might be advocated in some settings, the risk of contaminating the aortic graft would be excessive. Resection of the offending organ with ileotransverse colostomy would be the procedure of choice.

344. The answer is d. *(Case Records, N Engl J Med 317:1209–1218, 1987.)* Hydatid cysts secondary to echinococcal infection are most common in the liver in adults. Up to 25% of patients with hepatic cysts also have cysts in their lungs. In general, serologic tests are more likely to be positive the longer the lesion has been present, but false negativity occurs with sufficient frequency that results should not influence the decision to treat hepatic hydatid cysts. Spontaneous rupture of the cyst or leakage of cyst fluid during diagnostic or therapeutic aspiration may cause anaphylactic reactions or peritoneal dissemination of the disease. Definitive treatment requires surgical resection, enucleation, or evacuation of the cysts. Agents such as 0.5% silver nitrate or hypertonic saline are introduced into the cyst at the time of surgery, and efforts are made to avoid spillage and contamination of the peritoneal cavity. Treatment of patients with liver cysts with mebendazole or albendazole has not been effective enough to replace the need for surgery.

345. The answer is a. (*Mahmoodian, South Med J 85:19–24, 1992.*) Appendicitis complicates approximately 1 in 1700 pregnancies at an incidence comparable with that in nonpregnant women matched for age. It is the most prevalent extrauterine indication for laparotomy in pregnancy. The duration of gestation does not influence the severity of the disease, but the diagnosis does become more difficult as the pregnancy progresses. By the twentieth week of gestation the appendix often lies at the level of the umbilicus and more lateral than usual. Pregnancy should not delay surgery if appendicitis is suspected; appendiceal perforation greatly increases the chance of premature labor and fetal mortality (approximately 20% for each). In contrast, negative laparotomy under general anesthesia and non-perforated appendicitis are associated with very low risk to both the fetus and mother (less than 1% and 5%, respectively).

346. The answer is b. (*Schwartz, 7/e, pp 1161–1169.*) Normal respiration creates negative pressure in the thoracic cavity. As a result of the pressure gradient, blood enters the chest via the venae cava and air via the trachea; both are life-sustaining results of this pressure gradient. The pathophysiologic consequence of a hole in the diaphragm is that eventually abdominal viscera will be aspirated into the thorax. The sliding hernia, contained in the lower mediastinum by intact pleura, may rarely cause symptoms of reflux that would justify surgical attention, but such patients are in no danger of vascular compromise or of obstructive displacement of hollow viscera. The paraesophageal hernia, on the other hand, leaves the patient at substantial risk for both strangulation and obstruction. Either result would be a surgical catastrophe; with rare exceptions, paraesophageal hernias should be surgically repaired whenever diagnosed. A traction diverticulum is usually caused by inflammatory contraction around mediastinal nodes, is rarely of any symptomatic consequence, and need not be repaired. Neither the Schatzki's ring nor the esophageal web justifies esophageal surgery. They can be ignored or dilated as symptoms demand.

347. The answer is d. (*Greenfield, 2/e, pp 1092–1093.*) As classically described, Olgilvie syndrome was associated with the rare occurrence of malignant infiltration of the colonic sympathetic nerve supply in the region of the celiac plexus. The eponym is now applied to the condition in which massive cecal and colonic dilation is seen in the absence of mechanical obstruction. Other terms used to describe this condition are *acute colonic pseudo-obstruction, colonic ileus,* and *functional colonic obstruction.* It tends to occur in elderly patients in the setting of cardiopulmonary insufficiency, in other systemic disorders that require prolonged bed rest, and in the postoperative state. The diagnosis of Olgilvie syndrome cannot be confirmed until mechanical obstruction of the distal colon is excluded by colonoscopy or contrast enema. Anticholinergic agents and narcotics need to be discontinued, but any delay in decompressing the dilated cecum is inappropriate since colonic ischemia and perforation become a distinct hazard as the cecum reaches this degree of dilation. Cautious endoscopic colonic decompression has been demonstrated recently to be a safe and effective form of treatment. Endoscopy should be combined with rectal tube placement, correction of metabolic abnormalities, and the discontinuation of medications that diminish gastrointestinal motility. The high complication rate in this population notwithstanding, a direct surgical approach to decompression becomes necessary when colonoscopic decompression fails; a perforated cecum is a catastrophic event in such patients.

348. The answer is c. (*Schwartz, 7/e, p 1125.*) Zenker's diverticulum is an acquired abnormality. Premature contraction of the cricopharyngeus muscle on swallowing, which leads to partial obstruction, is believed to be the cause of this pulsion-type diverticulum of the pharyngoesophageal junction. High intraluminal pressure results in an outpouching of mucosa through the oblique fibers of the pharyngeal constrictors. Dysphagia is common and is the usual presenting symptom. The diagnosis is established by barium swallow. Treatment is surgical: diverticulectomy or suspension of the diverticulum is usually recommended. Because the diverticulum is located above the superior esophageal sphincter, no mechanism exists to prevent aspiration of the contents of the diverticulum. Pulmonary complications are common.

349. The answer is a. (*Merrell, West J Med 155:621–625, 1991.*) The classic Quincke triad of abdominal pain in the right upper quadrant, jaundice, and gastrointestinal bleeding is present in 30–40% of patients with hemobilia. With more frequent use of percutaneous liver procedures (e.g., transhepatic cholangiogram, transhepatic catheter drainage), iatrogenic injury has replaced other trauma as the most common cause of bloody bile. Other causes include spontaneous bleeding during anticoagulation, gallstones, parasitic infections/abscesses, and neoplastic lesions. Angiography and endoscopy are useful diagnostic studies and intrahepatic bleeding can be controlled by angiographic embolization in up to 95% of cases. Surgical treatment is advocated for bleeding from extrahepatic bile ducts or the gallbladder or in cases of penetrating trauma in which associated injuries might need attention.

350. The answer is d. (*Podolosky, N Engl J Med 325:928–937, 1991.*) The patient depicted in this question has Crohn's disease of the colon (Crohn's colitis). Crohn's colitis is characterized by linear mucosal ulcerations, discontinuous ("skip") lesions, a transmural inflammatory process, and noncaseating granulomata in up to 50% of patients. Because their clinical features and management differ, Crohn's colitis must be distinguished from ulcerative colitis. Ulcerative colitis is usually found in the rectum, although in rare cases the rectum is spared involvement. The entire colon, from cecum to rectum, may be involved ("pancolitis"). Ulcerative colitis typically presents as a grossly continuous inflammatory process (without skip lesions) that microscopically is confined to the mucosa and submucosa of the colon. In addition, crypt abscesses and superficial ulcerations are common in ulcerative colitis.

351. The answer is c. (*Podolosky, N Engl J Med 325:928–937, 1991.*) Patients with Crohn's disease can develop fistulas between the colon and other segments of intestine, the bladder, urethra, vagina, skin, and prostate in the male. Intestinal perforation can occur in about 5% of patients. Toxic megacolon can occur in patients with Crohn's disease, ulcerative colitis, or any severe inflammatory process of the large intestine. Extraintestinal manifestations are usually associated with active disease. Finally, patients with Crohn's colitis have a 5.6-fold increased risk of colon cancer relative to an age-matched population.

352. The answer is c. (*Schwartz, 7/e, pp 1161–1169.*) The condition demonstrated is a paraesophageal hernia. It is encountered much less frequently (approximately 5%) than is the sliding hiatal hernia and it has completely different therapeutic implications. Paraesophageal hernias are acquired, rarely present before middle age, and are most common in patients in their seventh decade. The position of the gastroesophageal junction distinguishes the two types of hernias, which occur near the esophageal hiatus of the diaphragm. In the more common sliding hernia, the gastroesophageal junction protrudes above the diaphragm; in the paraesophageal hernia, the anatomic junction between the esophagus and the stomach is anchored in its normal position below the diaphragm. The gastric cardia or fundus and occasionally other viscera herniate into the thorax within a true peritoneal sac alongside the gastroesophageal junction. Surgical repair is indicated as soon as the patient can be properly prepared for the procedure, as bleeding, ulceration, obstruction, necrosis of the stomach wall, and perforation are common.

353. The answer is b. (*Schwartz, 7/e, pp 1488–1492.*) The vast majority of pancreatic carcinomas are located in the head of the gland. Patients may present with painless jaundice by virtue of the carcinoma's obstruction of the intrapancreatic portion of the common bile duct. It is in this group of patients that resection is possible, although most tumors will be unresectable. Tumors in the body or tail of the gland are universally unresectable. The cause of pancreatic cancer is not known. There is a very strong association with diabetes mellitus (but not diabetes insipidus), but the nature of this relationship is not known. Prognosis is uniformly dismal whether resection is done or not, and only an anecdotal survivor will be alive at 5-year follow-up.

354. The answer is b. (*Schwartz, 7/e, pp 1732–1734.*) Intussusception is the result of invagination of a segment of bowel into distal bowel lumen. The most common type is ileocolic, which typically appears as a "coiled spring" on barium enema. Ileoileal and colocolic intussusceptions occur less commonly and are not easily diagnosed on barium enema. If bloody mucus, peritonitis, or systemic toxicity have not developed, hydrostatic reduction by barium enema is the appropriate initial treatment. Most patients are successfully managed this way and do not require surgical intervention. Immediate treatment should be instituted to avert the danger of bowel infarction. Recurrence is surprisingly uncommon after either surgical or nonsurgical treatment.

355. The answer is d. *(Schwartz, 7/e, pp 1244–1246.)* Carcinoid tumors arise from the neuroectoderm and are a type of apudoma. The most common site of carcinoid tumors is the small bowel, although appendiceal carcinoids are also common. Carcinoid syndrome, which is characterized by flushing, diarrhea, and cardiac valvular disease, occurs in a small percentage of patients with carcinoid tumors; it is rarely seen with appendiceal carcinoids. It occurs when serotonin is released into the systemic circulation and thus avoids breakdown by the liver. The appropriate therapy for a small carcinoid (less than 2 cm) of the appendix is simple appendectomy.

356. The answer is b. *(Schwartz, 7/e, pp 1586–1604.)* Direct inguinal hernias occur medial to the inferior epigastric vessels and are best repaired by reapproximating the transversalis fascia to Cooper's ligament and thus reconstructing the floor of the inguinal canal or by a tension-free Lichtenstein-type repair. The hernia sac is opened and ligated routinely during indirect hernia repair but not during direct hernia repair. The most common inguinal hernia in women is an indirect hernia. Direct hernias rarely present with a scrotal component and are less likely to present with incarceration than indirect hernias.

357. The answer is b. *(Cosentino, Surgery 112:740–748, 1992.)* Choledochal cysts are congenital cystic dilations of the extrahepatic biliary ducts. Intrahepatic cystic dilation can coexist (Caroli's disease), but it represents a distinct problem and is managed differently. Patients may present with symptoms at any age, but the classic triad of epigastric pain, abdominal mass, and jaundice is not frequently seen. Rather, most patients present with other conditions such as cholecystitis, cholangitis, or pancreatitis. Ultrasonography or endoscopic retrograde cholangiopancreatography (ERCP) is helpful in demonstrating cysts. Nonsurgical treatment of these cysts results in high morbidity and mortality, and therefore surgery is advised in all cases. The present recommendation is for complete resection of the cyst and Roux-en-Y choledochojejunostomy. Since malignant changes in choledochal cysts have been frequently described, complete resection rather than the performance of an internal drainage procedure is preferred whenever the resection can be done safely.

358. The answer is d. (*Schwartz, 7/e, pp 1062–1065.*) Stress ulceration refers to acute gastric or duodenal erosive lesions that occur following shock, sepsis, major surgery, trauma, or burns. These lesions tend to be superficial and can involve multiple sites. McClelland and associates showed that patients subjected to trauma and subsequent hemorrhagic shock do not have increased gastric secretion, but rather show decreased splanchnic blood flow. Ischemic damage to the mucosa may therefore play a role. Unlike chronic benign gastric ulcers, which are generally found along the lesser curvature and in the antrum, acute erosive lesions usually involve the body and fundus and spare the antrum.

359. The answer is b. (*Schwartz, 7/e, pp 1454–1455.*) Cholangitis is suggested by the presence of the Charcot triad: fever, jaundice, and pain in the right upper quadrant. These symptoms are usually caused by choledocholithiasis, but they can also occur in association with obstructing neoplasms and choledochal cysts. The disease occurs primarily in the elderly. Therapy is aimed at decompression of the common bile duct. In patients with suppurative cholangitis who fail to respond to intravenous antibiotics initially and fluid resuscitation, the nonoperative approach is the preferred intervention either via percutaneous or endoscopic drainage of the obstructed common bile duct. If the nonoperative approach fails, surgery is indicated. This is usually best accomplished by surgical placement of a T tube into the duct. Percutaneous transhepatic catheter drainage is an acceptable alternative in select patients. This procedure can often provide effective decompression during the acute septic phase of the disease. Cholecystostomy will be effective only if there is free flow of bile into the gallbladder via the cystic duct and in general should not be depended on to secure drainage of the common bile duct.

360. The answer is a. (*Schwartz, 7/e, pp 1459–1460.*) High-risk, critically ill patients with multisystem disease and cholecystitis experience a significant increase in morbidity and mortality following operative intervention. Tube cholecystostomy can be performed under local anesthesia in the operating room or via a percutaneous approach in the radiology suite. Open or laparoscopic procedures would carry the same general anesthetic risk whether done urgently or in a delayed (elective) fashion. Lithotripsy has no role in the treatment of acute cholecystitis.

361. The answer is a. *(Schwartz, 7/e, pp 1485–1487.)* Pancreatic pseudocysts can develop in the setting of acute and chronic pancreatitis. They are cystic collections that do not have an epithelial lining and therefore have no malignant potential. Most pseudocysts spontaneously resolve. Therapy should not be considered for 6 wk to allow for the possibility of spontaneous resolution as well as to allow for maturation of the cyst wall if the cyst persists. Complications of pseudocysts include gastric outlet and extrahepatic biliary obstructions as well as spontaneous rupture and hemorrhage. Pseudocysts can be excised, externally drained, or internally drained into the gastrointestinal tract (most commonly the stomach or a Roux-en-Y limb of jejunum).

362. The answer is d. *(Reilly, Dig Dis Sci 36:1702–1707, 1991.)* Dieulafoy's lesion has been identified more frequently recently as a source of gastrointestinal bleeding. It is characteristically located within 6 cm distal to the gastroesophageal junction. Dieulafoy's lesion typically consists of an abnormally large submucosal artery that protrudes through a small, solitary mucosal defect. The lesions may bleed spontaneously and massively for unclear reasons, in which case they require emergency intervention. Upper endoscopy is usually successful in localizing the lesion, and permanent hemostasis can be obtained endoscopically in most cases with injection sclerotherapy, electrocoagulation, or heater probe. If surgery is required, a gastrotomy and simple ligation or wedge resection of the lesion may be adequate. No large series have yet established the optimal surgical treatment for Dieulafoy's lesion; however, acid-reducing procedures have not been successful in preventing further bleeding.

363. The answer is b. *(Schwartz, 7/e, pp 1244–1246.)* Carcinoid tumors arise from enterochromaffin cells in the crypts of Lieberkühn. When they are encountered in the appendix and are less than 2 cm in size, simple appendectomy is the procedure of choice. When the tumors are larger than 2 cm, a right hemicolectomy should be performed. Carcinoid syndrome (hepatomegaly, diarrhea, cutaneous flushing, right heart valvular disease, and asthma) usually occurs in the presence of liver metastases but can also be seen when there are metastases to sites drained by systemic (as opposed to portal) veins or from primary carcinoids outside the portal system. Carcinoid syndrome is rare in patients with carcinoid of the appendix because the tumors are usually discovered before metastases occur.

364. The answer is d. *(Schwartz, 7/e, p 1374.)* Rectal carcinoids are slowly growing tumors, but they can be locally invasive and metastasize in up to 15% of patients. Patients manifest systemic signs of the carcinoid syndrome only in the rare circumstance where hepatic metastases have occurred. The malignant potential is low in carcinoid tumors when they are less than 2 cm in diameter, as is typically the case when diagnosed. The tumors are curable by wide, local transanal resection that includes the muscle layer. Endoscopic treatment leaves tumor cells near the margin of resection and is felt to increase the risk of recurrence. Whether more aggressive resection (abdominoperineal or low anterior resection) improves the prognosis in larger tumors remains controversial. The prognosis is excellent for patients with local disease.

365. The answer is b. *(Reilly, Dig Dis Sci 36:1702–1707, 1991.)* Polypoid lesions of the gallbladder are found most often in the third through fifth decades of life and are increasingly being detected by ultrasonography. These are generally small lesions that typically do not show a shadow on ultrasound. Ninety percent are benign lesions, such as cholesterol polyps (pseudotumors). True adenomas constitute about 10% of these benign lesions, but they can undergo malignant transformation. The indications for operative intervention remain controversial. Recent reviews suggest that the vast majority of malignant polypoid lesions are solitary, larger than 1.0 cm, and much more common in patients greater than 50 years of age. There is also an increased incidence of malignancy if the lesions are associated with gallstones. Symptomatic lesions should be removed regardless of their size. Asymptomatic small lesions can probably be safely followed by ultrasonography.

366. The answer is a. *(Greenfield, 2/e, p 912.)* The metabolic consequences of total pancreatectomy are manifold. They include weight loss, malabsorption attended by hypocalcemia and hypophosphatemia, diabetes mellitus, diarrhea, and both iron deficiency and pernicious anemia. In theory, total pancreatectomy should provide good surgical treatment for pancreatic carcinoma; in reality, the severe metabolic problems that result from total removal of the pancreas make partial pancreaticoduodenectomy a frequently preferred treatment for most cases of pancreatic carcinoma that are resectable. Because of the frequently multicentric nature of pancreatic cancers, however, some surgeons would rather perform a total pancreatectomy and accept the more complicated postoperative metabolic management entailed by the loss of pancreatic endocrine function.

367. The answer is d. (*Greenfield, 2/e, pp 1156–1157.*) Cecal diverticula must be differentiated from the more common variety of diverticula that are usually found in the left colon. Cecal diverticula are thought to be a congenital entity. The cecal diverticulum is often solitary and involves all layers of the bowel wall; therefore, cecal diverticula are true diverticula. Diverticula elsewhere in the colon are almost always multiple and are thought to be an acquired disorder. These acquired diverticula are really herniations of mucosa through weakened areas of the muscularis propria of the colon wall. The preoperative diagnosis in the case of cecal diverticulitis is "acute appendicitis" about 80% of the time. If there is extensive inflammation involving much of the cecum, an ileocolectomy is indicated. If the inflammation is well localized to the area of the diverticulum, a simple diverticulectomy with closure of the defect is the procedure of choice. To avoid diagnostic confusion in the future, the appendix should be removed whenever an incision is made in the right lower quadrant, unless operatively contraindicated.

368. The answer is c. (*Schwartz, 7/e, pp 1407–1408.*) Hepatic hemangiomata are the most common of all liver tumors. The infantile forms are highly vascular and occasionally cause hepatomegaly or congestive cardiac failure that requires angiographic or surgical interruption. The diagnostic incidence of incidental cavernous hemangiomata in adults has increased in this era of noninvasive imaging of organs with MRI, ultrasonography, and CT. When this lesion is suspected, the diagnosis can be confirmed with sensitive and more specific imaging techniques such as labeled red blood cell scanning (not liver/spleen scans). The mean age of presentation in adults is about 50 years and the vast majority of these lesions are asymptomatic. There is no evidence that they undergo malignant transformation. They may enlarge and become symptomatic more readily in women after multiple pregnancies or during the use of estrogen or oral contraceptives. The risk of rupture and severe hemorrhage into or from hemangiomata is extremely low; when it does occur, it is usually iatrogenic (following attempted biopsy). Given the typically benign and static nature of these lesions, management by angiographic embolization or resection should be reserved for the rare patient with symptomatic or complicated hemangioma.

369. The answer is d. (*Greenfield, 2/e, pp 1138, 1144.*) CEA is a tumor marker that was described in 1965 by Gold and Freedman. It is a nonspecific tumor marker that is elevated in only about one-half of patients with colorectal tumors and is often elevated in patients with lung, pancreatic, gastric, and gynecologic malignancies. CEA is also elevated in cigarette smokers. Patients in whom the primary colon tumor produced CEA and in whom the level falls below 2–3 ng/mL after resection have an excellent prognosis for disease control. In such patients, a subsequent rise in CEA has been demonstrated to be a very sensitive marker of the presence and extent of recurrent disease. Many surgeons follow CEA levels and perform "second-look" operations to resect local disease or possibly isolated metastatic disease if the levels become elevated postoperatively. Some surgeons recommend exploration in that circumstance even in the absence of other evidence (CT scan, colonoscopy) of recurrence. The long-term survival seems to be improved following this aggressive approach in some patients. Very high elevations of CEA, however, suggest extensive liver disease or peritoneal spread, which is unresectable.

370–373. The answers are 370-b, 371-d, 372-c, 373-a. (*Greenfield, 2/e, pp 785–787.*) Gastric ulcers have been classified as type I (incisura or most inferior portion of lesser curvature), type II (gastric and duodenal), type III (pyloric and prepyloric), and type IV (juxtacardial). Indications for surgery are intractability, perforation, obstruction, and bleeding. A patient with an intractable type I ulcer can be treated with an antrectomy alone or with a proximal gastric vagotomy. If done properly, antrectomy offers slightly lower recurrence rates and a higher incidence of postoperative sequelae as compared with proximal gastric vagotomy. However, significant scarring along the lesser curvature makes a proximal gastric vagotomy technically unfeasible.

Gastric outlet obstruction and severe inflammation around the pylorus and duodenum make resection a difficult and dangerous option. Similarly, pyloroplasty is often not adequate in the setting of gastric outlet obstruction to provide adequate drainage. Vagotomy and gastrojejunostomy, although associated with the highest recurrence rate, offers the best choice in the described setting.

In an elderly patient with a bleeding duodenal ulcer, recurrence rates are less of a consideration and thus the simplest and most expedient operation offers the best surgical outcome. Vagotomy and pyloroplasty with oversewing of the ulcer is the best choice in this setting.

Finally, in a young patient with intractable type III ulcers, antrectomy with vagotomy offers the best long-term outcome. Recurrence rates following this procedure are about 2–3%, as compared with 7.4% for vagotomy and drainage and 10–31% in patients receiving a proximal gastric vagotomy only.

374–376. The answers are 374-d, 375-d, 376-e. *(Schwartz, 7/e, pp 1161–1167.)* Paraesophageal hernias, generally thought to be acquired, involve herniation of any portion or all of the stomach into the thoracic cavity via the esophageal hiatus. These hernias are usually repaired electively because of a high incidence of complications. In these dangerous hernias, the cardioesophageal junction is in its normal position below the diaphragm.

Diaphragmatic ruptures usually affect adults and result from blunt trauma to the abdomen. Unless such ruptures are repaired, the negative intrathoracic pressure associated with each respiratory effort tends to such the abdominal contents into the chest with consequent loss of necessary space for lung expansion and substantial risk of damage to the intrathoracic bowel.

Sliding hiatal hernias, the most frequent type of hernia found in adults, are generally acquired. The significance of this type of hernia rests in its association with gastroesophageal reflux, a condition that may lead to reflux esophagitis. Because sliding hiatal hernias frequently do not exhibit significant gastroesophageal reflux, it is likely that other factors may be more important in the pathophysiology of that disorder.

The foramen of Bochdalek hernia is a congenital hernia of the posterolateral aspect of the diaphragm in which abdominal viscera enter the thorax and cause acute respiratory distress in infants. This hernia requires emergency repair.

The foramen of Morgagni hernia, although also congenital, is not usually detected until adulthood. It is usually an incidental finding on chest x-ray, where it appears as a low anterior mediastinal mass. However, on rare occasions it can produce acute respiratory distress in infants.

377–378. The answers are 377-b, c, h, i; 378-f. *(Schwartz, 7/e, pp 1529–1530, 1275–1277.)* The radiograph demonstrates pneumoperitoneum. Only a perforated viscus can produce this radiographic appearance in conjunction with diffuse peritonitis. A perforated gastric ulcer, perforated diverticulum, perforated transverse colon carcinoma, or strangulated hernia with necrotic bowel would all produce this clinical picture.

A sigmoid volvulus appears radiographically on plain film of the abdomen as an upside-down U or "bent inner tube." Acute sigmoid volvulus presents in the elderly with nausea, vomiting, abdominal distention, colicky abdominal pain, and obstipation. The first diagnostic and often therapeutic maneuver should be a sigmoidoscopy.

379–380. The answers are 379-d, e, f; 380-c. *(Schwartz, 7/e, pp 1168, 1156–1158.)* Patients with Mallory-Weiss syndrome typically present with a massive, painless hematemesis after severe vomiting or retching. The majority of tears (87%) occur just below the gastroesophageal junction. These tears occur 3 times more commonly in cirrhotics than in the normal population. Most of the time (90%), bleeding will stop without any intervention. When bleeding persists, balloon tamponade, endoscopic control of the bleeding, and surgical intervention with gastrotomy and oversewing of the tear have all been successful. Both intravenous and intraarterial infusion of vasopressin are also useful in controlling bleeding but are contraindicated in patients with coronary artery disease.

The patient presents with Boerhaave syndrome (spontaneous perforation of the esophagus following sudden increase in intraabdominal pressure). Unlike Mallory-Weiss tears, these tears are transmural perforations. Typical presentation is that of severe retrosternal or left chest or shoulder pain following an episode of retching; therefore, the symptoms can sometimes mimic a myocardial or pulmonary infarction. However, a good history can usually distinguish a Boerhaave perforation from these other entities. A Gastrografin swallow is helpful in cases that are diagnostically challenging. Treatment consists of left thoracotomy, repair of the transmural tear, and adequate drainage.

CARDIOTHORACIC PROBLEMS

Questions

DIRECTIONS: Each item below contains a question or incomplete statement followed by suggested responses. Select the **one best** response to each question.

381. Among the cardiovascular anomalies of newborns, the one most likely to present with cyanosis is

a. Patent ductus arteriosus
b. Coarctation of the aorta
c. Atrial septal defect
d. Ventricular septal defect
e. Transposition of the great vessels

382. The superior vena cava syndrome is most frequently seen in association with

a. Histoplasmosis (sclerosing mediastinitis)
b. Substernal thyroid
c. Thoracic aortic aneurysm
d. Constrictive pericarditis
e. Bronchogenic carcinoma

383. During endoscopic biopsy of a distal esophageal cancer, perforation of the esophagus is suspected when the patient complains of significant new substernal pain. An immediate chest film reveals air in the mediastinum. You would recommend

a. Placement of a nasogastric tube to the level of perforation, antibiotics, close observation
b. Spit fistula (cervical pharyngostomy), gastrostomy
c. Left thoracotomy, pleural patch oversewing of perforation, drainage of mediastinum
d. Esophagogastrectomy via celiotomy and right thoracotomy
e. Transhiatal esophagogastrectomy with cervical esophagogastrostomy

Items 384–385

384. A noncyanotic 2-day-old child has a systolic murmur along the left sternal border; the examination is otherwise normal. Chest x-ray and electrocardiogram are normal. These findings are most closely associated with which of the following congenital cardiac anomalies?

a. Tetralogy of Fallot
b. Ventricular septal defect
c. Tricuspid atresia
d. Transposition of the great vessels
e. Patent ductus arteriosus

385. A 3-year-old child with congenital cyanosis is most probably suffering from

a. Tetralogy of Fallot
b. Ventricular septal defect
c. Tricuspid atresia
d. Transposition of the great vessels
e. Patent ductus arteriosus

386. A stockbroker in his midforties consults you with complaints of episodes of severe, often incapacitating chest pain on swallowing. The diagnostic studies on the esophagus you have ordered yield the following: endoscopic examination and biopsy—mild inflammation distally; manometry—prolonged high-amplitude contractions from the arch of the aorta distally, lower esophageal sphincter (LES) pressure 20 mm Hg with relaxation on swallowing; barium swallow—2-cm epiphrenic diverticulum. You would recommend

a. Myotomy from level of aortic arch to distal sphincter; no disruption of LES
b. Diverticulectomy, myotomy from level of aortic arch to fundus, fundoplication
c. Diverticulectomy, cardiomyotomy of distal 3 cm of esophagus and proximal 2 cm of stomach with antireflux fundoplication
d. A trial of calcium channel blockers
e. Pneumatic dilation of LES

387. A 4-year-old boy is seen 1 h after ingestion of a lye drain cleaner. No oropharyngeal burns are noted, but the patient's voice is hoarse. Chest x-ray is normal. Of the following, which is the most appropriate therapy?

a. Immediate esophagoscopy
b. Parenteral steroids and antibiotics
c. Administration of an oral neutralizing agent
d. Induction of vomiting
e. Rapid administration of a quart of water to clear remaining lye from the esophagus and dilute material in stomach

388. A previously healthy 20-year-old man is admitted to a hospital with acute onset of left-sided chest pain. The electrocardiographic findings are normal but chest x-ray shows a 40% left pneumothorax. Treatment consists of which of the following procedures?

a. Observation
b. Barium swallow
c. Thoracotomy
d. Tube thoracostomy
e. Thoracostomy and intubation

389. A 50-year-old salesman is on a yacht with a client when he has a severe vomiting and retching spell punctuated by a sharp substernal pain. He arrives in your emergency room 4 h later and has a chest film in which the left descending aorta is outlined by air density. Optimum strategy for care would be

a. Immediate thoracotomy
b. Serial ECGs and CPKs to rule out myocardial ischemia
c. Left chest tube and spit fistula (cervical esophagostomy)
d. Flexible esophagogastroscopy to establish diagnosis
e. Nasogastric tube, antibiotics, close monitoring

Items 390–391

A 26-year-old man is brought to the emergency room after being extricated from the driver's seat of a car involved in a head-on collision in which the patient was not wearing his seat belt. His ECG is shown below.

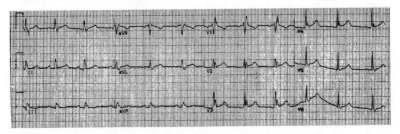

390. The ECG is most consistent with

a. Preexisting disease
b. Myocardial ischemia that caused the accident
c. Myocardial contusion that resulted from the accident
d. Chagas disease
e. Normal variant

391. The best test for establishing the diagnosis and the degree of myocardial dysfunction is

a. Serial ECGs
b. Creatine phosphokinase (CPK-MB) fractionation
c. Echocardiography
d. Radionuclide angiography
e. Coronary angiography

Items 392–393

Several days following esophagectomy a patient complains of dyspnea and chest tightness. A large pleural effusion is noted on chest radiograph and thoracentesis yields milky fluid consistent with chyle.

392. Initial management of this patient consists of which of the following procedures?

a. Immediate operation to repair the thoracic duct
b. Immediate operation to ligate the thoracic duct
c. Tube thoracostomy and low-fat diet
d. Observation and low-fat diet
e. Observation and antibiotics

393. Two weeks following the initial management of this patient's chylothorax there is persistent accumulation of chyle in the pleural space. Appropriate management at this time includes which of the following procedures?

a. Neck exploration and ligation of the thoracic duct
b. Subdiaphragmatic ligation of the thoracic duct
c. Thoracotomy and repair of the thoracic duct
d. Thoracotomy and ligation of the thoracic duct
e. Thoracotomy and abrasion of the pleural space

394. A 56-year-old woman was treated for 3 years for wheezing on exertion, which was diagnosed as asthma. The chest radiograph below is obtained, which reveals a midline mass compressing the trachea. The most likely diagnosis is

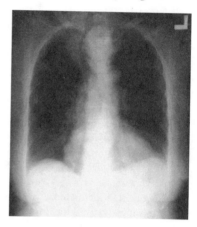

a. Lymphoma
b. Neurogenic tumor
c. Lung carcinoma
d. Goiter
e. Pericardial cyst

395. A full-term male newborn experiences respiratory distress immediately after birth. A prenatal sonogram had been read as normal. An emergency radiograph is shown below. The patient was intubated and placed on 100% O_2. The arterial blood gas revealed pH 7.24; P_{O_2} 60 kPa; P_{CO_2} 52 kPa. The baby has sternal retractions and a scaphoid abdomen. Which of the following statements correctly refers to this condition?

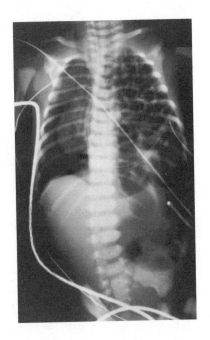

a. The most likely cause of this problem is in utero traumatic rupture of the diaphragm
b. The most important aspect in management would be immediate exploration and repair of the defect
c. The size of the defect directly correlates with severity of the disease
d. The defect is usually anteromedial in location
e. Any abdominal organ can be involved

396. An 89-year-old man has lost 30 lb over the past 2 years. He reports that food frequently sticks when he swallows. He also complains of a chronic cough. Pulmonary function tests show a vital capacity of 60% of expected, and forced expiratory volume is 50% of predicted. Barium swallow is shown below. Which of the following statements is true?

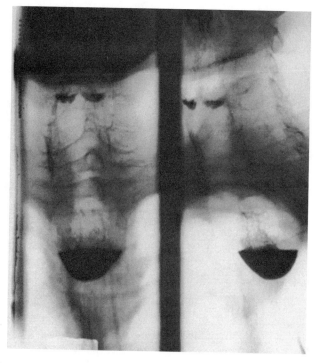

a. Radiation therapy and stenting can be expected to produce the same long-term survival as would surgery
b. Esophagoscopy and biopsy should be performed to confirm the x-ray findings
c. This patient is atypical in that the lesion usually appears in the second or third decade of life
d. The patient should be treated with antituberculous medications before any surgical intervention is considered
e. The carotid bifurcation lies adjacent to the lesion

397. Which of the following statements is true concerning aortocoronary bypass grafting?

a. It is indicated for crescendo (pre-infarction) angina
b. It is indicated for congestive heart failure
c. It is not indicated for chronic disabling angina
d. It is associated with a 10% operative mortality
e. It is only indicated if significant triple vessel disease is documented angiographically

398. Which of the following statements is true regarding the thoracic outlet syndrome?

a. It is associated with cervical spine disk disease
b. It is reliably diagnosed by positional obliteration of the radial pulse
c. If conservative measures fail, it is best treated by surgical decompression of the brachial plexus
d. It most commonly affects the median nerve
e. It can be reliably ruled out by angiography

399. A 35-year-old man presents with a history of 4 days of severe substernal pain and fever to 38.89°C (102°F). He has a past medical history of peptic ulcer disease that resulted in a Billroth II procedure 5 years earlier. On admission, the chest film below is obtained. A true statement regarding this patient's case is which of the following?

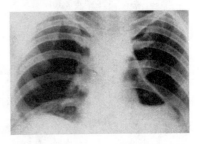

a. Pericardial effusion is present
b. The condition may be managed with antibiotics and close observation if the patient remains hemodynamically stable
c. The condition could have resulted from recurrent peptic ulcer disease
d. The condition could have resulted from a myocardial infarction
e. The previous Billroth II procedure effectively rules out peptic ulcer as the cause of the condition

400. Superior pulmonary sulcus carcinomas (Pancoast tumors) are bronchogenic carcinomas that typically produce which of the following clinical features?

a. Atelectasis of the involved apical segment
b. Horner syndrome
c. Pain in the T4 and T5 dermatomes
d. Nonproductive cough
e. Hemoptysis

401. A 2-year-old asymptomatic child is noted to have a systolic murmur, hypertension, and diminished femoral pulses. Which of the following is true about this child's disorder?

a. The life expectancy without surgery is about 5 years
b. Immediate surgery is indicated
c. Rib notching is often seen on x-ray
d. Claudication is frequently noted
e. Operative mortality approaches 10%

402. A correct statement concerning bronchial carcinoid tumors is that

a. They frequently metastasize
b. They most commonly arise in peripheral terminal bronchioles
c. They rarely produce the carcinoid syndrome
d. They are radiosensitive
e. Five-year survival is less than 50%

Items 403–404

Six months ago at the time of lumpectomy for breast cancer, a 60-year-old female attorney quit a 30-year smoking habit of two packs per day. She had the chest radiograph below as part of her routine follow-up examination.

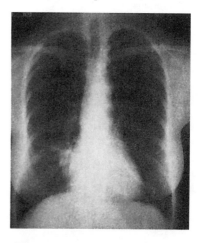

403. True statements about the lesion visualized on the film include which of the following?

a. It is more apt to be metastatic breast carcinoma than primary lung carcinoma
b. There is a 90% chance that this mass is malignant
c. Since the diagnosis can only be established with certainty by resection, the mass should be excised
d. If the mass is malignant, the possibility for cure with excision is remote
e. The mass is most likely benign

404. At the time of operation on the patient in the preceding question, a firm, rubbery lesion in the periphery of the lung is discovered. It is sectioned in the operating room to reveal tissue that looks like cartilage and smooth muscle. The most likely diagnosis is

a. Fibroma
b. Chondroma
c. Osteochondroma
d. Hamartoma
e. Aspergilloma

405. The condition shown in the x-rays below is compatible with which of the following manifestations?

a. Difficulty swallowing solids but not liquids
b. Higher-than-normal incidence of esophageal carcinoma
c. Failure of the upper esophageal sphincter to relax in response to swallowing
d. Normal pressure in the body of the esophagus
e. Normal esophageal motility

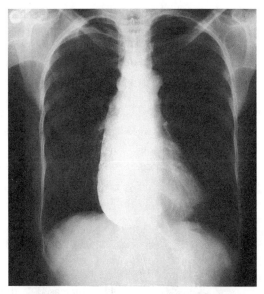

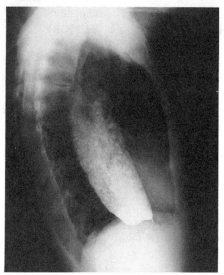

DIRECTIONS: Each group of questions below consists of lettered options followed by numbered items. For each numbered item, select the appropriate lettered option(s). Each lettered option may be used once, more than once, or not at all. **Choose exactly the number of options indicated following each item.**

Items 406–410

For each physical finding or group of physical findings below, select the cardiovascular disorder with which it is most likely to be associated.

a. Massive tricuspid regurgitation
b. Aortic regurgitation
c. Coarctation of the aorta
d. Thoracic aortic aneurysm
e. Myocarditis

406. Argyll Robertson pupil **(SELECT 1 DISORDER)**

407. Exophthalmos **(SELECT 1 DISORDER)**

408. Quincke pulse **(SELECT 1 DISORDER)**

409. Conjunctivitis, urethral discharge, and arthralgia **(SELECT 1 DISORDER)**

410. Short stature, webbed neck, low-set ears, and epicanthal folds **(SELECT 1 DISORDER)**

Items 411–415

For each pathologic sign below, select the mediastinal tumor with which it is most likely to be associated.

a. Thymoma
b. Hodgkin's disease
c. Neuroblastoma
d. Parathyroid adenoma
e. Cystic teratoma

411. Increased urinary catecholamine level **(SELECT 1 TUMOR)**

412. Red blood cell aplasia **(SELECT 1 TUMOR)**

413. Renal stones **(SELECT 1 TUMOR)**

414. T-cell deficiency **(SELECT 1 TUMOR)**

415. Ectopic hair **(SELECT 1 TUMOR)**

Items 416–420

Match the appropriate pharmacologic agent with each description.

a. Epinephrine
b. Norepinephrine
c. Isoproterenol
d. Dopamine
e. Dobutamine
f. Amrinone
g. Digitalis
h. Nitroprusside
i. Nitroglycerin
j. Milrinone

416. Balanced arterial and venous dilation **(SELECT 1 AGENT)**

417. Action as an inotrope and vasodilator by inhibiting endogenous phosphodiesterase **(SELECT 2 AGENTS)**

418. Pure beta agonist with profound chronotropic properties **(SELECT 1 AGENT)**

419. Endogenous catecholamine secreted into the circulation under normal conditions **(SELECT 2 AGENTS)**

420. Inotropic and antiarrhythmic properties **(SELECT 1 AGENT)**

CARDIOTHORACIC PROBLEMS

Answers

381. The answer is e. (*Schwartz, 7/e, pp 812–826.*) With the exception of coarctation, in which no shunt (or cyanosis) exists, the anomalies listed cause a shunting of blood between the systemic and lower-pressure pulmonary circulation. Transposition of the great vessels is a right-to-left shunt that leads to cyanosis. Except where there is persistent congenital pulmonary hypertension, patent ductus arteriosus and atrial septal defects cause a shunting of oxygenated blood from the aorta and left atrium, respectively, back into the pulmonary artery and right atrium. These anomalies cause "recirculation" of oxygenated blood within the cardiopulmonary circuit but not cyanosis. When a ventricular septal defect is combined with pulmonary artery atresia (tetralogy of Fallot), the resulting undercirculation in the pulmonary system joins transposition as a cause of cyanosis. Other less common congenital lesions in which the pulmonary arterial blood flow is relatively decreased include tricuspid atresia, Ebstein's anomaly, and hypoplastic right ventricle.

382. The answer is e. (*Schwartz, 7/e, p 784.*) Superior vena cava obstruction is almost always due to malignancy and, in three out of four cases, results from invasion of the vena cava by bronchogenic carcinoma. Lymphomas account for most of the remaining cases of the superior vena cava syndrome. Fibrosing mediastinitis as a complication of histoplasmosis or ingestion of methysergide may occur but is rare. Rarely a substernal thyroid or thoracic aortic aneurysm may be responsible for the obstruction. Although constrictive pericarditis may decrease venous return to the heart, it does not produce obstruction of the superior vena cava. Whatever the cause of the superior vena cava syndrome, the resultant increased venous pressure produces edema of the upper body, cyanosis, dilated subcutaneous collateral vessels in the chest, and headache. Cervical lymphadenopathy may also be present as a result of either stasis or metastatic involvement. When carcinoma is the cause of the superior vena cava syndrome, the treatment is usually palliative and consists of diuretics and radiation.

383. The answer is d. *(Schwartz, 7/e, pp 1156–1158.)* Perforation of the esophagus in the chest is a surgical catastrophe that requires aggressive intervention in virtually all circumstances. While that intervention can usually consist of efforts to patch the perforation and drain the mediastinum, concomitant obstructive esophageal disease, whether inflammatory stenosis or cancer, mandates removal or bypass of the obstruction if control of the leak and its consequent persisting mediastinal and pleural contamination is to be accomplished. For distal esophageal cancers, many thoracic surgeons would use the classic Ivor-Lewis operation, which consists of mobilizing the stomach in the abdomen and then performing a right thoracotomy with mediastinal cleanout, esophagectomy, and esophagogastrostomy. In some circumstances, and by some surgeons' preference, a left thoracotomy approach might be used. The transhiatal approach would probably be avoided in this situation where an unknown amount of mediastinal contamination has taken place.

384–385. The answers are 384-b, 385-a. *(Schwartz, 7/e, pp 812–826.)* Ventricular septal defect accounts for 20–30% of all congenital cardiac anomalies. It may lead to cardiac failure and pulmonary hypertension if the defect is larger than 1 cm; or it may be asymptomatic if the defect is small. Surgery is not indicated for the asymptomatic patient with a small defect since a substantial number of these anomalies close spontaneously during the first few years of life. Operation is indicated in infants with congestive heart failure or rising pulmonary vascular resistance (owing to the left-to-right shunt). When symptoms are mild and can be controlled medically, operation is usually delayed until age 4–6 years. Operative mortality ranges from less than 5% to more than 20% depending on the degree of pulmonary vascular resistance.

Tetralogy of Fallot, transposition, and tricuspid atresia are cyanotic lesions. Congenital cyanosis that persists beyond the age of 2 years is associated, in the vast majority of cases, with a tetralogy of Fallot. Patent ductus arteriosus is associated with the characteristic continuous machinery murmur.

386. The answer is a. *(Schwartz, 7/e, pp 1103–1121.)* The diagnostic studies listed reveal minimal reflux esophagitis, normal LES relaxation and pressure, and an incidental small epiphrenic diverticulum. None of these findings justifies treatment and none explains the patient's symptoms. On the other hand, the finding of prolonged high-amplitude contractions in the body of the esophagus in a highly symptomatic patient is diagnostic of diffuse esophageal spasm. The cause of this hypermotility disorder is unknown, but its symptoms can be disabling. The recommended treatment for this relatively rare disorder is a long myotomy guided by the manometric evidence. If the LES is functioning properly, most surgeons would now recommend stopping the myotomy short of the normal lower sphincter. It should continue upward at least to the level of the aortic arch—higher if manometric findings of spasm are noted above that level. Eighty to 90% of patients treated in this fashion will experience acceptable relief of symptoms.

387. The answer is b. (*Schwartz, 7/e, pp 1158–1161.*) Corrosive injuries of the esophagus most frequently occur in young children due to accidental ingestion of strong alkaline cleaning agents. Significant esophageal injury occurs in 15% of patients with no oropharyngeal injury, while 70% of patients with oropharyngeal injury have no esophageal damage. Signs of airway injury or imminent obstruction warrant close observation and possibly tracheostomy. The risk of adding injury, particularly in a child, makes esophagoscopy contraindicated in the opinion of most surgeons. Administration of oral "antidotes" is ineffective unless given within moments of ingestion; even then, the additional damage potentially caused by the chemical reactions of neutralization often makes use of them unwise. A barium esophagogram is usually done within 24 h unless evidence of perforation is present. In most reports, steroids in conjunction with antibiotics reduce the incidence of formation of strictures from about 70% to about 15%. Vomiting should be avoided, if possible, to prevent further corrosive injury and possible aspiration. It is probably wise to avoid all oral intake until the full extent of injury is ascertained.

The most helpful ECG finding is the presence of a new right bundle branch block, which occurs because of damage to the anterior portion of the interventricular septum; ST-segment and T-wave changes and even the development of new Q waves may be seen. CPK-MB fractions are useful if they are positive; however, frequent false negatives may be seen because of the release of CPK-MM from other contused organs, such as the pectoralis muscles, which can dilute the cardiac CPK-MB to nondiagnostic levels. Echocardiography may be helpful, but the right ventricle is often poorly visualized. Radionuclide angiography is most useful because it suggests the degree of myocardial impairment caused by decreased compliance.

Therapy of myocardial contusion is directed at inotropic support of the ventricle; usually, the coronary arteries are intact after the injury and so there is little role for coronary vasodilators and less for coronary artery bypass grafting.

388. The answer is d. *(Schwartz, 7/e, pp 711–713, 781.)* Spontaneous pneumothorax usually results from the rupture of subpleural blebs in young men (age 20–40), which is often signaled by a sudden onset of chest and shoulder pain. Pneumothorax of more than 25% requires placement of a chest tube; thoracotomy with bleb excision and pleural abrasion is generally recommended if spontaneous pneumothorax is recurrent. Small pneumothoraxes in patients with minimal symptoms usually resolve and therefore can be observed. A spontaneous perforation of the esophagus (Boerhaave syndrome) can result in hydropneumothorax as well as the more usual pneumomediastinum, but would not present with an isolated 40% pneumothorax. Barium swallow is an appropriate diagnostic test for evaluation of a suspected leaking esophagus.

389. The answer is a. *(Henderson, Am J Med 86:559–567, 1989.)* The presence of air in the mediastinum after an episode of vomiting and retching is virtually pathognomonic of spontaneous rupture of the esophagus (Boerhaave syndrome). The evidence is overwhelming that without prompt surgical exploration of the mediastinum by left thoracotomy, the patient has little chance for a short-term outcome of low morbidity. The aspiration of highly acidic gastric contents into the mediastinum creates havoc in the tissues exposed to it. The surgical procedure must include extensive opening of the mediastinal pleura and removal of any particulate debris that might have been aspirated into the thorax from the stomach. Closure of the esophageal laceration with reinforcement by a pleural flap and secure chest tube drainage of the pleural space are mandatory. If the operation is delayed beyond the first 8–24 h, the mortality rises sharply and survival will only follow prolonged intensive care and multiple operations. This catastrophic event is one of the few in which prompt diagnosis and intervention are crucial to success. Because the findings are classic and the diagnosis is so important, Boerhaave syndrome justifiably receives emphasis in educational programs for emergency physicians, internists, radiologists, and surgeons alike.

390–391. The answers are 388-c, 389-d. *(Schwartz, 7/e, pp 159–161.)* The incidence of myocardial contusion is about 25% in patients with severe blunt injury to the chest. The injury occurs as a result of direct compression of the heart between the sternum and the vertebral column. The right ventricle, being the most anterior portion of the heart, is the most commonly injured portion. The blow causes extravasation of blood into the myocardium and results in a progressive loss of ventricular compliance and decreased cardiac output, which usually peaks by 8–24 h after the injury.

392–393. The answers are 392-c, 393-b. *(Schwartz, 7/e, pp 706–709.)* Chylothorax may occur after intrathoracic surgery, or it may follow malignant invasion or compression of the thoracic duct. Intraoperative recognition of a thoracic duct injury is managed by double ligation of the duct. Direct repair is impractical owing to the extreme friability of the thoracic duct. Injuries not recognized until several days after intrathoracic surgery frequently heal following the institution of a low-fat diet and either repeated thoracentesis or tube thoracostomy drainage. A low-fat, medium-chain triglyceride diet often reduces the flow of chyle. Failure of this treatment modality requires direct surgical ligation of the thoracic duct. This is best approached from below the diaphragm, regardless of the site of intrathoracic injury.

394. The answer is d. *(Schwartz, 7/e, pp 771–780.)* The boundaries of the mediastinum are the thoracic inlet, the diaphragm, the sternum, the vertebral column, and the pleura bilaterally. The mediastinum itself is divided into three portions delineated by the pericardial sac: the anterosuperior and posterosuperior regions are in front of and behind the sac, respectively, while the middle region designates the contents of the pericardium. Mediastinal masses occur most frequently in the anterosuperior region (54%) and less often in the posterosuperior (26%) and middle (20%) regions. Cysts (either pericardial, bronchogenic, or enteric) are the most common tumors of the middle region; neurogenic tumors are the most common (40%) of the primary tumors of the posterior mediastinum. The primary neoplasms of the mediastinum in the anteroposterior region are thymomas (31%), lymphomas (23%), and germ-cell tumors (17%). More commonly, though, a mass in this area represents the substernal extension of a benign substernal goiter. Diagnosis may be made by visualization of an enhancing structure on CT; radioactive iodine scanning is useful in management because it may make the diagnosis if the mediastinal tissue is functional and will also document the presence of functioning cervical thyroid tissue to prevent removal of all functional thyroid tissue during mediastinal excision.

395. The answer is e. *(Schwartz, 7/e, pp 1719–1721.)* This radiograph of a child with a scaphoid abdomen and respiratory disease is characteristic of a congenital diaphragmatic hernia. These defects are posterolateral and occur from failure of the embryologic diaphragm to fuse between the eighth and twelfth weeks of intrauterine life. The size of the defect does not correlate with the symptoms. Even a large diaphragmatic hernia can be missed on prenatal sonogram if the abdominal contents have slipped back into the abdomen at the time of the study. Hernias of Morgagni are anteromedial and do not present as emergencies at birth. Any abdominal organ—pancreas, kidney, small and large intestine, stomach, liver, or spleen—can herniate into the chest. The abdominal organ acts as a space-occupying lesion and retards growth of the lung, which results in pulmonary hypoplasia. Respiratory problems at birth stem from primary pulmonary hypertension, the consequence of hypoplasia, rather than from compression of the lung by abdominal contents. Most experts recommend stabilizing the pulmonary hypertensive crisis medically or with extracorporeal membrane oxygenation (ECMO) prior to attempting repair.

396. The answer is e. *(Schwartz, 7/e, p 1125.)* Pharyngoesophageal (Zenker's) diverticulum is an outpouching of mucosa between the lower pharyngeal constrictor and the cricopharyngeus muscles. It is thought to result from an incoordination of cricopharyngeal relaxation with swallowing. These diverticula occur in elderly patients and more commonly on the left. The typical patient presents with complaints of dysphagia, weight loss, and choking. Other patients present with the effects of repeated aspiration, pneumonia, or chronic cough. A mass is sometimes palpable and a gurgle may be heard. Treatment is excision and division of the cricopharyngeus muscle, which can be done under local anesthesia in a cooperative patient. Esophagoscopy is dangerous because the blind pouch is easily perforated. Even though the pouch may extend down into the mediastinum, the origin of the diverticulum is at the cricopharyngeus muscle near the level of the bifurcation of the carotid artery.

397. The answer is a. *(Schwartz, 7/e, pp 865–867.)* Coronary artery bypass surgery was developed in the late 1960s and is now being regularly performed. Indications for surgery include chronic disabling angina and crescendo (or preinfarction) angina. Cardiac catheterization with selective coronary angiography defines the extent of disease, which generally is localized to the proximal segments of the vessels. Operative mortality is about 2%, and relief of angina is obtained in most affected patients. Patients with left main coronary artery disease as well as those with triple vessel disease and ventricular dysfunction have an increased longevity following successful bypass. Data regarding extension of life in other groups is conflicting. Coronary artery bypass is not indicated for congestive heart failure unless this condition is ischemic in origin and angiography identifies disease amenable to surgical revascularization.

398. The answer is c. (*Schwartz, 7/e, pp 977–980.*) The thoracic outlet syndrome designates a symptom complex whose precise cause is unknown. It is felt to result from compression of the brachial plexus or subclavian vessels, or both, in the anatomic space bounded by the first rib, the clavicle, and scalene muscles. Since objective determinants of disease may be lacking or imprecise, the diagnosis often is established by resectional surgery. Carpal tunnel syndrome (compression of the median nerve as it passes through the carpal tunnel of the wrist) and cervical disk disease are the two entities most commonly confused with the thoracic outlet syndrome, whose symptoms and signs include pain, paresthesias, edema, venous congestion, and digital vasospastic changes. Positional dampening or obliteration of the radial pulse is an unreliable finding since it is present in up to 70% of the normal population. Neurologic abnormalities may be documented by nerve conduction studies. Angiographic studies are often negative. Conservative management, which generally should precede surgery, consists of an exercise program to strengthen shoulder girdle muscles and decrease shoulder droop. Operative treatment includes division of the scalenus anticus and medius muscles, first rib resection, cervical rib resection, or a combination of all three.

399. The answer is c. (*Cummings, Ann Thorac Surg 37:511–518, 1984.*) This x-ray demonstrates an air-fluid level in the pericardium. Pneumopericardium can result from penetrating or blunt chest trauma, spontaneous formation of gas from anaerobic bacteria, iatrogenic causes, or direct extension into the pericardium by diseased adjacent organs. In this case, a patient with a high gastrojejunostomy developed a recurrent ulcer that eroded through the diaphragm and into the pericardium and thus caused a pneumopyopericardium. Often these patients have an unrecognized gastrinoma (Zollinger-Ellison syndrome) and therefore continue to have peptic ulcer disease despite aggressive surgical therapy. The presence of pneumopyopericardium as seen in this chest film should be treated as a surgical emergency in this setting. Inability to demonstrate a fistula on roentgenographic investigation should not preclude the diagnosis of this entity. If the cause of the pericardial fluid is not clearly diagnosed by available means, then a pericardial window should be performed for diagnostic as well as therapeutic reasons. The pericardial sac should be irrigated and adequate continuing drainage should be ensured. Although myocardial infarction may result in pericardial effusion or (rarely) tamponade, it does not cause pneumopericardium.

400. The answer is b. *(Schwartz, 7/e, p 1913.)* Pancoast tumors are peripheral bronchogenic carcinomas that produce symptoms by involvement of extrapulmonary structures adjacent to the cupula. These structures include the nerve roots of C8 and T1, as well as the sympathetic trunk. Interruption of the cervical sympathetic trunk leads to miosis, ptosis, and anhidrosis, the triad of signs that constitutes Horner syndrome. Involvement of the nerve roots causes pain along the corresponding dermatomes. The peripheral location of the neoplasm makes pulmonary signs, such as atelectasis, cough, and hemoptysis, unlikely.

401. The answer is c. *(Schwartz, 7/e, pp 802–805.)* Coarctation of the aorta is a congenital anomaly that usually causes aortic stenosis just distal to the left subclavian artery in the area of the ligamentum arteriosum. Collateral circulation develops around the obstruction by way of intercostal vessels and accounts for the classic x-ray appearance of rib notching. Without surgery, the average life span is about 30–40 years with eventual death from cardiac failure, rupture of aortic aneurysms or of a cerebral artery, and bacterial endocarditis. Surgery can be accomplished with less than a 1% mortality and should be performed around 5 years of age, when the aorta is sufficiently large to be operable but before it becomes fibrotic and calcified, conditions that increase the technical difficulty of the operation. Claudication is not a common feature of this disorder.

402. The answer is c. *(Schwartz, 7/e, p 759–761.)* Bronchial carcinoid tumors rarely produce the carcinoid syndrome. They are slow-growing, infrequently metastatic tumors that histologically resemble the carcinoid tumors of the small intestine. Over 80% arise in the major proximal bronchi, and their intraluminal growth is responsible for the frequent presentation of bronchial obstruction. The only therapy for this lesion is operative resection, because neither the primary tumor nor the infrequent lymph node metastasis is radiosensitive. The low malignant potential for this lesion is reflected by a long-term survival rate that approaches 90%.

403. The answer is c. *(Schwartz, 7/e, pp 758–759.)* "Coin lesions" have been defined as densities within the lung field of up to 4 cm, usually round, and free of signs of infections such as cavitation or surrounding infiltrates. Malignant solitary lesions may contain flecks of calcification, but heavy calcification or concentric rings of calcium generally suggest a benign etiology. The differential diagnosis for coin lesions includes primary pulmonary carcinomas, metastatic carcinomas to the lung, benign lung neoplasms such as chondromas and other benign lung processes such as granulomas, or vascular abnormalities such as arteriovenous malformations. The likelihood that a coin lesion is a primary lung malignancy increases linearly with age: 15% at age 40, 40% at age 55, 70% at age 75. With the diminishing frequency of granulomatous disease and the continued rise in lung cancers, such lesions should be removed because there is an excellent chance of cure if the lesion is a primary lung malignancy. If the patient has had a previous malignancy of tissue other than lung, the likelihood that the lesion represents a metastatic lesion depends on the tissue of origin of the previous malignancy. If all patients with a history of prior cancer are considered together, a lung nodule will be a new lung primary in 60%, a metastatic lesion in 25%, and a benign process in 15% of cases. However, 80% of solitary lesions in patients with melanoma represent metastatic disease, while only 40% of lesions in patients with breast cancer represent metastasis, and solitary lesions in patients with colon carcinoma are equally likely to be metastatic or primary lung cancers.

404. The answer is d. *(Schwartz, 7/e, pp 759–764.)* The term *hamartoma* denotes a tumor that arises from the disorganized arrangement of tissues normally found in an organ. Pulmonary hamartomas are solitary lesions of the pulmonary parenchyma and generally appear as asymptomatic peripheral nodules; they represent the most common benign epithelial and mesodermal elements. Pulmonary chondromas consist of mesodermal elements alone and arise centrally in major bronchi, where they produce signs and symptoms of bronchial obstruction. Fibromas are the most common benign mesodermal tumors found in the lung; they may occur either within the lung parenchyma or, more commonly, within the tracheobronchial tree. Osteochondromas are lesions of bone and are not found in the lung. Aspergillomas are due to infection with the fungus *Aspergillus* and most commonly appear in the upper lobes as oval, friable, necrotic gray or yellow masses often surrounded by evidence of preexisting parenchymal lung disease.

405. The answer is b. *(Schwartz, 7/e, pp 1126–1127.)* The x-rays presented in the question are consistent with a diagnosis of achalasia, a motility disorder of the esophagus that usually affects persons between 30 and 50 years of age. The x-rays show a classic beaklike narrowing of the distal esophagus and a large, dilated esophagus proximal to the narrowing. The diagnosis of achalasia is generally suspected on the basis of barium x-rays, but, because other esophageal disorders may mimic the condition, an esophageal motility study is usually required to confirm the diagnosis. The characteristic findings on a motility study are small-amplitude, repetitive, simultaneous postdeglutition contractions in the body of the esophagus, failure of the lower esophageal sphincter to relax after deglutition, and a higher-than-normal pressure in the body of the esophagus. Carcinoma of the esophagus is approximately 7 times more frequent in persons who have achalasia than in the general population. Patients usually describe difficulty in swallowing solids and liquids.

406–410. The answers are 406-d, 407-a, 408-b, 409-e, 410-c. *(Greenfield, 2/e, pp 1575–1577, 1506. Sabiston, 15/e, p 2139.)* Myocarditis, aortitis, and pericarditis all have been described in association with Reiter syndrome; the original description included conjunctivitis, urethritis, and arthralgias. Although its cause is unknown, Reiter syndrome is associated with HLA-B27 antigen, as are aortic regurgitation, pericarditis, and ankylosing spondylitis.

Short stature, webbed neck, low-set ears, and epicanthal folds are the classic features of patients who have Turner syndrome. Persons affected by the syndrome, which is commonly linked with aortic coarctation, are genotypically XO. However, females and males have been described with normal sex chromosome constitutions (XX, XY) but with the phenotypic abnormalities of Turner syndrome. Additional cardiac lesions associated with Turner syndrome include septal defects, valvular stenosis, and anomalies of the great vessels.

The Argyll Robertson pupil, a pupil that constricts with accommodation but not in response to light, is characteristic of central nervous system syphilis and is associated with vascular system manifestations of this disease. *Treponema pallidum* invades the vasa vasorum and causes an obliterative endarteritis and necrosis. The resulting aortitis gradually weakens the aortic wall and predisposes it to aneurysm formation. Once an aneurysm has formed, the prognosis is grave.

Massive isolated tricuspid regurgitation produces a markedly elevated venous pressure, usually manifested by a severely engorged (often pulsating) liver. If the venous pressure is sufficiently elevated, exophthalmos may result. Tricuspid regurgitation of rheumatic origin is almost never an isolated lesion, and the major symptoms of patients who have rheumatic heart disease are usually attributable to concurrent left heart lesions. Bacterial endocarditis from intravenous drug abuse is becoming an increasingly important cause of isolated tricuspid regurgitation.

A Quincke pulse, which consists of alternate flushing and paling of the skin or nail beds, is associated with aortic regurgitation. Other characteristic features of the peripheral pulse in aortic regurgitation include the water-hammer pulse (Corrigan pulse, caused by a rapid systolic upstroke) and pulsus bisferiens, which describes a double systolic hump in the pulse contour. The finding of a wide pulse pressure provides an additional diagnostic clue to aortic regurgitation.

411–415. The answers are 411-c, 412-a, 413-d, 414-b, 415-e.
(*Schwartz, 7/e, pp 771–780.*) Neuroblastoma, a highly malignant tumor of children, occurs along the distribution of the sympathetic nervous system. It is derived from ganglion cell precursors and thus usually causes an increased excretion of catecholamines and their metabolites. Because of its propensity to metastasize to bone and its histological resemblance to Ewing's sarcoma, its association with elevated catecholamine levels is a major factor in differential diagnosis.

Renal stones occur in about half the cases of hyperparathyroidism. Other disorders sometimes associated with hyperparathyroidism include peptic ulcers, pancreatitis, and bone disease; central nervous system symptoms may also arise in connection with hyperparathyroidism. Occasionally, parathyroid adenomas occur in conjunction with neoplasms of other endocrine organs, a condition known as multiple endocrine adenomatosis.

Cystic teratomas, or dermoid cysts, include endodermal, ectodermal, and mesodermal elements. They are characteristically cystic and contain poorly pigmented hair, sebaceous material, and occasionally teeth. Dermoid cysts occur in the gonads and central nervous system, as well as in the mediastinum. With rare exceptions, these lesions are benign. Thymomas are associated with myasthenia gravis, agammaglobulinemia, and red blood cell aplasia. These tumors are typically cystic and occur in the anterior mediastinum. Most thymic lesions associated with myasthenia gravis are hyperplastic rather than neoplastic.

Persons afflicted with Hodgkin's disease have impaired cell-mediated immunity and are particularly susceptible to mycotic infections and tuberculosis. The severity of the immune deficiency correlates with the extent of the disease. The nodular sclerosing variant of primary mediastinal Hodgkin's disease is the most common type.

416–420. The answers are 416-h; 417-f, j; 418-c; 419-a, d; 420-g. *(Schwartz, 7/e, pp 103–105, 114.)* Epinephrine is a circulating endogenous catecholamine, released mainly from the adrenal medulla, whose effects are mediated by binding of free circulating hormone to β_1- and β_2-receptors, with lesser effects on α-adrenoreceptors. Norepinephrine is also endogenously produced, but acts locally through release at nerve synapses. Isoproterenol is a synthetic sympathomimetic that acts as a pure beta agonist, resulting in profound vasodilator and chronotropic effects. Dopamine is an endogenous catecholamine that is released into the circulation and acts by binding to β_1-receptors as well as specific dopamine receptors in the renal, mesenteric, coronary, and intracerebral vascular beds, causing vasodilation. Dobutamine is a synthetic sympathomimetic structurally related to dopamine and is a potent inotrope but possesses only small chronotropic properties. Amrinone and milrinone are bipyridine derivatives that induce vasodilation and inotropy via inhibition of phosphodiesterase, thereby enhancing intracellular concentrations of cyclic AMP. Digitalis exerts positive inotropic effects by inhibition of Na-K-activated ATPase, resulting in increased intracellular sodium concentrations, which lead to increased intracellular calcium concentrations. Digitalis is also used in the management of arrhythmias, most commonly atrial fibrillation. Nitroprusside and nitroglycerin are systemic vasodilators, and while nitroprusside causes balanced arterial and venous dilation, the effects of nitroglycerin are less pronounced in the arterial than the venous system, often resulting in venous pooling.

PERIPHERAL VASCULAR PROBLEMS

Questions

DIRECTIONS: Each item below contains a question or incomplete statement followed by suggested responses. Select the **one best** response to each question.

421. Patients with phlebographically confirmed deep vein thrombosis of the calf

a. Can expect asymptomatic recovery if treated promptly with anticoagulants
b. May be effectively treated with low-dose heparin
c. May be effectively treated with pneumatic compression stockings
d. May be effectively treated with acetylsalicylic acid
e. Are at risk for significant pulmonary embolism

422. For the first 6 h following surgical repair of a leaking abdominal aortic aneurysm in a 70-year-old man, oliguria (total urinary output of 25 mL since the operation) has become a concern. Of most diagnostic help would be

a. Renal scan
b. Aortogram
c. Left heart preload pressures
d. Urinary sodium concentration
e. Creatinine clearance

423. Following aortic reconstruction, the viability of the sigmoid colon can most reliably be evaluated by

a. Intraoperative measurement of inferior mesenteric artery stump pressure
b. Intraoperative Doppler arterial signal in the sigmoid mesentery
c. Intraoperative observation of bowel peristalsis
d. Postoperative sigmoidoscopy
e. Postoperative barium enema

424. A 25-year-old woman presents to the emergency room complaining of redness and pain in her right foot up to the level of the midcalf. She reports that her right leg has been swollen for at least 15 years, but her left leg has been normal. On physical examination she has a temperature of 39°C (102.2°F). The left leg is normal. The right leg is not tender, but it is swollen from the inguinal ligament down and there is an obvious cellulitis of the right foot. The patient's underlying problem is

a. Popliteal entrapment syndrome
b. Acute arterial insufficiency
c. Primary lymphedema
d. Deep venous thrombosis
e. None of the above

425. A 76-year-old woman is admitted with back pain and hypotension. A CT scan (shown below) is obtained, and the patient is taken to the operating room. Three days after resection of a ruptured abdominal aortic aneurysm, she complains of severe, dull left flank pain and passes bloody mucus per rectum. The diagnosis that must be immediately considered is

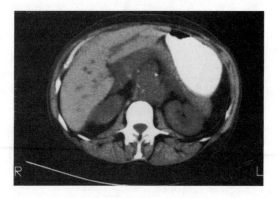

a. Staphylococcal enterocolitis
b. Diverticulitis
c. Bleeding AV malformation
d. Ischemia of the left colon
e. Bleeding colonic carcinoma

426. The angiogram depicted below is most typical of the patient whose history includes

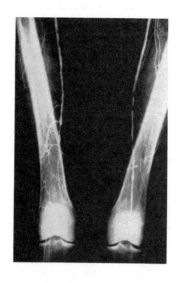 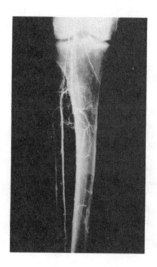

a. Cigarette smoking
b. Alcoholism
c. Hypertension
d. Diabetes
e. Type I hyperlipoproteinemia

427. An 80-year-old man is found to have an asymptomatic abdominal mass. An arteriogram is obtained, which is pictured below. This patient should be advised that

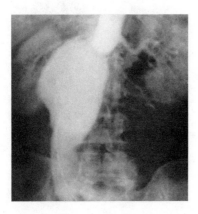

a. Surgery should be performed, but a mortality of 20% is to be anticipated
b. Surgery should be performed only if symptoms develop
c. Surgery will improve his 5-year survival
d. Surgery this extensive should not be performed in a patient of his age
e. Surgery should be performed only if follow-up ultrasound demonstrates increasing size

Items 428–429

428. A 75-year-old man is found by his internist to have an asymptomatic carotid bruit. The best initial diagnostic examination would be

a. Transcranial Doppler studies
b. Doppler ultrasonography (duplex)
c. Spiral CT angiography
d. Arch aortogram with selective carotid artery injections
e. Magnetic resonance arteriogram (MRA)

429. An arteriogram on the above patient is shown below. The patient has mild hypertension and mild COPD. The current recommendation for this man would be

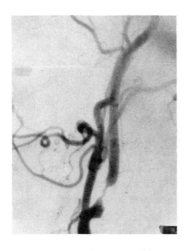

a. Medical therapy with aspirin 325 mg/day and medical risk factor management
b. Medical therapy with warfarin
c. Angioplasty of the carotid lesion followed by carotid endarterectomy if the angioplasty is unsuccessful
d. Carotid endarterectomy
e. Medical risk factor management and carotid endarterectomy if neurologic symptoms develop

430. A 55-year-old man with recent onset of atrial fibrillation presents with a cold, pulseless left lower extremity. He complains of left leg paresthesia and is unable to dorsiflex his toes. Following a successful popliteal embolectomy, with restoration of palpable pedal pulses, the patient is still unable to dorsiflex his toes. The next step in management should be

a. Electromyography (EMG)
b. Measurement of anterior compartment pressure
c. Elevation of the left leg
d. Immediate fasciotomy
e. Application of a posterior splint

431. Conservative management rather than reconstructive arterial surgery is generally recommended for patients with which of the following symptoms or signs of arterial insufficiency?

a. Ischemic ulceration
b. Ischemic neuropathy
c. Claudication
d. Nocturnal foot pain
e. Toe gangrene

432. Correct statements concerning antiplatelet therapy include

a. Aspirin has been shown to be an effective antiplatelet agent
b. Most antiplatelet agents work by enhancing prostaglandin synthesis
c. Antiplatelet agents have not been shown to increase patency rates of coronary artery bypass grafts
d. Aspirin can be used to treat deep venous thrombophlebitis
e. The antiplatelet effect of aspirin will last for the life of the platelet, which is generally 20–25 days

433. The subclavian steal syndrome is associated with which of the following hemodynamic abnormalities?

a. Antegrade flow through a vertebral artery
b. Venous congestion of upper extremities
c. Occlusion of the carotid artery
d. Occlusion of the vertebral artery
e. Occlusion of the subclavian artery

434. Symptoms or signs of atherosclerotic occlusive disease of the bifurcation of the abdominal aorta (Leriche syndrome) include

a. Claudication of the buttock and thigh
b. Causalgia of the lower leg
c. Retrograde ejaculation
d. Gangrene of the feet
e. Dependent rubor of the feet

435. Among patients with suspected (occult) coronary artery disease, the occurrence of postoperative ischemic cardiac events following peripheral vascular surgery correlates closely with abnormal preoperative

a. Exercise stress testing
b. Gated blood pool studies that demonstrate an ejection fraction of 50% or less
c. Coronary angiography
d. Dipyridamole-thallium imaging
e. Transesophageal echocardiography

436. A 64-year-old man is admitted 14 mo following a femoropopliteal bypass graft procedure with a cold foot and no graft pulse. Urokinase infusion is begun. Which of the following statements regarding management is true?

a. Clot lysis is accomplished in 25% of patients
b. After successful clot lysis, surgical revision of the opened graft should be considered only if early reocclusion occurs
c. With optimal treatment, a 20% reocclusion rate is expected within 1 year
d. Urokinase is less successful in lysing acute thromboses of prosthetic grafts than those of vein grafts
e. Streptokinase is the preferred thrombolytic agent when treating graft occlusions

437. A 60-year-old man is admitted to the coronary care unit with a large anterior wall myocardial infarction. On his second hospital day he begins to complain of the sudden onset of numbness in his right foot and an inability to move his right foot. On physical examination, the right femoral, popliteal, and pedal pulses are no longer palpable. Vascular consultation is obtained. Diagnosis of acute arterial embolus is made. Which of the following statements concerning this condition is true?

a. Appropriate management would be embolectomy of the right femoral artery under general anesthesia
b. Noninvasive hemodynamic testing is required
c. Prophylactic exploration of the contralateral femoral artery should be done despite the presence of a normal pulse
d. The source of the embolus is most likely the left ventricle
e. Arteriography is mandatory prior to operative intervention

438. Which of the following statements concerning the condition depicted on the arteriogram shown below is true?

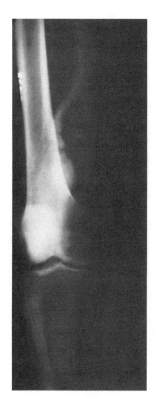

a. Surgery should be performed only if the patient is symptomatic
b. Limb loss is a definite risk in the untreated patient
c. The contralateral limb is affected in a similar fashion in over 75% of cases
d. Embolization is unlikely
e. Bleeding into the leg is the most common presentation

439. A 65-year-old male cigarette smoker reports onset of claudication of his right lower extremity approximately 3 wk previously. His walking radius is limited to three blocks before the onset of claudication. Physical examination reveals palpable pulses in the entire left lower extremity, but no pulses are palpable below the right groin level. Noninvasive flow studies are obtained, which are pictured below. Which of the following statements regarding this patient's condition is true?

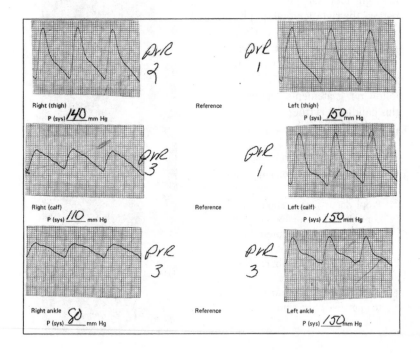

a. Femoropopliteal bypass is indicated on a relatively urgent basis in order to salvage the right leg
b. The occlusive process is in the right superficial femoral artery, with flow to the right foot supplied by the profunda femoris artery
c. About one-half of patients with similar symptoms will ultimately require amputation
d. The occlusive process is most likely caused by embolic disease
e. The noninvasive studies suggest iliac as well as superficial femoral occlusive disease on the right side

440. Indications for placement of the device pictured in the abdominal x-ray shown below include

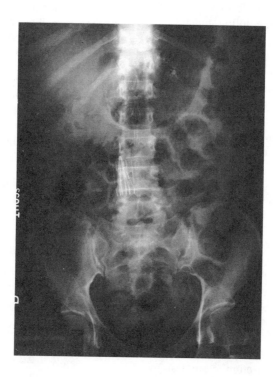

a. Recurrent pulmonary embolus despite adequate anticoagulation therapy
b. Axillary vein thrombosis
c. Pulmonary embolus in a patient with a perforated duodenal ulcer
d. Pulmonary embolus due to deep vein thrombosis of the lower extremity that occurs 2 wk postoperatively
e. Pulmonary embolus in a patient with metastatic pancreatic carcinoma

441. Two days after admission to the hospital for a myocardial infarction, a 65-year-old man complains of severe, unremitting midabdominal pain. His cardiac index is 1.6. Physical examination is remarkable for an absence of peritoneal irritation or distention despite the patient's persistent complaint of severe pain. Serum lactate is 9 (normal less than 3). In managing this problem you should

a. Perform computed tomography
b. Perform mesenteric angiography
c. Perform laparoscopy
d. Perform flexible sigmoidoscopy to assess the distal colon and rectum
e. Defer decision to explore the abdomen until the arterial lactate is greater than 10

442. During evaluation for the repair of an expanding abdominal aortic aneurysm, a patient is discovered to have a horseshoe kidney. The optimum surgical approach would be

a. Midline abdominal incision, preservation of the renal isthmus
b. Midline abdominal incision, division of the renal isthmus
c. Retroperitoneal approach, implantation of anomalous renal arteries
d. Nephrectomy, repair of aneurysm, chronic dialysis
e. Repair of aneurysm after autotransplantation of the kidney into the iliac fossa

443. Which statement regarding contrast venography is true?

a. It is more accurate than Doppler analysis and B-mode ultrasound (duplex scan) at detecting thrombi in the deep veins responsible for pulmonary emboli
b. It identifies incompetent deep, superficial, and perforating veins
c. It is totally noninvasive, painless, and safe
d. It is easily performed in a vascular laboratory or radiology suite or at the bedside
e. It is particularly sensitive in identifying the proximal extent of an iliofemoral thrombus

DIRECTIONS: The group of questions below consists of lettered options followed by numbered items. For each numbered item, select the appropriate lettered option(s). Each lettered option may be used once, more than once, or not at all. **Choose exactly the number of options indicated following each item.**

Items 444–445

The arteriogram below applies to both patients described on the following page. For each patient, select the appropriate options.

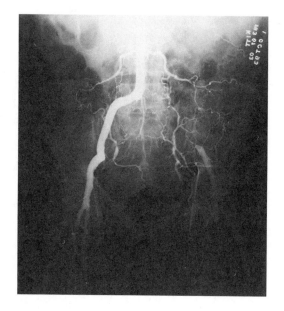

a. Femorofemoral bypass
b. Axillofemoral bypass
c. Femoropopliteal bypass
d. Common femoral and profunda femoral endarterectomies
e. Aorto-left-iliac bypass
f. Aortobifemoral bypass

444. A 52-year-old man presents with severe pain in his left hip and buttocks while walking about 50 yd. The pain is relieved shortly after resting. The patient is otherwise healthy. He claims to have stopped smoking, after a long history of cigarette abuse, approximately 1 year prior to presentation. **(SELECT 3 PROCEDURES)**

445. A 72-year-old woman with severe COPD that requires home oxygen is unable to ambulate inside her home without experiencing severe left hip pain. She was hospitalized 1 year ago for a viral pneumonia and was ventilator dependent at that time for 6 wk. **(SELECT 2 PROCEDURES)**

PERIPHERAL VASCULAR PROBLEMS

Answers

421. The answer is e. (*Schwartz, 7/e, pp 1007–1014.*) Low-dose heparin and pneumatic compression stockings have been shown to be effective prophylaxis against deep vein thrombosis; however, they are not effective against established thrombosis, the treatment for which is therapeutic heparinization. Salicylate has not been convincingly shown to have either a prophylactic or therapeutic role in the treatment of deep vein thrombosis. Even following prompt, aggressive treatment of deep vein thrombosis of the calf, as many as half of affected patients will develop symptoms of chronic venous hypertension, and a larger number will have abnormal venous hemodynamic findings. Untreated vein thrombosis of the calf may propagate into the larger popliteal veins and cause life-threatening pulmonary embolism.

422. The answer is c. (*Schwartz, 7/e, pp 947–948.*) By far the most likely cause of the oliguria observed in this patient is hypovolemia. Volume status would be best assessed by floating a Swan-Ganz catheter to measure the preload pressures in the left atrium (by inference from the pulmonary capillary wedge pressures). Patients who have had a leaking aneurysm and then a long, usually difficult operation with large surgical fields that collect "third-space" fluids may be intravascularly depleted despite large volumes of intravenous fluid and blood replacement. The proper management usually involves titrating the cardiac output by providing as much fluid as necessary to keep the wedge pressures near 15 mm Hg. The other studies listed might become useful if urinary flow remains depressed after optimal cardiac output has been achieved, but in view of the probability of hypovolemia, they are not indicated as a first diagnostic study.

423. The answer is d. (*Schroeder, Surg Gynecol Obstet 160:299–303, 1985. Schwartz, 7/e, p 948.*) Viability of the colon can be evaluated intraoperatively by Doppler auscultation of the bowel mesentery and serosa, observation of bowel peristalsis, and measurement of the IMA stump pressure. A strong, pulsatile Doppler signal in the mesentery; active sigmoid peristalsis; a chronically occluded IMA; or a patent IMA with stump pressure greater than 40 mm Hg presage viability of the sigmoid colon postoperatively. However, none of these observations excludes the possibility of late sigmoid ischemia. Serial postoperative sigmoidoscopic examination is the best predictor of ischemic colitis and in experienced hands allows assessment of the depth of ischemic injury before frank perforation has occurred. Barium enema is not as accurate as sigmoidoscopy in determining depth of injury and carries grave risks of contamination by barium and feces if perforation occurs.

424. The answer is c. *(Schwartz, 7/e, pp 1028–1030.)* This patient is at high risk for developing cellulitis of her right foot because her underlying problem is unilateral primary lymphedema. Hypoplasia of the lymphatic system of the lower extremity accounts for greater than 90% of patients with primary lymphedema. If edema is present at birth it is referred to as congenital; if it starts early in life (as in this woman) it is called praecox; and if it appears after age 35 it is tarda. The inadequacy of the lymphatic system accounts for the repeated episodes of cellulitis that these patients experience. Swelling is not seen with acute arterial insufficiency or with popliteal entrapment syndrome. Deep venous thrombophlebitis will result in tenderness and is generally not a predisposing factor for cellulitis of the foot.

425. The answer is d. *(Brewster, Surgery 109:447–457, 1991.)* The CT scan reveals a fractured ring of calcification in the abdominal aorta with significant density in the paraaortic area. The inferior mesenteric artery (IMA) is always at risk in patients with the changes in the vessel wall characteristic of abdominal aneurysms, but particularly so in the presence of rupture and retroperitoneal dissection of blood under systemic arterial pressures. The incidence of ischemic colitis following abdominal aortic resection is about 2%. Blood flow to the left colon normally derives from the IMA with collateral flow from the middle and inferior hemorrhoidal vessels. The superior mesenteric artery (SMA) may also contribute via the marginal artery of Drummond. If the SMA is stenotic or occluded, flow to the left colon will be primarily dependent on an intact IMA. The IMA is usually ligated at the time of aneurysmorrhaphy. Those patients at highest risk for diminished flow through collateral vessels are those with a history of visceral angina, those found to have a patent IMA at the time of operation, patients who have suffered an episode of hypotension following rupture of an aneurysm, those in whom preoperative angiograms reveal occlusion of the SMA, and those in whom Doppler flow signals along the mesenteric border cease following occlusion of the IMA. Recognition of bowel ischemia at the time of operation should be treated by reimplantation of the IMA into the graft to restore flow.

426. The answer is a. *(Schwartz, 7/e, pp 957–964.)* The angiogram presented in the question demonstrates an isolated segment of atherosclerotic occlusion of the superficial femoral artery. Patients who have isolated femoropopliteal disease tend to be smokers, whereas those who have isolated tibioperoneal disease frequently are diabetic. Hypertension and hyperlipidemia predispose to accelerated atherosclerosis. On the other hand, type I hyperlipoproteinemia (hyperchylomicronemia), which is associated with dramatic levels of plasma triglyceride and formation of xanthomas, does not cause accelerated vascular disease.

427. The answer is c. *(Schwartz, 7/e, pp 941–944.)* Most abdominal aortic aneurysms are asymptomatic and are discovered on palpation by a physician. A radiograph of the abdomen is useful in demonstrating the aneurysm if there is calcification in the walls. Ultrasound is generally the first diagnostic procedure in confirming the presence of an aneurysm, with arteriography being performed if the aneurysm is considered large enough to require resection (greater than 5 cm in diameter). Recently CT scan has been found to be useful as a preoperative study in patients suspected of having aneurysms. Surgery should be performed despite the absence of symptoms and can be carried out with a mortality of less than 5%. With leaking or ruptured aneurysms, the operative mortality associated with this emergency situation is upward of 75%. The patient's age is not a contraindication to surgery, because several studies have demonstrated a low mortality (less than 5%) and satisfactory long-term survival and quality of life in elderly, even octogenarian, patients.

428. The answer is b. *(Greenfield, 2/e, pp 1751–1752.)* Doppler ultrasonography (duplex) has become the best initial test for screening patients with carotid disease. It has become a highly accurate test, often obviating the need for carotid arteriography prior to carotid endarterectomy. Carotid arteriography remains the "gold standard" when quantifying the degree of carotid stenosis, but it is usually performed after noninvasive testing suggests significant stenosis. Spiral CT angiography is a new noninvasive modality that has been used to evaluate many segments of the vascular tree, but as yet its accuracy does not approach that of standard arteriography and it would certainly not be used in the initial evaluation of a patient with an asymptomatic bruit. Magnetic resonance arteriography (MRA) is also a relatively new modality that has enjoyed moderate success in the investigation of carotid disease. Although not quite as accurate as standard arteriography, it has been used in conjunction with the duplex as a complementary study. Once again, because of its cost, MRA would not be used as the primary screening modality. Transcranial Doppler studies are used to assess the intracranial vasculature.

429. The answer is d. (*Executive Committee, JAMA 273:1421–1428, 1995.*) In a recent prospective, randomized, multicenter trial involving 1662 patients in a study known as the Asymptomatic Carotid Atherosclerosis Study, patients with asymptomatic carotid artery stenosis of 60% or greater reduction in diameter and whose general health made them good candidates for elective surgery were found to have a significant reduction in the 5-year risk for ipsilateral stroke with surgery compared with medically treated cohorts (5.1 vs. 11.0%). Medically treated patients were treated with aspirin on a daily basis. Warfarin has not been shown to be effective in the management of patients with carotid disease. Angioplasty of carotid stenoses is being performed in some institutions on a purely investigational basis and to date has not replaced surgery as the treatment for high-grade carotid stenoses.

430. The answer is d. (*Greenfield, 2/e, pp 1640–1642.*) This case illustrates two (among many) conditions that lead to the anterior compartment syndrome, namely, acute arterial occlusion without collateral inflow and rapid reperfusion of ischemic muscle. Treatment for a compartment syndrome is prompt fasciotomy. Assessing a compartment syndrome and proceeding with fasciotomy are generally based on clinical judgment. Inability to dorsiflex the toes is a grave sign of anterior compartment ischemia. EMG studies and compartment pressure measurements would probably be abnormal, but are unnecessary in view of the known findings and would delay treatment. Mere elevation of the leg would be an ineffective means of relieving compartment pressure, although elevation should accompany fasciotomy. Application of a splint has no role in the acute management of this problem.

431. The answer is c. *(Greenfield, 2/e, pp 1715–1718.)* The major threat to patients with arterial occlusive disease is limb loss. Ischemic ulceration, neuropathy, rest pain, and gangrene represent advanced stages of arterial insufficiency and warrant reconstructive surgery whenever clinically feasible. Claudication, in most cases, reflects mild ischemia; the majority of affected patients are successfully managed without surgery (only 2.5% develop gangrene). Most will stabilize or improve with development of increased collateral blood flow following institution of a program of daily exercise, cessation of smoking, and weight loss. Vasodilator drugs have been shown to have little benefit in the conservative management of intermittent claudication.

432. The answer is a. *(Willerson, Am J Cardiol 67:12A–18A, 1991.)* Aspirin exerts an antiplatelet effect that will last for the life of the platelet (approximately 7–10 days). Patients who take aspirin will experience its effect for 7–10 days after stopping the medication. Aspirin interferes with platelet function by inhibiting the synthesis of thromboxane A_2 and the subsequent production of prostaglandins. The platelet does not have a nucleus and thus cannot remanufacture the prostaglandins necessary for its functioning. Antiplatelet agents are generally used to prevent thrombotic and embolic events on the arterial side of the circulation. The Canadian Cooperative Study has shown antiplatelet therapy to be effective in preventing strokes in men with carotid artery disease, but it is not used to treat thrombophlebitis in the deep venous system. Antiplatelet therapy has been shown to increase graft patency rates following coronary artery bypass grafting if the medication is started preoperatively and continued postoperatively.

433. The answer is e. *(Schwartz, 7/e, pp 965, 971.)* Atherosclerotic occlusion of the subclavian artery proximal to the vertebral artery is the anatomic situation that results in the subclavian steal syndrome. On being subjected to exercise, the involved extremity (usually left) develops relative ischemia, which gives rise to reversal of flow through the vertebral artery with consequent diminished flow to the brain. The upper extremity symptom is intermittent claudication. Venous occlusive disease is not a feature of the syndrome. The operative procedure for treating the subclavian steal syndrome consists of delivering blood to the extremity by creating either a carotid-subclavian bypass or a subclavian-carotid transposition.

434. The answer is a. (*Schwartz, 7/e, pp 957–961.*) The slow progression of aortoiliac atherosclerotic occlusive disease is usually associated with the development of collateral flow through the lumbar branches of the aorta, anastomosing via retroperitoneal branches of the gluteal arteries with the profunda femoris arteries in the legs. This network of collateral vessels provides sufficient blood flow to nourish the extremities at rest but cannot prevent claudication of the upper and lower muscle groups of the leg during exercise. Sexual impotence, also part of the Leriche syndrome, is believed to be a result of bilateral stenosis or occlusion of the hypogastric (internal iliac) arteries. Retrograde ejaculation can occur after disruption of the sympathetic chain overlying the distal aorta and left iliac and can occur after dissection around these vessels during vascular reconstructions. Gangrene of the feet or toes is rarely seen unless distal embolization of atherosclerotic material from the aorta occludes the pedal or digital arteries. Dependent rubor is usually a sign of significant ischemia resulting from lower extremity occlusive and not aortoiliac disease. Causalgia or reflex sympathetic dystrophy is a disorder of the sympathetic nervous system that can affect the upper or lower extremities.

435. The answer is d. (*Boucher, N Engl J Med 312:389–394, 1985. Pasternack, Circulation 72:13–17, 1985.*) The occurrence of perioperative ischemic cardiac events among patients undergoing peripheral vascular reconstruction has been found to correlate with gated blood pool ejection fractions of 35% or less and with reversible perfusion defects (thallium redistribution) on dipyridamole-thallium imaging. Ischemic rest pain or early onset of claudication after minimal exercise limits the effectiveness of stress testing as a screening procedure for occult coronary artery disease in this group of patients. Screening coronary angiography, followed by angioplasty or bypass of asymptomatic lesions, had an adverse effect on patient survival in a large prospective study of patients who had peripheral vascular surgery. Transesophageal echocardiography has no role in the preoperative screening of peripheral vascular patients.

436. The answer is c. *(Belkin, Surgery 212:769–773, 1986. Eisbud, Am J Surg 160:160–165, 1990.)* Management of acute graft occlusion must include both reestablishment of peripheral perfusion and correction of any underlying hemodynamic problem. Urokinase is associated with fewer allergic reactions than streptokinase and is the preferred thrombolytic agent. Treatment results in total clot lysis in 75% of patients. However, high reocclusion rates are observed (20% within 1 year) even if angioplasty or anastomotic revision is performed after successful lysis. Without surgical revision following clot lysis, a 50% reocclusion rate is expected within 3 mo. Urokinase has proved equally successful in opening both vein and prosthetic graft thromboses.

437. The answer is d. *(Schwartz, 7/e, pp 953–954.)* The heart is the most common source of arterial emboli and accounts for 90% of cases. Within the heart, sources include diseased valves, endocarditis, the left atrium in patients with unstable atrial arrhythmias, and mural thrombus on the wall of the left ventricle in patients with a myocardial infarction. The diagnosis in this patient is clear, and therefore neither noninvasive testing nor arteriography is indicated. Arteriography in fact may also prove to be too stressful for a patient undergoing an acute myocardial infarction. Embolectomy of the femoral artery can be performed under local anesthesia with minimal risk to the patient. Emboli typically lodge in one femoral artery; contralateral exploration is not indicated in the absence of signs or symptoms. One should always prepare the contralateral groin in case flow is not restored via simple thrombectomy and femoral-femoral bypass is needed to provide inflow to the affected limb.

438. The answer is b. *(Schwartz, 7/e, pp 949–950.)* Popliteal aneurysms are usually due to atherosclerosis, are bilateral 25% of the time, and require excision even if asymptomatic. Because of the risk of embolization (60–70%) and thrombosis with resultant gangrene, as well as the lesser risk of rupture, all of which lead to substantial likelihood of limb loss, even relatively small, asymptomatic aneurysms should be excised when discovered. Rupture of the aneurysm can occur but is an uncommon presentation compared with embolization.

439. The answer is b. *(Schwartz, 7/e, pp 961–964.)* This patient has occlusion of the right superficial femoral artery caused by atherosclerosis, and this is confirmed by both the physical examination and the flow study findings, which indicate a sharp decrease in the blood pressure below the level of the common femoral artery. Fewer than 10% of patients with claudication progress to gangrene and the need for amputation. Operative therapy would not be suggested at this time because it is quite likely that with cessation of cigarette smoking and adherence to an exercise program, the patient could markedly improve his walking radius as collateral vessels enlarge to deliver more blood to the affected tissues. Operative therapy (femoropopliteal bypass) would be indicated at this time in this patient only if symptoms of rest pain or ischemic ulceration were present. Physical examination and flow studies indicate disease distal to the aortoiliac distribution.

440. The answer is a. (*Schwartz, 7/e, p 1014.*) The Greenfield filter pictured on the x-ray is used to interrupt migration of emboli to the lungs from the veins below the level of the filter. It is indicated in patients who sustain a recurrent pulmonary embolus despite adequate anticoagulant therapy or in patients with pulmonary emboli who cannot receive anticoagulants because of a contraindication (e.g., bleeding ulcer, intracranial hemorrhage). The filter is not used in patients who sustain a single pulmonary embolus. It is placed in the inferior vena cava just below the renal veins and therefore would not be effective for emboli that arise cephalad to its position. Despite the hypercoagulable state seen in some patients with metastatic pancreatic cancer, anticoagulation can still be used as a first-line defense.

441. The answer is b. (*Schwartz, 7/e, pp 966–968.*) Abdominal pain out of proportion to findings on physical examination is characteristic of intestinal ischemia. The etiology of ischemia may be embolic or thrombotic occlusion of the mesenteric vessels or nonocclusive ischemia due to a low cardiac index or mesenteric vasospasm. Differentiation among these etiologies is best made by mesenteric angiography. While not without serious risks, angiography also offers the possibility of direct infusion of vasodilators into the mesenteric vasculature in the setting of nonocclusive ischemia. This patient, with a recent myocardial infarction and a low cardiac index, is at risk for embolism of clot from a left ventricle mural thrombus as well as "low-flow" mesenteric ischemia. If embolism or thrombosis is found angiographically (usually involving the superior mesenteric artery), operative embolectomy or vascular bypass is indicated to restore flow. If occlusive disease cannot be demonstrated, efforts should be made to simultaneously increase cardiac output with inotropic agents and dilate the mesenteric vascular bed by angiographic instillation of papaverine, nitrates, or calcium channel blockers. Computed tomography is not helpful in delineating the cause of intestinal ischemia because it does not provide a sufficiently detailed image of the mesenteric vessels. Laparoscopy might secure the diagnosis of intestinal ischemia, but requires administering general anesthesia and would shed no light on the etiology of this patient's problem. Flexible sigmoidoscopy, while useful in patients with ischemic colitis, has no role in the workup of mesenteric ischemia, which primarily involves the small intestine and right colon. Serum lactate is helpful in raising the suspicion of intestinal ischemia, but no absolute level should be used to decide whether or not to explore a patient.

442. The answer is c. (*O'Hara, J Vasc Surg 17:940–947, 1993.*) A horseshoe kidney is a fused kidney that occupies space on both sides of the vertebral column. The fusion is ordinarily at the lower poles with the isthmus anterior to the aorta. The ureters run anterior to the isthmus and the kidney frequently has an anomalous blood supply. The arterial supply to the kidney is highly variable with vessels arising not only from the normal position in the aorta but also from a variable number of accessory segmental end-arteries from the lower aorta and iliac arteries. Most cases of abdominal aortic aneurysm associated with a horseshoe kidney can be successfully resected, but these anomalies make the repair challenging. When the horseshoe kidney is recognized preoperatively, an arteriogram helps to define the vascular anatomy. The preferred operative approach is then via a retroperitoneal dissection. This allows the kidney and its collecting system to be swept anteromedially and provides relatively unobstructed access to the aneurysm. All anomalous renal arteries should be implanted into the graft after the aneurysm sac is opened since the proportionate contribution from each may be hard to determine.

The renal isthmus and collecting system restrict access to the aneurysm and make the anterior approach less desirable. Though division of the isthmus can be accomplished, there is high risk of calyceal or ureteral injury. Given the numerous arterial, venous, and collecting system anomalies, autotransplantation of the kidney is not a good option. The presence of the fresh intravascular foreign body (aortic graft) contraindicates dialysis because of the excessive risk of infecting the graft.

443. The answer is b. (*Schwartz, 7/e, p 1009.*) Doppler analysis and B-mode ultrasonography (duplex scan) has virtually replaced venography as the first diagnostic test in the evaluation of deep venous thrombosis. The duplex scanning device is portable and therefore the study is easily performed at the bedside, in a vascular laboratory, or in a radiology suite. It is completely noninvasive, painless, and safe. Venography, however, must be performed in a radiology suite, and requires the use of an intravenous contrast medium that is painful upon injection and is itself thrombogenic. Incompetent deep, superficial, and perforating veins can be accurately identified by either venography or duplex scan. Both venography and duplex scan are highly accurate in diagnosing deep venous thrombi that may result in pulmonary embolism. But, significantly, contrast venography does not provide information regarding the proximal extent of an iliofemoral thrombus when it fails to fill the deep femoral system due to total occlusion by blood clot.

444–445. The answers are 444-a, e, f; 445-a, b. (*Schwartz, 7/e, pp 957–961.*) The arteriogram shown demonstrates a left iliac artery occlusion. In a patient with severe symptoms that are interfering with his lifestyle, intervention is indicated. In the young healthy patient with iliac artery occlusive disease, when angioplasty is not a treatment option, femorofemoral and aortoiliac bypasses offer excellent long-term relief. Femorofemoral bypass offers the additional benefit of not disturbing sexual function. Both bypasses provide similar long-term patencies. Aortobifemoral bypass, while clearly the most risky of the treatment options offered, provides the best long-term patency.

In the elderly patient with severe COPD, so-called extraanatomic bypasses (femorofemoral or axillofemoral bypasses) offer fair long-term patencies while not subjecting the patient to the risks of general anesthesia.

UROLOGY

Questions

DIRECTIONS: Each item below contains a question or incomplete statement followed by suggested responses. Select the **one best** response to each question.

446. Initial management of a patient who has a flaccid neurogenic bladder may include which of the following measures?

a. Surgical bladder augmentation
b. Self-catheterization
c. Supravesical urinary diversion
d. Limiting fluid intake to less than 300 mL/day
e. Transurethral resection of the bladder neck

447. Which of the following statements regarding hypospadias is correct?

a. It is often associated with chordee (ventral curvature of the penis)
b. It is associated with undescended testes in more than 50% of cases
c. It is a rare fusion defect of the posterior male urethra
d. It occurs sporadically, without evidence of familial inheritance
e. The most common location is penoscrotal

448. The recommended treatment for stage A (superficial and submucosal) transitional cell carcinoma of the bladder is

a. Local excision
b. Radical cystectomy
c. Radiation therapy
d. Topical (intravesicular) chemotherapy
e. Systemic chemotherapy

449. A 36-year-old man presents to the emergency room with renal colic. A radiograph reveals a 1.5-cm stone. Which of the following statements regarding this disorder is correct?

a. Conservative treatment including hydration and analgesics will not result in a satisfactory outcome
b. Serial kidney, ureter, bladder (KUB) radiographs should be used to follow this patient
c. The urinalysis will nearly always reveal microhematuria
d. When the acute event is correctly treated, this disease seldom recurs
e. Elevated BUN and creatinine are expected

450. Optimal management of bilateral undescended testicles in an infant is

a. Immediate surgical placement into the scrotum
b. Chorionic gonadotropin therapy for 1 mo; operative placement into the scrotum before age 1 if descent has not occurred
c. Observation until the child is 2 years old because delayed descent is common
d. Observation until age 5; if no descent by then, plastic surgical scrotal prostheses before the child enters school
e. No therapy; reassurance of the parent that full masculinization and normal spermatogenesis are likely even if the testicle does not fully descend

451. Seminoma is accurately described by which of the following statements?

a. It is the most common type of testicular cancer
b. Metastases to liver and bone are frequently found
c. It does not respond to radiation
d. The 5-year survival rate approaches 50%
e. Common presentation is that of a painful lump that transilluminates

452. A 10-year-old boy presents to the emergency room with testicular pain of 5 h duration. The pain was of acute onset and woke the patient from sleep. On physical examination, he is noted to have a high-riding, indurated, and markedly tender left testis. Pain is not diminished by elevation. Urinalysis is unremarkable. Which of the following statements regarding the patient's diagnosis and treatment is true?

a. There is a strong likelihood that this patient's father or brother has had or will have a similar event
b. Operation should be delayed until a technetium scan clarifies the diagnosis
c. The majority of testicles that have undergone torsion can be salvaged if surgery is performed within 24 h
d. If torsion is found, both testes should undergo orchiopexy
e. The differential diagnosis includes spermatocele

453. Genitourinary tuberculosis in a male patient is suggested by which of the following findings?

a. Microscopic hematuria
b. Bacteriuria without pyuria
c. Unilateral renal cysts
d. Painful swelling of the epididymis
e. Pneumaturia

454. Which of the following statements regarding carcinoma of the prostate is true?

a. It has a higher incidence among American blacks than other American ethnic groups
b. A single microscopic focus of prostate cancer discovered on transurethral resection of the prostate (TURP) is an indication for radical prostatectomy
c. It arises initially in the gland's central portion
d. It commonly produces osteoclastic bony metastases
e. Screening for prostate-specific antigen, although easily done, offers no advantage over simple rectal examination in the detection of the disease

455. Which of the following statements regarding benign prostatic hyperplasia (BPH) is true?

a. The fibrostromal proliferation of BPH occurs mainly in the outer portion of the gland
b. Assuming a voided volume greater than 100 mL, a peak urine flow rate of 30 mL/s or less is good evidence of outflow obstruction
c. Suprapubic prostatectomy for BPH involves enucleation of the entire prostate and eliminates the risk of future prostate cancer
d. Indications for surgery include acute urinary retention and recurrent urinary tract infections (UTIs)
e. BPH is a risk factor for the development of prostatic cancer

456. During the course of an operation on an unstable, critically ill patient, the left ureter is lacerated through 50% of its circumference. If the patient's condition is felt to be too serious to allow time for definitive repair, alternative methods of management include

a. Ligation of the injured ureter and ipsilateral nephrostomy
b. Ipsilateral nephrectomy
c. Placement of a catheter from the distal ureter through an abdominal wall stab wound
d. Placement of a suction drain adjacent to the injury without further manipulation that might convert the partial laceration into a complete disruption
e. Bringing the proximal ureter up to the skin as a ureterostomy

457. A pedestrian is hit by a speeding car. Radiologic studies obtained in the emergency room, including a retrograde urethrogram, are consistent with a pelvic fracture with a rupture of the urethra superior to the urogenital diaphragm. Management should consist of

a. Immediate percutaneous nephrostomy
b. Immediate placement of a Foley catheter through the urethra into the bladder to align and stent the injured portions
c. Immediate reconstruction of the ruptured urethra after initial stabilization of the patient
d. Immediate exploration of the pelvis for control of hemorrhage from pelvic fracture and drainage of the pelvic hematoma
e. Immediate placement of a suprapubic cystostomy tube

UROLOGY

Answers

446. The answer is b. (*Schwartz, 7/e, pp 1759, 1768–1769.*) Patients who have a lower motor neuron lesion (flaccid neurogenic bladder) can usually be managed by conservative measures that prevent the development of a large residual urine volume in the bladder. These measures include intermittent self-catheterization and scheduled voiding with increased abdominal pressure provided by the Valsalva maneuver or manual pressure on the abdomen. Detrusor contractions can sometimes be strengthened by parasympathomimetic agents such as bethanechol chloride (Urecholine). Bladder augmentation to increase capacitance, bladder neck resection to reduce outlet obstruction, and supravesicle ureteral diversion are indicated only in the presence of deterioration of bladder compliance or gross ureterocalyxectasis that resists the foregoing measures and threatens the loss of renal function or debilitating urinary incontinence. Severely restricting fluid intake is impractical and may promote formation of calculi.

447. The answer is a. (*Schwartz, 7/e, pp 1813–1815.*) Hypospadias is a common congenital anomaly of the penis resulting from incomplete development of the anterior urethra. It occurs in about 1 in 300 live births and is believed to have a multifactorial genetic mode of inheritance. Of those with hypospadias, about 7% have a father with the disorder, 14% a brother, and 20% a second family member. Hypospadias occurs in the corona in about 75% of cases, where it is often accompanied by chordee. Undescended testes occur in about 10% of cases of hypospadias, as do inguinal hernias. Hypospadias in the scrotal area is associated with bilateral undescended testes and infertility and must be differentiated from pseudohermaphroditism and adrenogenital syndrome.

448. The answer is d. (*Schwartz, 7/e, pp 1792–1793.*) Bladder cancer represents 2% of all cancers, and 90% of bladder cancers are of transitional cell origin. It is most prevalent among men with a heavy smoking history and is usually multifocal and superficial, even when recurrent. When the disease is still superficial, transurethral resection of visible lesions and intravesicular chemotherapy are most often recommended. More radical surgical extirpation is reserved for advanced stages of the disease.

449. The answer is a. *(Schwartz, 7/e, pp 1774–1784.)* Initial management should include hydration and analgesics. However, as the stone is larger than 1 cm, it is unlikely to pass spontaneously, though stones smaller than 0.5 cm usually do pass spontaneously. The size of the stone also makes a high-grade obstruction more likely; therefore an intravenous pyelogram (IVP) must be urgently performed. A high-grade obstruction will require nephrostomy or the passage of a ureteral stent. If the stone is completely occluding the lumen of the ureter, the urinalysis may not show microhematuria and thus may be misleading. Approximately 15% of patients will have a recurrence within 1 year, and almost 50% may have a recurrence within 4 years. Elevated BUN and creatinine are expected only in the setting of an obstructed single functioning kidney.

450. The answer is b. *(Schwartz, 7/e, pp 1744–1745, 1810–1811.)* By the second year, a testicle not in the cooler environment of the scrotal sac will begin to undergo histologic changes characterized by reduced spermatogonia. Testicles left longer in the undescended state not only have a higher incidence of malignant degeneration, but are inaccessible for examination. If a malignancy should occur, diagnosis will be delayed. There is also a substantial psychological burden when children reach school age or are otherwise subjected to exposure of their deformed genitalia. Gel-filled prostheses are generally inserted when a testicle cannot be placed in the scrotum. Close follow-up by a physician until the late teens is indicated in all patients who have had an undescended testicle. Since these patients may be at increased risk for malignancy throughout life, careful training should be given in self-examination.

451. The answer is a. *(Schwartz, 7/e, pp 1794–1795.)* Seminomas tend to grow slowly and metastasize late. They usually present as a nonpainful lump that does not transilluminate. They represent about 40% of malignant testicular tumors; embryonal cell carcinoma and teratocarcinoma each represent about 25%. Because most tumors have mixed elements, they are usually classified according to the most malignant cell type encountered, whatever the predominant cell type. When metastases occur, they are usually along the regional lymphatic drainage pathways to the iliac, aortic, and renal lymph nodes. Because of their slow growth and radiosensitivity, seminomas are associated with a 90% 5-year survival rate. Therapy generally consists of removing the affected testis and sampling the lymph nodes (usually external iliac) for evidence of metastasis. If metastases are present, radiation therapy is given locally to areas of known involvement. Radiation therapy is highly effective in seminoma, and metastatic disease may be palliated for extended periods.

452. The answer is d. *(Schwartz, 7/e, pp 1812–1813.)* Testicular torsion occurs commonly in adolescents. The underlying pathology is secondary to an abnormally narrowed testicular mesentery with tunica vaginalis surrounding the testis and epididymis in a "bell-clapper" deformity. As the testis twists, it comes to lie in a higher position within the scrotum. Urinalysis is usually negative. Elevation will not provide a decrease in pain (negative Prehn sign); a positive Prehn sign might indicate epididymitis. A ^{99m}Tc pertechnetate scan may be helpful in clarifying a confusing case; however, operation should not be delayed beyond 4 h from the time of onset of symptoms in order to maximize testicular salvage. This patient's presentation warrants immediate operation. The salvage rate for delay greater than 12 h is less than 20%. Both the affected and unaffected testes should undergo orchiopexy. The differential diagnosis between torsion of the testicle and epididymitis is sometimes quite difficult. On occasion, one has to explore a patient with epididymitis just to rule out a torsion of the testicle. Epididymitis usually occurs in sexually active males. Urinalysis is usually positive for inflammatory cells, and urethral discharge is often present. Spermatocele is a cyst of an efferent ductule of the rete testis. It presents as a painless transilluminable cystic mass that is separate from the testes.

453. The answer is a. *(Schwartz, 7/e, pp 1773–1774.)* Genitourinary tuberculosis develops from reactivation of foci in the renal cortex or prostate that were hematogenously seeded during the primary (usually asymptomatic) pulmonary infection. Local spread from the renal and prostatic sites can lead to involvement of the calyx, ureter, bladder, vas deferens, epididymis, and (rarely) the testis. A low-grade inflammatory response results in hematuria or pyuria without bacteriuria. Whenever pus cells are seen on routine urine culture without bacteria on smear or culture plate, genitourinary tuberculosis should be considered. The end result of focal caseation necrosis in the kidney may be scarring and dystrophic calcification. Genital tract infection often causes an asymptomatic swelling in the epididymis; secondary infection or formation of a sinus tract to the scrotal skin may cause more dramatic signs and symptoms. Epididymal tuberculosis is usually managed by chemotherapy, with surgery reserved for refractory cases. Pneumaturia is associated with a colovesical fistula and not with genitourinary tuberculosis.

454. The answer is a. (*Schwartz, 7/e, pp 1793–1795.*) One of the most frequent causes of male cancer deaths, prostate cancer has an incidence of more than 75,000 new cases per year in the United States. American blacks appear to have a 50% higher incidence and mortality. Prostate cancer (adenocarcinoma) arises initially in the periphery of the gland. Therefore, one of the best screening tests is careful rectal examination. However, the use of screening for prostate-specific antigen (PSA) has increased the detection rate fourfold. Spread is by direct local extension and by lymphatic and vascular channels. The most common locations of distant metastases are in the axial skeleton with osteoblastic bony lesions. A single focus of disease discovered on TURP or simple prostatectomy is considered stage A_1. Only 2% of patients have unsuspected nodes (i.e., only 2% 5- to 10-year mortality). Therefore, no definitive therapy is required except possibly in patients less than 60 years old. Follow-up should be undertaken and progression of disease may be treated as necessary. Several foci or diffuse disease is considered stage A_2 and surgery or radiation therapy is generally indicated.

455. The answer is d. (*Schwartz, 7/e, pp 1784–1788.*) In contrast to prostate cancer, BPH arises first in the periurethral prostate tissue as a fibrostromal proliferation. As the periurethral prostate grows, the outer prostate glands are compressed against the true prostatic capsule, which results in a thick pseudocapsule. As the prostate enlarges, it encroaches on the urethra and causes urinary outflow obstruction. Obstructive symptoms include decreased force of stream, hesitancy, recurrent UTIs, and occasionally acute urinary retention; the latter two are indications for surgery. Uroflow is the best noninvasive method of estimating the degree of outlet obstruction. Flow less than 10 mL/s is good evidence of significant obstruction. The major treatments for BPH are surgical. Simple prostatectomy involves shelling out the prostate adenoma and leaving the pseudocapsule (true prostate) behind. Therefore, these patients are still at risk of developing prostate cancer although BPH in and of itself is not a risk factor for prostatic cancer.

456. The answer is a. _(Schwartz, 7/e, pp 1800–1801.)_ If time and the patient's condition permit, primary ureteral reconstruction should be carried out. In the middle third of the ureter, this will usually consist of ureteroureterostomy using absorbable sutures over a stent. If the injury involves the upper third, ureteropyeloplasty may be necessary. In the lower third, ureteral implantation into the bladder using a tunneling technique is preferred. If time does not permit definitive repair, suction drainage adjacent to the injured segment alone is inadequate; either ligation and nephrostomy or placement of a catheter into the proximal ureter is an acceptable alternative that would allow reconstruction to be performed later. The creation of a watertight seal is difficult and nephrectomy may be required if the injury occurs during a procedure in which a vascular prosthesis is being implanted (e.g., an aortic reconstructive procedure) and contamination of the foreign body by urine must be avoided.

457. The answer is e. _(Schwartz, 7/e, pp 1804–1807.)_ If a rupture of the urethra is suspected, a retrograde urethrogram should be obtained before any attempts are made to place a Foley catheter, as efforts to do so may result in the creation of multiple false passages or conversion of a partial laceration into complete rupture. Previously, treatment had included attempts to realign the urethra immediately through the placement of interlocking sounds and traction using either a catheter passed over the sounds or perineal traction sutures through the bladder neck. Preferred treatment currently avoids both dissection into the pelvic hematoma surrounding the disruption and manipulation of the urethra; instead, only a suprapubic tube is placed immediately with delayed reconstruction after 3–6 mo, at which time the hematoma will have resolved and the prostate will have descended into the proximity of the urogenital diaphragm. Percutaneous nephrostomy has no role in the management of this problem.

ORTHOPEDICS

Questions

DIRECTIONS: Each item below contains a question or incomplete statement followed by suggested responses. Select the **one best** response to each question.

458. Meniscal tears usually result from which of the following circumstances?

a. Hyperextension
b. Flexion and rotation
c. Simple hyperflexion
d. Compression
e. Femoral condylar fracture

459. Volkmann's ischemic contracture is associated with

a. Intertrochanteric femoral fracture
b. Supracondylar fracture of the humerus
c. Posterior dislocation of the knee
d. Traumatic shoulder separation
e. Colles "silver fork" fracture

460. In an uncomplicated dislocation of the glenohumeral joint, the humeral head usually dislocates primarily in which of the following directions?

a. Anteriorly
b. Superiorly
c. Posteriorly
d. Laterally
e. Medially

461. The most severe epiphyseal growth disturbance is likely to result from which of the following types of fracture?

a. Fracture dislocation of a joint adjacent to an epiphysis
b. Fracture through the articular cartilage extending into the epiphysis
c. Transverse fracture of the bone shaft on the metaphyseal side of the epiphysis
d. Separation of the epiphysis at the diaphyseal side of the growth plate
e. Crushing injury compressing the growth plate

462. Which of the following fractures is most commonly seen in healthy bones subjected to violent falls?

a. Colles fracture
b. Femoral neck fracture
c. Intertrochanteric fracture
d. Clavicular fracture
e. Vertebral compression fracture

463. Which nerve is most at risk in the injury in the accompanying radiograph?

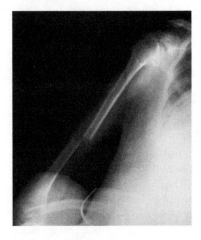

a. Median nerve
b. Radial nerve
c. Posterior interosseous nerve
d. Ulnar nerve
e. Ascending circumflex brachial nerve

464. In a failed suicide gesture, a depressed student severs her radial nerve at the wrist. The expected disability is

a. Loss of ability to extend the wrist
b. Loss of ability to flex the wrist
c. Wasting of the intrinsic muscles of the hand
d. Sensory loss over the thenar pad and the thumb web
e. Palmar insensitivity

465. Which of the following statements regarding compartment syndromes following orthopedic injuries is true?

a. The first sign is usually loss of pulse in the extremity
b. Passive flexion of the extremity proximal to the involved compartment will aggravate the pain
c. Surgical decompression (fasciectomy) is necessary only as a last resort
d. These syndromes are most commonly associated with supracondylar fractures of the humerus and tibial shaft
e. The syndrome is often painless

466. In contrast to closed reduction, open reduction of a fracture

a. Produces a shorter healing time
b. Decreases trauma to the fracture site
c. Produces a higher incidence of nonunion
d. Reduces the risk of infection
e. Requires longer periods of immobilization

DIRECTIONS: Each group of questions below consists of lettered options followed by numbered items. For each numbered item, select the appropriate lettered option(s). Each lettered option may be used once, more than once, or not at all. **Choose exactly the number of options indicated following each item.**

Items 467–470

For each description below, select the type of fracture or dislocation with which it is most likely to be associated.

a. Navicular (scaphoid) fracture
b. Monteggia's deformity
c. Greenstick fracture
d. Spiral fracture
e. Posterior shoulder dislocation

467. Epileptiform convulsion may be a cause. (**SELECT 1 INJURY**)

468. Avascular necrosis is not uncommon. (**SELECT 1 INJURY**)

469. The radial head is dislocated and the proximal third of the ulna is fractured. (**SELECT 1 INJURY**)

470. Tenderness in the anatomist's snuffbox may be observed. (**SELECT 1 INJURY**)

Items 471–474

For each description below, select the type of bone disease with which it is most likely to be associated.

a. Osteogenesis imperfecta
b. Osteopetrosis
c. Osteitis fibrosa cystica
d. Osteomalacia
e. Osteitis deformans

471. Association with hyperparathyroidism (**SELECT 1 DISEASE**)

472. A defect in the mineralization of adult bone secondary to abnormalities in vitamin D metabolism (**SELECT 1 DISEASE**)

473. Genetically determined disorder in the structure or processing of type I collagen (**SELECT 1 DISEASE**)

474. Synonym for Paget's disease (**SELECT 1 DISEASE**)

Items 475–477

For each description below, select the type of bone lesion with which it is most likely to be associated.

a. Osteoma
b. Osteoid osteoma
c. Osteoblastoma
d. Osteosarcoma
e. Paget's disease
f. Ewing's sarcoma

475. An 11-year-old boy presents with pain in his right leg. A radiograph shows a "sunburst" appearance with bone destruction, soft tissue mass, new bone formation, and sclerosis limited to the metaphysis of the lower femur. **(SELECT 1 LESION)**

476. A 25-year-old man presents with severe pain in the left femur. The pain is relieved by aspirin. On plain film, a 0.5-cm lucent lesion, which is surrounded by marked reactive sclerosis, is seen. **(SELECT 1 LESION)**

477. A 12-year-old boy complains of pain in his left leg that is worse at night. He has been experiencing fevers and also has a 9-lb weight loss. X-ray demonstrates an aggressive lesion with a permeative pattern of bone lysis and periosteal reaction. There is an associated large soft tissue mass as well. Pathology demonstrates the tumor to be of the round cell type. **(SELECT 1 LESION)**

ORTHOPEDICS

Answers

458. The answer is b. (*Schwartz, 7/e, pp 1979–1980.*) Most meniscal tears are produced by flexion and rapid rotation. A classic example ("football knee") involves a player who is hit while running. The knee, supporting all the player's weight, usually is slightly flexed, and the foot is anchored to the ground by cleats. Impact from an opposing player usually causes rotation almost entirely restricted to the knee. The injury involves rapid rotation of the flexed femoral condyles about the tibial plateau, which most frequently tears the medial meniscus. (Less frequently, the lateral meniscus is torn.) A tear in the inner free border of the cartilage is also common whenever excessive rotation without flexion or extension occurs. Early surgical removal of the displaced menisci is usually recommended to prevent further damage to the cartilage or ligaments.

459. The answer is b. (*Schwartz, 7/e, pp 1959, 2052–2053.*) Compromise of blood supply to the muscles of the forearm can lead to a compartment syndrome and permanent serious functional deformity of the arm. Any patient with a compressive dressing or cast of the upper extremity can experience this potential catastrophe. Whenever a patient has increasing pain in the presence of a circular dressing around the arm or forearm, the dressing should be removed immediately. If there is tenderness in the forearm on either the ulnar or dorsal aspect, a fasciotomy should be considered.

460. The answer is a. (*Schwartz, 7/e, pp 1963–1964.*) The glenohumeral joint is bounded posteriorly by the teres minor and infraspinatus muscles and partially by the long head of the triceps. It is bounded laterally by the powerful deltoid muscle; superiorly, the acromion process precludes upward dislocation. However, anteriorly and inferiorly the pectoralis major and the long head of the biceps do not completely stabilize the glenohumeral joint; in this region the articular ligaments and joint capsule provide the major structural support. Thus, the joint is not strongly supported in its anteroinferior aspect, and consequently anterior (or anteroinferior) dislocations are the most common glenohumeral dislocations. The humeral head is driven anteriorly, which tears the shoulder capsule, detaches the labrum from the glenoid, and produces a compression fracture of the humeral head. Most glenohumeral dislocations result from a posteriorly directed force on an arm that is partially abducted. Posterior dislocation is much rarer and should raise the possibility of a seizure as the precipitating cause.

461. The answer is e. (*Schwartz, 7/e, pp 1958–1959.*) Longitudinal growth of bone follows ossification of cartilage that forms at the epiphyseal plate. Fractures that involve separation of the growth plate (type I) (almost always on the diaphyseal side) may be realigned; normal growth usually follows epiphyseal separation because the proliferative cells are still attached to their blood supply in the bone epiphysis. Fractures that extend perpendicular to and through the epiphysis (types II, III, IV) may result in the formation of bony bridges across the epiphysis that can disrupt later growth. Though all the fractures listed in the question place the epiphyseal growth plate in some jeopardy, crushing injuries to the epiphysis (type V) have the worst prognosis; numerous bony bridges may form and prevent longitudinal growth.

462. The answer is d. (*Schwartz, 7/e, pp 1948–1949.*) Postmenopausal osteoporosis is responsible for a large number of fractures in elderly women. Though bone mineralization is normal in osteoporosis, total bone mass and trabecular volume are decreased. Common fracture sites are the vertebrae, distal radius, and hip. Vertebral compression fractures are often sustained by elderly men and women even without trauma. A minor fall on the outstretched hand can lead to a Colles' fracture when the distal radius is weakened by osteoporosis. Similarly, either a femoral neck fracture or an intertrochanteric fracture can follow a fall on the hip. Clavicular fractures are less likely to result from osteoporosis. While these fractures occur in both children and adults, they are common in healthy children and young adults after violent falls onto an outstretched hand.

463. The answer is b. (*Schwartz, 7/e, pp 1964–1965.*) The radiograph demonstrates a transverse fracture of the distal half of the humeral shaft. The radial nerve runs in a groove on the posterior aspect of the humerus as it courses into the forearm compartment and is therefore at high risk of injury. If the nerve injury is apparent before any manipulation has been done, the fracture should be reduced; the nerve injury should be observed since the nerve function will likely improve with time. If the nerve injury is only present after reduction, immediate surgical exploration is warranted because the nerve might be trapped in the fracture site. At this level of the arm, the ulnar and median nerves are well protected by muscle. The posterior interosseous nerve is a distal branch of the radial nerve and may be injured in fractures near the radial head, but it is in no danger from injuries at the level seen in this radiograph. There is no "ascending circumflex brachial nerve."

464. The answer is d. *(Schwartz, 7/e, p 2068.)* An injury to the radial nerve at the wrist would cause primarily sensory abnormalities. The dorsum of the hand from the radial aspect of the fourth digit over the thumb, including the thenar pad and thumb web, becomes insensate after severance of the radial nerve at the wrist. Radial injuries more proximally would impair extension of the wrist and digits as well as forearm supination.

465. The answer is d. *(Schwartz, 7/e, pp 1959, 2052–2053.)* Compartment syndromes result from increasing pressures in the fascial compartments of the arm or leg. When the pressure in the muscles is greater than that of the capillaries, ischemia and necrosis of the muscles occur even though the arterial pressure is still high enough to produce pulses; pulselessness is an unreliable sign. Extreme pain (out of proportion to the injury), pain on passive extension of the fingers or toes, pallor of the extremity, motor paralysis, and paresthesias are all components of the syndrome. The patient will usually hold the injured part in a position of flexion to maximally relax the fascia and reduce the pain; passive extension will usually produce severe pain. The diagnosis can be confirmed by measuring intracompartmental pressures, but whenever physical findings or symptoms are suspicious, immediate surgical decompression by fasciectomy is indicated since delay is likely to lead to irreversible damage.

466. The answer is c. *(Schwartz, 7/e, pp 1973–1978.)* Open reduction of a fracture involves the restoration of normal bone alignment under direct observation at surgery. In effect, open reduction converts a simple fracture into a compound (or open) fracture and thereby increases the risk of infection. Operative manipulation also increases trauma at the fracture site and may consequently add to the probability of infection. Hematomas at the site of fracture may be important for early healing; open reduction, which usually involves removing the clots in the field, could contribute to a delay in bone healing and to nonunion. The major advantage of open reduction is the shorter period of immobilization it allows, an advantage that often outweighs all the disadvantages previously mentioned, as in the open reduction of femoral neck fractures in the elderly. This allows these patients to get out of bed much sooner than if they were treated with several weeks of traction.

467–470. The answers are 467-e, 468-a, 469-b, 470-a. (*Schwartz, 7/e, pp 1963–1964, 1968–1971, 1981–1982.*) Fractures of the navicular bone of the wrist should be suspected in anyone, particularly a young person, who falls on an outstretched hand. Although x-rays are mandatory, it is important to realize that the fracture may not be seen on the initial x-ray and that a presumptive diagnosis can and should be made on clinical grounds alone. Typically, there will be tenderness to palpation over the navicular tuberosity and limitation of wrist flexion and extension. Immobilization of the wrist for about 16 wk and sometimes up to 6 mo is required. Nonunion or avascular necrosis is not uncommon and may require bone grafting for correction.

Dislocation of the radial head with a fracture of the proximal third of the ulna is known as Monteggia's deformity. Usually, the radial head is dislocated anteriorly. The injury is usually caused by forced pronation. The injury can be treated by reduction and stabilization of the ulna followed by reduction of the radial head via supination and direct pressure.

Anterior shoulder dislocations occur more frequently than posterior dislocations. However, posterior dislocations are seen in special situations, such as during an epileptiform convulsion and during electroshock therapy. Closed reduction followed by immobilization is usually sufficient therapy.

A spiral fracture, frequently seen in the tibia in skiers, results from the application of torque to a long bone. Greenstick fractures are common in children. The bones of young children are able to bend to a greater degree than those of adults; the fracture may occur only at the site of maximal cortical stress but not at the opposite cortex, the site of maximal longitudinal compression.

471–474. The answers are 471-c, 472-d, 473-a, 474-e. (*Schwartz, 7/e, pp 1946–1951.*) Osteitis fibrosa cystica is commonly associated with hyperparathyroidism. Hemorrhagic cystic lesions (brown tumors) usually occur in the long bones. Treatment is parathyroidectomy. Osteomalacia is defined as a defect in mineralization of adult bone that results from abnormalities in vitamin D metabolism. Treatment generally involves vitamin D supplementation. Osteogenesis imperfecta is a genetically determined disorder in the structure or processing of type I collagen. Treatment is surgical and involves orthoses to prevent fractures and correction of deformities by multiple osteotomies. Osteitis deformans is also known as Paget's disease. Osteopetrosis is a rare skeletal deformity associated with increased density of the bones.

475–477. The answers are 475-d, 476-b, 477-f. *(Schwartz, 7/e, pp 2008–2011, 2014.)* Osteosarcoma, or osteogenic sarcoma, usually is seen in patients between the ages of 10 and 25 years. The distal femur is the site most frequently involved. The radiograph has a blastic, or sunburst, appearance. The tumor is not sensitive to radiation but does respond well to combination chemotherapy followed by surgical resection or amputation.

An osteoid osteoma typically presents with severe pain that is characteristically relieved by aspirin. On radiograph, the lesion appears as a small lucency (usually <1.0 cm) within the bone that is surrounded by reactive sclerosis. These lesions gradually regress over 5–10 years, but most are excised to relieve symptoms. Surgical extirpation is usually curative.

Ewing's sarcoma is a round cell–type tumor. This is a highly malignant tumor that affects children (age range 5–15 years) and tends to occur in the diaphyses of long bones. The spine and pelvis can also be primary sites. There is a permeative pattern of bone lysis and periosteal reaction often associated with a large soft tissue mass. Fever and weight loss are common. The pain is often more pronounced at night. Treatment usually involves a combination of radiation and systemic chemotherapy, with 5-year survivals around 50%. Adjuvant surgery in combination with radiation and chemotherapy improves the 5-year survival to about 75%.

NEUROSURGERY

Questions

DIRECTIONS: Each item below contains a question or incomplete statement followed by suggested responses. Select the **one best** response to each question.

478. Which of the following statements regarding the Glasgow coma scale is true?

a. It serves as a scale to assess the long-term sequelae of head trauma
b. A high score correlates with a high mortality
c. It includes measurement of intracranial pressure
d. It includes measurement of pupillary reflexes
e. It includes measurement of verbal response

479. Controlled hyperventilation (induced hypocapnia) is frequently recommended following head trauma. The therapeutic consequences of this therapy include

a. Reduction of endogenous catecholamines
b. Reduction of intracellular potassium levels
c. Increase in cerebrovascular resistance
d. Induction of compensatory metabolic alkalosis
e. Requirement of monitoring the intracranial pressure

480. Which of the following statements regarding glioblastoma multiforme is true?

a. It is a neuronal cell tumor
b. It arises from the malignant degeneration of an astrocytoma
c. With aggressive treatment, most patients can live up to 10 years with this disease
d. It is the most common childhood intracranial neoplasm
e. With combined surgery, chemotherapy, and radiation therapy, cure rates now approach 50%

481. A 60-year-old woman presents to her physician with a 3-wk history of severe headaches. A contrast CT scan reveals a small, circular, hypodense lesion with ringlike contrast enhancement. The most likely diagnosis is

a. Brain abscess
b. High-grade astrocytoma
c. Parenchymal hemorrhage
d. Metastatic lesion
e. Toxoplasmosis

482. Which of the following statements regarding skull fractures is true?

a. Depressed fractures are those in which the patient's level of consciousness is diminished or absent
b. Compound fractures are those in which the skull is fractured and the underlying brain is lacerated
c. Any bone fragment displaced more than 1 cm inwardly should be elevated surgically
d. Drainage of cerebrospinal fluid via the ear or nose requires prompt surgical treatment
e. Most skull fractures require surgical treatment

483. A 39-year-old man presents to his physician with the complaint of loss of peripheral vision. The subsequent magnetic resonance imaging (MRI) scan below demonstrates

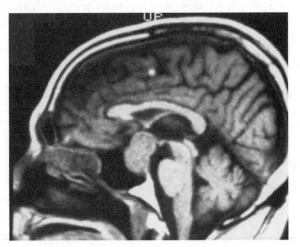

a. Cerebral atrophy
b. Pituitary adenoma
c. Optic glioma
d. Pontine hemorrhage
e. Multiple sclerosis plaque

484. An 18-year-old man is admitted to the emergency room following a motorcycle accident. He is alert and fully oriented, but witnesses to the accident report an interval of unresponsiveness following the injury. Skull films disclose a fracture of the left temporal bone. Following x-ray, the patient suddenly loses consciousness and dilation of the left pupil is noted. This patient should be considered to have

a. Ruptured berry aneurysm
b. Acute subdural hematoma
c. Epidural hematoma
d. Intraabdominal hemorrhage
e. Ruptured arteriovenous malformation

485. Which of the following statements regarding the cerebral angiogram below is true?

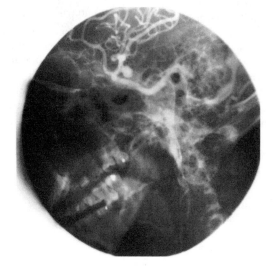

a. The aneurysm arises from an arteriovenous malformation
b. The lesion is a giant aneurysm
c. There is a basilar artery lesion
d. Initial treatment includes aggressive fluid hydration
e. Surgical clipping of this lesion is curative

486. An acute increase in intracranial pressure is characterized by which of the following clinical findings?

a. Respiratory irregularities
b. Decreased blood pressure
c. Tachycardia
d. Papilledema
e. Compression of the fifth cranial nerve

487. Which of the following statements about schwannomas is true?

a. They represent central nerve tumors
b. Treatment is via excision
c. They arise most frequently in motor nerves
d. They often degenerate to malignancy
e. The most common presentation is a painful mass

488. Which of the following statements about craniopharyngiomas is true?

a. The tumors are uniformly solid
b. The tumors are usually malignant
c. Children with these tumors often develop signs and symptoms of acromegaly
d. The tumors may cause compression of the optic tracts and visual symptoms
e. The primary mode of treatment is radiation therapy

489. Which of the following statements regarding cerebral contusions is true?

a. They occur most frequently in the occipital lobes
b. They may occur opposite the point of skull impact
c. They are rarely accompanied by parenchymal bleeding
d. They may occur spontaneously in patients receiving anticoagulants
e. Anticonvulsants have no role in the early management of this disorder

490. True statements regarding meningiomas include that they

a. Are malignant in 50% of cases
b. Occur predominantly in men
c. Are treated primarily by surgical excision
d. Are cured, when properly treated, in nearly 95% of cases
e. Arise from the dura

DIRECTIONS: The group of questions below consists of lettered options followed by numbered items. For each numbered item, select the appropriate lettered option(s). Each lettered option may be used once, more than once, or not at all. **Choose exactly the number of options indicated following each item.**

Items 491–492

For each description below, select the type of vascular event with which it is most likely to be associated.

a. Subdural hematoma
b. Epidural hematoma
c. Carotid dissection
d. Brain contusion
e. Ruptured intracranial aneurysm

491. While watching a golf tournament, a 37-year-old man is struck on the side of the head by a golf ball. He is conscious and talkative after the injury, but several days later he is noted to be increasingly lethargic, somewhat confused, and unable to move his right side. (**SELECT 1 DIAGNOSIS**)

492. A 42-year-old woman complains of the sudden onset of a severe headache, stiff neck, and photophobia. She loses consciousness. She is later noted to have a dilated pupil. (**SELECT 1 DIAGNOSIS**)

NEUROSURGERY

Answers

478. The answer is e. (*Schwartz, 7/e, pp 1880–1881.*) The Glasgow coma scale was developed to enable an initial assessment of the severity of head trauma. It is now also used to standardize serial neurologic examinations in the early postinjury period. It measures the level of consciousness using three parameters: verbal response (5 points), motor response (6 points), and eye opening (4 points). The score is the sum of the highest number achieved in each category. The fully oriented and alert patient will receive a maximum score of 15. A score of less than 5 is associated with a mortality of over 50%.

479. The answer is c. (*Schwartz, 7/e, pp 1878, 1880–1881.*) Controlled hyperventilation to a Pa_{CO_2} of 25 kPa raises tissue pH, increases cerebrovascular resistance, decreases cerebral blood flow, and consequently reduces intracerebral pressure (ICP). In the effort to avoid brain swelling by lowering cerebral blood flow and ICP, the clinician must be wary of causing ischemic brain damage through hypoperfusion. The metabolic compensation to induced hypocapnia leads to normalization of the pH by loss of bicarbonate (metabolic acidosis), and over 8–24 h the beneficial effects of the hypocapnia will have been lost. The partial pressures of carbon dioxide should be allowed to slowly return to normal and should be held in reserve in case unanticipated increases in ICP require another pulse of short-term reduction. It is important to monitor the patient while the Pa_{CO_2} is rising because untoward or rapid increases in ICP may occur in response to the rising cerebral blood flow.

480. The answer is b. (*Schwartz, 7/e, pp 1886–1887.*) Glioblastoma multiforme is the most common form of primary intracranial neuroepithelial tumor. It represents 25% of all intracranial tumors and 50% of tumors originating in the central nervous system. It is a heterogeneous glial cell tumor derived from the malignant degeneration of an astrocytoma or anaplastic astrocytoma. These tumors are most commonly found in the cerebral hemispheres during the fifth decade of life. CT and MRI scans typically reveal an irregular lesion with hypodense central necrosis, peripheral ring enhancement of the highly cellular tumor tissue, and surrounding edema and mass effect. Curative resections are rare. Therapy consists of diagnostic biopsy followed by radiotherapy to slow the tumor growth. The course of the disease progresses rapidly after presentation, with few patients living more than 2 years.

481. The answer is d. (*Schwartz, 7/e, p 1890.*) The CT findings are consistent with any of the suggested lesions. However, the most likely diagnosis is metastatic disease. Almost 50% of intracranial neoplasms are metastatic lesions. Roughly 20–25% of cancer patients develop intracranial metastases during the course of their disease. Cancers of the lung and breast and melanomas frequently metastasize to the brain parenchyma. Leukemia shows a predilection for the leptomeninges. A large majority of these lesions become symptomatic owing to mass effect from white matter edema. Palliation is the primary goal for most patients and involves corticosteroids and radiation. Surgery is employed for the 25% of patients with a solitary brain metastasis and cured or arrested systemic disease.

482. The answer is c. (*Schwartz, 7/e, pp 1879–1880.*) Most skull fractures do not require surgical treatment unless they are depressed or compound. A general rule is that all depressed skull fractures, defined as fractures in which the cranial vault is displaced inward, should be surgically elevated, especially if they are depressed more than 1 cm, if a fragment is over the motor strip, or if small, sharp fragments are seen on x-ray (as they may tear the underlying dura). Compound fractures, defined as fractures in which the bone and the overlying skin are broken, must be cleansed and debrided and the wound must be closed. When a skull fracture occurs in an area of the paranasal sinuses, the mastoid air cells, or the middle ear, a tear in the meninges may result in cerebrospinal fluid drainage from the ear or nose. The presence of rhinorrhea or otorrhea requires observation and prophylactic antibiotics, because meningitis is a serious sequel. Otorrhea usually heals within a few days. Persistent cerebrospinal fluid from the nose or ear for more than 14 days requires surgical repair of the torn dura.

483. The answer is b. (*Schwartz, 7/e, pp 1620–1628.*) This T1-weighted sagittal MRI scan reveals a dumbbell-shaped homogeneous mass involving the sella turcica and the suprasellar region. This lesion is most consistent with a pituitary adenoma, a benign tumor arising from the adenohypophysis. Pituitary adenomas are the most common sellar lesion and constitute 10–15% of all intracranial neoplasms. Macroadenomas (>10 mm) are generally nonsecreting tumors. Microadenomas (<10 mm) become clinically apparent from hormonal secretion. They may secrete prolactin (amenorrhea or galactorrhea), growth hormone (gigantism or acromegaly), or ACTH (Cushing syndrome). The tumor pictured is a macroadenoma. Its dumbbell shape results from impingement on the adenoma by the diaphragm of the sella turcica. The suprasellar extension seen here makes a frontal craniotomy rather than a transsphenoidal approach more appropriate.

484. The answer is c. (*Schwartz, 7/e, p 1881.*) Epidural hematomas are typically caused by a tear of the middle meningeal artery or vein or a dural venous sinus. Ninety percent of epidural hematomas are associated with linear skull fractures, usually in the temporal region. Only 2% of patients admitted with craniocerebral trauma suffer epidural hematomas. The lesion appears as a hyperdense biconvex mass between the skull and brain on CT scan. Clinical presentation is highly variable and outcome largely depends on promptness of diagnosis and surgical evacuation. The typical history is one of head trauma followed by a momentary alteration in consciousness and then a lucid interval lasting for up to a few hours. This is followed by a loss of consciousness, dilation of the pupil on the side of the epidural hematoma, and then compromise of the brainstem and death. Treatment consists of temporal craniectomy, evaluation of the hemorrhage, and control of the bleeding vessel. The mortality of epidural hematoma is approximately 50%.

485. The answer is e. (*Schwartz, 7/e, pp 1893–1895.*) This digital subtraction cerebral angiogram is an oblique view of the anterior circulation of the brain. Dye injected in the internal carotid reveals an aneurysm at the bifurcation of the internal carotid and the posterior communicating artery. A giant aneurysm is generally regarded as a lesion greater than 24 mm in cross-section. Surgical clipping of this aneurysm would be curative. Only after the risk of rebleeding is eliminated by clipping can the patient undergo volume expansion if vasospasm arises. The vertebrobasilar system is not visualized here.

486. The answer is a. *(Schwartz, 7/e, pp 1878, 1895–1896.)* The onset of irregular respirations, bradycardia, and finally increased blood pressure with increasing intracranial pressure (ICP) is termed the *Cushing response.* These physiologic alterations are caused by brainstem compression. Slow rises in ICP are, by contrast, autoregulated by the brain's compensatory mechanisms and lead to a late onset of neurologic sequelae. A mass lesion is more apt to compromise local cerebral blood flow and increase cerebral edema and ICP. The vector of the mass effect may lead to herniation of brain parenchyma through the tentorial incisura or foramen magnum with resultant brainstem compression. Herniation usually causes compression of the third cranial nerve and thus leads to a fixed and dilated pupil on that side. Papilledema is a finding with chronic increases in ICP.

487. The answer is b. *(Schwartz, 7/e, pp 1888–1889, 1892.)* Peripheral nerve tumors include lesions of peripheral nerves, the adrenal gland nerve tissue, and the sympathetic chain. Schwannomas are peripheral nerve sheath tumors that arise from perineural fibroblasts (Schwann cells). They are usually painless. Malignant schwannomas are rare. Treatment is via surgical excision. The nerve of origin can usually be preserved. Because schwannomas have virtually no malignant potential, if a major nerve would have to be sacrificed in order to extirpate the tumor, the nerve is spared and a small portion of the tumor is left in situ. Intracranial schwannomas most frequently originate in the vestibular branch of the eighth cranial nerve and represent 10% of all intracranial neoplasms. Symptoms include hearing loss, tinnitus, and vertigo. Neurofibromas are also Schwann cell tumors but are histologically distinguishable from schwannomas. Neurofibromatosis (von Recklinghausen's disease) involves multiple peripheral nerve neoplasms. Neuronal tumors of peripheral nerves include ganglioneuroma, neuroblastoma, chemodectoma, and pheochromocytoma.

488. The answer is d. *(Schwartz, 7/e, pp 1628–1629.)* Craniopharyngiomas are cystic tumors with areas of calcification and originate in the epithelial remnants of Rathke's pouch. These usually benign tumors are found in the sellar and suprasellar region and lead to compression of the pituitary, optic tracts, and third ventricle. As a result they show up on radiographic imaging as an area of sellar erosion with calcification within or above the sella. Craniopharyngiomas are most commonly found in children but may also present in adulthood. In children they can cause growth retardation because of hypothalamic-pituitary dysfunction. Treatment consists of subfrontal or transsphenoidal excision with adjuvant radiotherapy if total removal is not possible.

489. The answer is b. *(Sabiston, 15/e, pp 1355–1358.)* Cerebral contusions are bruises of neural parenchyma that most commonly involve the convex surface of a gyrus. The most frequent sites of cerebral contusion are the orbital surfaces of the frontal lobes and the anterior portion of the temporal lobes. The etiology of the contusion is always traumatic, and subsequent neurologic impairment, such as epilepsy, is common if the original injury was significant. Patients deemed to have a substantial contusion should receive anticonvulsive medication in the early posttraumatic period.

490. The answer is c. *(Schwartz, 7/e, pp 1887–1888.)* Meningiomas are relatively benign tumors that arise from the arachnoid layer of the meninges. They occur predominantly in women (65%) and are treated primarily by surgical excision. Despite their relatively benign nature, the 15-year survival rate for nonmalignant meningiomas is only 68%.

491–492. The answers are 491-a, 492-e. *(Sabiston, 15/e, pp 1349–1352, 1360.)* Subdural hematomas usually arise from tears in the veins bridging from the cerebral cortex to the dura or venous sinuses, often after only minor head injuries. They can become apparent several days after the initial injury. Treatment is with drainage of the hematoma through a burr hole; a formal craniotomy may be required if the fluid reaccumulates. Significant brain contusions due to blunt trauma are usually associated with at least transient loss of consciousness; similarly, epidural hematomas result in a period of unconsciousness, although a "lucid interval" may follow during which neurologic findings are minimal.

Subarachnoid hemorrhage (SAH) in the absence of antecedent trauma most commonly arises from a ruptured intracranial aneurysm, which typically is found at the bifurcation of the major branches of the circle of Willis. Other less frequent causes include hypertensive hemorrhage, trauma, and bleeding from an arteriovenous malformation. Patients present with the sudden onset of an excruciating headache. Complaints of a stiff neck and photophobia are common. Loss of consciousness may be transient or evolve into frank coma. Cranial nerve palsies are seen as a consequence both of increased intracranial pressure due to hemorrhage and pressure of the aneurysm on adjacent cranial nerves. CT scans followed by cerebral arteriography help to confirm the diagnosis as well as to identify the location of the aneurysm. Treatment consists of surgical ligation of the aneurysm by placing a clip across its neck. Early surgical intervention (within 72 h of SAH) may prevent aneurysmal rebleeding and allow aggressive management of posthemorrhage vasospasm.

OTOLARYNGOLOGY

Questions

DIRECTIONS: Each item below contains a question or incomplete statement followed by suggested responses. Select the **one best** response to each question.

493. Which of the following statements concerning nasopharyngeal cancer is true?

a. It has an unusually high incidence among Chinese
b. It occurs primarily after the sixth decade of life
c. It undergoes early metastasis to the lungs
d. The treatment of choice is wide surgical excision of the primary tumor
e. Initial evaluation should involve a biopsy of the primary tumor and neck nodes

494. Severe maxillofacial trauma is often the result of high-velocity impact sustained in automobile or motorcycle accidents. Regarding these injuries, which of the following statements is true?

a. Evaluation of the cervical spine should precede that of the facial injuries
b. Severe hemorrhage from the nasopharynx rarely occurs with LeFort fractures
c. Direct oral or nasotracheal intubation should be performed promptly to prevent airway obstruction
d. Standard facial x-ray series are preferable to computed tomography to assess facial fractures because they may be obtained in the emergency department, are performed faster, and are equally accurate
e. Definitive management of fractures of facial bones should not be delayed

495. Which of the following statements regarding squamous cell carcinoma of the head and neck is true?

a. Squamous cancers of the head and neck are caused by smoking tobacco rather than chewing tobacco

b. Chemotherapy rarely produces a response with pharyngeal carcinoma and is not employed

c. Squamous cancers of the nasopharynx are best treated by radiotherapy; surgery is reserved for lymph node metastases that have not responded to radiation

d. Squamous cancers of the oropharynx are best treated by radiotherapy; surgery is not recommended

e. For squamous cancers of the hypopharynx, radical neck dissection is performed only if lymph nodes are enlarged

496. Pleomorphic adenomas (mixed tumors) of the salivary glands are characterized by which of the following?

a. They occur most commonly on the lips, tongue, and palate

b. They grow rapidly

c. They rarely recur if simply enucleated

d. They present as rock-hard masses

e. They have no malignant potential

497. Which of the following statements about branchial cleft anomalies is true?

a. A fistula that lies between the external auditory canal and the submandibular region originates from the second branchial cleft

b. The course of the first branchial cleft fistula is through the bifurcation of the carotid artery

c. Injury to the hypoglossal nerve may occur during excision of a second branchial cleft fistula

d. The internal opening of the second branchial cleft fistula is usually found in the maxillary sinus

e. The internal opening of the first branchial cleft cyst is just underneath the base of the tongue

498. Which of the following statements regarding symptomatic thyroglossal duct cysts is true?

a. Over 90% manifest themselves before age 12

b. Treatment includes resection of the hyoid bone

c. They usually present as a painful swelling in the lateral neck

d. Approximately 10–15% contain malignant elements

e. They rarely become infected

499. Which of the following statements regarding cancer of the tongue is true?

a. Carcinomas at the base of the tongue are best treated by irradiation alone rather than surgery

b. Stage I and stage II cancers of the mobile tongue are treated more effectively by irradiation than by surgery

c. Cancer of the tongue is usually advanced to stage III by the time it is diagnosed

d. Prophylactic irradiation of the neck nodes is indicated in patients whose primary cancer of the tongue is treated by irradiation

e. Cancer of the tongue is the third most common malignancy of the oral cavity

500. Verrucous carcinoma of the buccal mucosa is identified with which of the following characteristics?

a. It is faster growing than the epidermoid form

b. It is not associated with tobacco chewing

c. It has a predilection for the gingivobuccal gutter

d. It rarely extends to the mandible

e. It has a dark-brown, flat, smooth border on presentation

OTOLARYNGOLOGY

Answers

493. The answer is a. *(Schwartz, 7/e, pp 645–648.)* There is an unusually high incidence of carcinoma of the nasopharynx among Chinese. In the early stages of the disease, metastases remain confined to the neck. Diagnosis of nasopharyngeal cancer, which tends to arise in relatively young people, should be made by biopsy of the primary tumor. Biopsy of the neck nodes should be avoided because implantation of the tumor in skin and subcutaneous tissue may occur. Radiation therapy is the treatment of choice for the primary nasopharyngeal cancer. Cervical metastases that remain clinically evident should be removed by a radical neck dissection.

494. The answer is a. *(Greenfield, 2/e, pp 298–308.)* In patients with severe facial or mandibular trauma, airway difficulties may develop secondary to the effects of massive hemorrhage, tissue swelling, or associated laryngeal trauma. A cricothyroidotomy is preferred over direct oral or nasotracheal intubation because it can be performed quickly without manipulation of the cervical spine or injured parts. If prolonged postoperative airway problems are anticipated, the cricothyroidotomy may convert to a tracheostomy. Evaluation of the cervical spine is a top priority and should be performed in any patient with head trauma prior to further facial studies. Although most facial fractures can be diagnosed easily with a standard "facial series," computed tomography (CT) is more accurate and allows assessment of areas (e.g., intracerebral contents) that cannot be evaluated by conventional techniques. Therefore, in most centers, CT is presently the preferred method of evaluation for patients with severe maxillofacial trauma. Maxillary fractures are categorized by the LeFort classification, and, unlike other facial fractures, are frequently associated with severe nasal and nasopharyngeal hemorrhage. This may be treated with head elevation and ice compresses. Nasal packing also affords good control of hemorrhage, and in extreme cases ligation or embolization of the internal maxillary artery may be necessary. Definitive reduction and fixation of fractures may be delayed while other injuries and medical problems are addressed. In addition to control of hemorrhage, initial management of facial fractures may include temporary stabilization, wound closure, and oral lavage with solutions containing antibiotics.

495. The answer is c. (*Greenfield, 2/e, pp 637–651.*) Squamous cell cancers of the head and neck appear to arise as a response to tobacco in general (including chewing tobacco), rather than just to cigarette smoking, especially when used in combination with alcohol ingestion. Chemotherapy for squamous cell pharyngeal cancer has been used very successfully in childhood and adolescence, although its role in adult pharyngeal cancer is uncertain. Treatment of nasopharyngeal squamous cell carcinoma is by radiation, followed by radical neck dissection if lymph node metastases have not been controlled. Oropharyngeal cancers have responded equally well to surgery and radiation, and both treatments are routinely employed. In the hypopharynx surgery is the optimal treatment, often supplemented by postoperative radiation therapy. Surgery for hypopharyngeal cancers includes radical neck dissection because lymph node metastases occur frequently and are not well controlled by radiation alone.

496. The answer is a. (*Schwartz, 7/e, pp 656–662.*) There are approximately 400–700 minor salivary glands in the oral cavity. Pleomorphic adenomas (mixed tumors) can occur in any of them. These round tumors have a rubbery consistency and are slow-growing; all are potentially malignant. Unless adequately excised, they tend to recur locally in a high percentage of cases. The sites most commonly affected by pleomorphic adenomas of the salivary glands are the lips, tongue, and palate.

497. The answer is c. (*Greenfield, 2/e, pp 1995–1998.*) Branchial cleft cysts, sinuses, and fistulas are remnants of the first and second branchial pouches. The internal opening of the first is the external auditory canal; for the second, it is the posterolateral pharynx below the tonsillar fossa. The facial nerve may be injured during dissection of the first fistula. The second fistula passes between the carotid bifurcation and adjacent to the hypoglossal nerve. In childhood most branchial cleft anomalies present as a painless nodule along the lateral border of the sternocleidomastoid muscle. In adults, superinfection of the cyst or fistulous drainage via an orifice in the supraclavicular region may occur. Treatment is surgical excision.

498. The answer is b. (*Greenfield, 2/e, pp 1998–1999.*) Thyroglossal duct cysts result from retention of an epithelial tract between the thyroid and its embryologic origin in the foramen cecum at the base of the tongue. This tract usually penetrates the hyoid bone. There is no sex predilection, and although these cysts are more frequently detected in children, up to 25% do not become symptomatic until adulthood. The most common presentation is a painless swelling in the midline of the neck that moves with protrusion of the tongue or swallowing. The cysts are prone to infection and progressive enlargement. Although rare (less than 1%), epidermoid or papillary carcinomas do occur within thyroglossal duct cysts. Surgical resection is the standard therapy. The Sistrunk procedure, which involves local resection of the cyst and the central portion of the hyoid bone, is the operation of choice. Simple excision of the cyst results in an unacceptably high recurrence rate.

499. The answer is d. (*Schwartz, 7/e, pp 635–639.*) Cancer of the tongue is the most common malignant tumor in the oral cavity and accounts for slightly less than one-third of the malignancies in the area. About two-thirds of cases present as early lesions in the mobile anterior portion of the tongue. Most workers in the field agree that for these stage I and stage II lesions, surgery and irradiation give equivalent results (45% 5-year survival), and the treatment should therefore be tailored to the patient. Failures are almost always due to supraclavicular recurrence and many recommend excision of the radiation scar and prophylactic irradiation of the neck nodes, particularly in the stage II and stage IV tumors in the base of the tongue, which have a poorer prognosis.

500. The answer is c. (*Schwartz, 7/e, pp 631–632.*) Verrucous carcinoma is a less aggressive form of locally invasive buccal cancer than the usual epidermoid form. Its frequency is increased in people who chew tobacco. The tumor usually grows very slowly, occurs chiefly in the gingivobuccal gutter, and has a tendency to invade bone. It is identified by its characteristic exophytic, white, shaggy appearance. Wide excision is the best initial treatment for this neoplasm. Even though the tumor may regress in response to radiation, it tends to recur in a more malignant form with metastases. Cervical metastases usually are not present when the lesion is first diagnosed; it is only for the most highly malignant grades of verrucous carcinoma that radical neck dissection and block excision of the cheek are indicated.

BIBLIOGRAPHY

ANDERSON RJ, ET AL: Unrecognized adult salicylate intoxication. Ann Intern Med 85:745–748, 1976.

BARNAVON Y, WALLACK MK: Management of the pregnant patient with carcinoma of the breast. Surg Gynecol Obstet 171:347–352, 1990.

BELKIN M, ET AL: Intra-arterial fibrinolytic therapy. Efficacy of streptokinase vs urokinase. Arch Surg 121:769–773, 1986.

BERCI: Am J Surg 161:332–335, 1991.

BOUCHER CA, ET AL: Determination of cardiac risk by dipyridamolethallium imaging before peripheral vascular surgery. N Engl J Med 312:389–394, 1985.

BREWSTER DC, FRANKLIN DP, CAMBRIA RP, ET AL: Intestinal ischemia complicating abdominal aortic surgery. Surgery 109:447–454, 1991.

BUNT TJ, ET AL: Frequency of vascular injury with blunt trauma-induced extremity injury. Am J Surg 160:226–228, 1990.

CAMERON JL: Current Surgical Therapy, 5th ed. St Louis, Mosby, 1995.

CASE RECORDS OF THE MASSACHUSETTS GENERAL HOSPITAL. Weekly Clinicopathological Exercises. Case 45-1987: A 16-year-old girl with hepatic and pulmonary masses. N Engl J Med 317:1209–1218, 1987.

CASS AS: Renovascular injuries from external trauma. Diagnosis, treatment, and outcome. Urol Clin North Am 16:213–220, 1989.

CHARLSON ME, ET AL: The preoperative and intraoperative hemodynamic predictors of postoperative myocardial infarction or ischemia in patients undergoing noncardiac surgery. Ann Surg 210:637–648, 1989.

COSENTINO CM, ET AL: Choledochal duct cyst: Resection with physiologic reconstruction. Surgery 112:740–748, 1992.

CUMMINGS RA, ET AL: Pneumopericardium resulting in cardiac tamponade. Ann Thorac Surg 37:511–518, 1984.

DIETTRICH NA, ET AL: A growing spectrum of surgical disease in patients with human immunodeficiency virus/acquired immunodeficiency syndrome. Experience with 120 major cases. Arch Surg 126:860–866, 1991.

DUBROW TJ, ET AL: Myocardial contusion in the stable patient. Surgery 106:267–273, 1989.

DUTKY PA, STEVENS SL, MAULL KI: Factors affecting rapid fluid resuscitation with large-bore introducer catheters. J Trauma 29:856–860, 1989.

EISBUD DE, ET AL: Treatment of acute vascular occlusions with intraarterial urokinase. Am J Surg 160:160–165, 1990.

ERWIN TJ, CLARK JR, WEICHSELBAUM RR: Multidisciplinary treatment of advanced squamous carcinoma of the head and neck. Semin Oncol 12:71–82, 1985.

Executive Committee for the Asymptomatic Carotid Atherosclerosis Study: JAMA 273:1421–1428, 1995.

FLINT L, ET AL: Definitive control of mortality from severe pelvic fracture. Ann Surg 211:703–707, 1990.

GAJRAJ H, YOUNG AE: Adrenal incidentaloma. Br J Surg 80:422–426, 1993.

GOBBI PG: Cancer 65(11):2528–2536, 1990

GOLDMAN: J Cardiothorac Anesth 1:237, 1987.

GOODNOUGH LT, SHUCK JM: Risks, options, and informed consent for blood transfusion in elective surgery. Am J Surg 159:602–609, 1990.

GRAHAM DY, GO MF: Helicobacter pylori: Current status. Gastroenterology 105:279–282, 1993.

GREENFIELD L, ET AL (EDS): Surgery: Scientific Principles and Practice, 2d ed. Philadelphia, Lippincott-Raven, 1997.

HARRIS J, ET AL: Diseases of the Breast. Philadelphia, Lippincott-Raven, 1996.

HENDERSON JA, PELOQUIN AJ: Boerhaave revisited: Spontaneous esophageal perforation as a diagnostic masquerader. Am J Med 86:559–567, 1989.

HEYS SD, ET AL: Nutrition and malignant disease: Implications for surgical practice. Br J Surg 79:614–623, 1992.

LANDERCASPER J, ET AL: Perioperative stroke risk in 173 consecutive patients with a past history of stroke. Arch Surg 125:986–989, 1990.

LIPSETT PA, ET AL: Pseudomembranous colitis: A surgical disease? Surgery 116:491–496, 1994.

MAHMOODIAN S: Appendicitis complicating pregnancy. South Med J 85:19–24, 1992.

MCQUAID KR, ISENBERG JI: Medical therapy of peptic ulcer disease. Surg Clin North Am 72:285–316, 1992.

MERRELL SW, SCHNEIDER PD: Hemobilia: Evolution of current diagnosis and treatment. West J Med 155:621–625, 1991.

MILLER FB, SHUMATE CR, RICHARDSON JD: Myocardial contusion. When can the diagnosis be eliminated? Arch Surg 124:805–808, 1989.